Preliminary Edition Notice

You have been selected to receive a copy of this book in the form of a preliminary edition. A preliminary edition is used in a classroom setting to test the overall value of a book's content and its effectiveness in a practical course prior to its formal publication on the national market.

As you use this text in your course, please share any and all feedback regarding the volume with your professor. Your comments on this text will allow the author to further develop the content of the book, so we can ensure it will be a useful and informative classroom tool for students in universities across the nation and around the globe. If you find the material is challenging to understand, or could be expanded to improve the usefulness of the text, it is important for us to know. If you have any suggestions for improving the material contained in the book or the way it is presented, we encourage you to share your thoughts.

Please note, preliminary editions are similar to review copies, which publishers distribute to select readers prior to publication in order to test a book's audience and elicit early feedback; therefore, you may find inconsistencies in formatting or design, or small textual errors within this volume. Design elements and the written text will likely undergo changes before this book goes to print and is distributed on the national market.

This text is not available in wide release on the market, as it is actively being prepared for formal publication. Accordingly, the book is offered to you at a discounted price to reflect its preliminary status.

If you would like to provide notes directly to the publisher, you may contact us by e-mailing studentreviews@cognella.com. Please include the book's title, author, and 7-digit SKU reference number (found below the barcode on the back cover of the book) in the body of your message.

D1531539

Good Taste

A Reader on Dietary Factors Affecting
Global Cuisines

Revised Preliminary Edition

Edited by Mary S. Willis

University of Nebraska–Lincoln

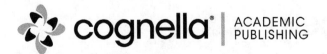
cognella® | ACADEMIC PUBLISHING

Bassim Hamadeh, CEO and Publisher
Natalie Piccotti, Director of Marketing
Kassie Graves, Vice President of Editorial
Jamie Giganti, Director of Academic Publishing
Kristina Stolte, Senior Field Acquisitions Editor
Tony Paese, Project Editor
Casey Hands, Associate Production Editor
Jess Estrella, Senior Graphic Designer
Danielle Gradisher, Licensing Associate

ISBN: 978-1-5165-2284-2 (pbk) / 978-1-5165-2285-9 (br)

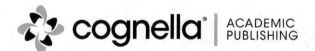

Table of Contents

Topic VII: The Future of Food and Nutrition   317

Introduction

The concept of what tastes good most certainly has a biological component, but more than anything else, one's preferences for food and drink are *culture*-bound. Specifically, we *learn* what is good to eat as we grow up in a specific time, place, and context. Etkin (2006;36) writes that, "Biological hunger is culturally reconfigured into appetites called *cuisines*, which represent complex cycles of pattern and social process." Thus, to explore these complex biological and cultural aspects of food and nutrition, one must consider the four pillars of food security; the availability, accessibility, use-ability, and sustainability of food. The articles selected for *Good Taste!* cover seven general themes within 21 individual documents. Students can consider a food-related topic, in more depth and detail, supplementing what they know and learn in an introductory course on food, nutrition, and culture. They can also gain a new perspective on food and the way in which particular aspects of culture guide and constrain food production, processing, preparation, and consumption.

In many ways, we are what we eat. It for this reason that an understanding of food, and all food-related culture, must be a significant part of working toward individual, but also population health and well-being. Yet in Western countries such as the US, where few of us are involved in any aspect of food-related work, from farm all the way to table, we simply give little thought to what we eat and how it has been produced. Furthermore, there is a clear disconnect with the environment; most of us no longer have any contact with, or knowledge of, the natural resources that are essential for producing food and maintaining health. No longer do we link health issues to the food we consume, thus, in contrast to what was true for Hippocrates, food is no longer an automatic form of medicine. We no longer consider that nutrition will be enhanced or diminished based upon the way in which food has been grown, harvested, and processed. We have lost an understanding of how agriculture works and the many steps required in producing what appears on the shelf of a grocery store. This is in stark contrast to those who produce as much as 85% of the world's food in developing countries, the small-holder farming families. Small-holder families, who farm around two acres of land, have an intimate knowledge of the soil, water, climate, plants, insects, and both wild and domestic animals. They depend on the ecosystem. Their success is directly connected to knowing and understanding how climatic factors, natural resources, and pest species, for example, will impact the growth of the plants and animals they produce for human consumption.

Although we cannot all be expected to return to farming, and regain the lost knowledge related to food production and the importance of natural resources, we can work to understand what the term 'culture' means and how it applies to food. We can become familiar with the way in which all food-related behaviors and patterns are entangled in our own cultural 'bundle.' In addition, we can rediscover how our own food production system or systems, processing techniques, and consumption patterns will affect our health and the health of others. For these reasons, this reader emphasizes cultural aspects of food and nutrition, but also considers some of the biological aspects too, within parts one and two, respectively. Part three includes selections on some of the sociocultural aspects of food and nutrition; one is based in the archaeology of Mesopotamia, one concerns the social aspects of coffee, and another illustrates how religion, and in this case Judaism, can shape food culture. Parts four through six focus on regions, countries, and foods found within or indigenous to the continents of Africa, the Americas, and Asia. The articles that are part of these sections detail foods and food products that are indigenous to or arising from each continental land mass. Most of these foods or food items have made their way around the world to become an integral part of thousands of cuisines. There is also discussion of traditional and newly emerging mechanisms or processes for growing, processing, preparing, and consuming foods, regardless of their origin. Lastly, there are inclusions across each of the continental section readings that discuss traditional protein sources, e.g., termites in Africa, and changing patterns in protein consumption types based upon changing economies, e.g. increased meat consumption in China. The final article describes the future of food and food production, particularly in the face of climate change.

In sum, each general topic and article should strengthen an understanding of food and nutrition, and reinforce the way in which culture shapes, and perhaps dictates, everything one does when it comes to food.

References

Etkin, N. L. (2008). *Edible Medicines: An Ethnopharmacology of Food.* University of Arizona Press.

Topic I: Defining Culture

Culture is one of the most difficult concepts to understand and apply, in any realm and for any topic. Therefore, "What is Culture, Where Does it Come From?" describes culture in a comprehensive way, breaking down the concept into smaller components, and outlining the way one acquires culture throughout a life time. Terms such as 'culture shock' and 'ethnocentrism' are included in the essay and help to deconstruct the culture concept. If you can grasp the culture concept, you will begin to understand how and why people around the world eat the way they do and label or identify a food as one that tastes good. You will also begin to realize that there is no superior way to live, when comparing countries and cultures, and that what tastes good, to one population or culture, may not taste good to another. There is no objective way to define food that tastes good. Rather this idea of 'good' is subjective, an artifact of enculturation.

What Is Culture, Where Does It Come From?

Lawrence A. Beer

Culture is the core determinant of all we are. It is the filter of our senses and therefore the chief controlling agent of life's values, its perceptions, and decisions. Inspection to determine how and why people act the way they do is a far ranging field of learning. Housed in the arena of sociology and psychology the scientific discipline of anthropology studies humans across two interlinked scopes of inquiry—history and geography. The field is divided into four distinct but related subfields that impact, borrow, and therefore influence each other. They are:

1. *archaeology*: studying ancient and prehistoric societies;
2. *physical anthropology*: examining the biological make-up of human beings;
3. *anthropological linguistics*: a comparative inquiry into languages and communication;
4. *cultural anthropology*: the search for similarities and differences among contemporary peoples of the world.

Cultural anthropology looks to identify and describe how people's thought processes produce a set of values upon which they construct their life, the choices they make, and the actions undertaken driven by varied mind-sets. While the world shares many similarities, it differs in many others. There is a marked tendency to assume that we are all alike, for example, in terms of basic human nature. This comes from the fact that most of us draw such conclusions from our limited observations of the immediate society around us. When confronted with an alien or foreign society whose people act differently from us, we think of them as weird, strange, or exhibiting downright wrong behavior. Culture is not positive or negative, it just exists. It is our judgments of culture that contain such judicial dispositions.

Our assumptions of reality are culturally bound because we practice cultural monotheism. This natural tendency disqualifies all of us to act as empathetic arbitrators of differences as we are all strongly anchored in and held back by the chains of our own culture. To unlock this judgmental stranglehold one needs to embrace the idea that cultural pluralism, in masked form, resides in all of us. We possess, although hidden from our consciousness, dormant cultural traits that mirror to an extent those people who on the surface are perceived as different from us, and vice versa—what is called the duality factor.

Exploring the Meaning of Culture

When one thinks of culture, a mirage of defining terms and examples appears. To be "cultured" is to have received an introduction to the classy things in life. We often think one who is cultured possesses a superior education or at least an awareness of such things as the fine arts and classical literature, is knowledgeable about the philosophies of great teachers, and appreciative of the music of the great masters.

When describing the culture of a society, we normally address surface attributes—those characteristics that we can physically sense as stimulating our eyes, ears, smell, and touch. But below the illustrated surface or *folk culture* lies a host of hidden or *deep cultural* attributes. They are recessed in the mind-sets of people, exercising control over their thoughts and behavior and are responsible for their core beliefs and values—how people rationalize and think. Figure 1.1 illustrates the multisurface aspects of the cultural minutiae. Like an iceberg, most of a group's perceived cultural attitudes, the overt, lie on the top layer while those below the surface, the covert, are revealed only when people are engaged in relationships with others and the curtain of familiarity is drawn.

Even our own cultural knowledge of ourselves is often masked as rarely does one take the time to examine, much less classify one's personal tendencies, why we behave and act in a certain way. Our deep cultural identity is only challenged when we encounter an alien society and begin to perhaps question our own values in the face of differences.

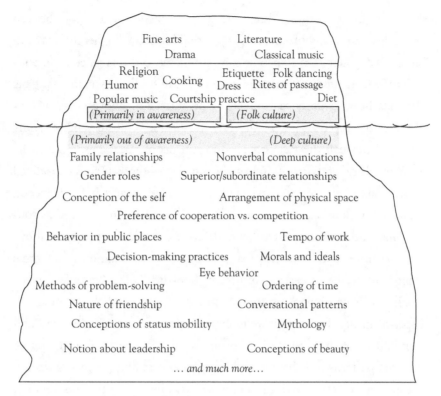

Figure 1.1. The cultural iceberg.

Defining Culture

There may be no single acceptable definition of what is meant by the all encompassing term culture. In his book *The Cultural Dimension of International Business*, Gary Ferraro notes that two early researchers in the field "A. L. Kroeber and Clyde Kluckhohn in 1952 identified more than 160 different definitions of culture."[1] In its simplest description culture is a design system for living. Edward Tylor, writing over a century ago, described culture as "that complex whole which includes knowledge, belief, art, morals, law, custom and any other capabilities and habits acquired by man as a member of society."[2] M. J. Herskovits depicted culture as mental, "the man made part of the environment" as opposed to the material or physical created by nature.[3] Geert Hofstede referred to the process as the "collective programming of the mind which distinguishes the members of one group from another."[4] Hofstede described a series of habitual thinking patterns made up of shared values, beliefs, symbols, behaviors, and assumptions that define the group. Technically, culture is an abstraction that cannot be seen or touched, an intangible mental process that Hofstede further defines as an intellectual system to help people solve problems. But it is reflected in one's activities, so it produces material examples, physically observable tangible elements from artifacts to language—the surface or above water aspects of the cultural iceberg (see Figure 1.1). In the end, culture is most vividly expressed through the values it produces in people and is exemplified by what people do and do not do in a given society—that which is considered as acceptable behavior and that which is deemed unacceptable behavior. Prevailing or dominant actions and/or reactions to life are regarded as conventional and tend to be classified to describe the culture of a given group.

It is important to remember this point when examining all these approaches to the subject of culture, as the word "collective" refers to the fact that it is contingent on the combined reflections of the members of a specific group. Hence culture is shared by two or more individuals and is indicative of their repetitive, normative, demonstrative, and therefore expected patterns of behavior—allowing one to qualify these as a deductive generalized characterization of a society. However, this consideration is both positive and negative. If we can classify a specific culture via a set of applied research-based determinants, those of oneself and others, we may learn in advance how to form relationships with them, by concentrating on the similarities but keeping in mind the differences. On the other hand, such a classification approach induces prejudices, a prejudgment that may not allow for a cultural free space to exist where one first observes before forming opinions to guide their action and reaction. Edward T. Hall warns those studying culture that it often hides more that it reveals and what it obscures most effectively is an appreciation and understanding of one's own culture.[5] Culture can therefore be a minefield of contradictions, misplaced assumptions, false observations, and tainted conclusions but its value as a relationship building tool should not be dismissed or understated. One is instructed to just tread lightly in the illuminated path it provides. The numerous sets of cross-cultural determinants, as reviewed in chapter 3, can result in a labyrinth whose positive metaphorical intent is meant to hone one's focus and provide a pathway of understanding. But to many the vast collections turn into a maze, perverting the ability to comprehend, often confusing and trapping the cross-cultural traveler.

Where Does Culture Come From?

In the end, culture can be summarized as "everything that people have, think and do as members of their society"[6]; a total way of life. With representative examples of culture both above and below the surface of inspection and with defined parameters of what it is, it is valuable in understanding how it works to consider where it comes from. If culture is the sum total of one's observations and indoctrinations it follows that it is a learned experience that begins at birth. While the hardware of our brain is biologically constructed the loaded software is placed in the mental system by interaction via our sensory mechanisms with one's environment—the material world and relationships with its inhabitants. Unlike the genetic construction of the physical brain which is internal, cultural learning is external. This simple axiom is universal and while cultures differ around the world the process of acquiring culture is similarly reproduced in all societies.

Cultural indoctrination is the sum of all one is exposed to as we emerge from the womb, and hence it continues to death. During life it never stops. The process is composed of inputs beginning with the family unit and like the proverbial pebble thrown into a pond it radiates outward growing wider and wider as new segments of exposure are engaged. This mechanism of learning is socialization. It starts with family/kinship relationships conferring upon us our first introduction to our cultural heritage. It is influenced by the physical environment in which we live as we view how others who went before us have adapted to it. Our cultural identity is more formally built on the educational system one is placed in. It is molded on the ethical and moral teachings encountered in a society that morph into secular laws as well as spiritual guidance based on religious doctrines and philosophical approaches defining expected behavior. It is also prejudiced by unwritten customs and traditions that are followed. Hence one often hears the refrain "this just isn't done" or "this is how we do it" without pointing to a specific educational indoctrination or authoritative prescribed written code of conduct. While one's cultural programming includes formal and informal training it is absorbed from mere observation via general immersion in society as well as through trial and error as one is punished for unacceptable actions. It emerges from problem solving of everyday matters.

Cultural Steps: Levels of Associations Contributing to Cultural Self-Identity Building

Cultural indoctrination is a journey of steps or building levels that one goes through in a given society (see Figure 1.2). The first step is birthright cultural indoctrination initially acquired via the family one emerges from the womb or is adopted into. It is this first primary group that provides the initial level of cultural indoctrination and includes the collateral influence of a clan or tribe of common ethnic, racial, or religious/philosophical principles that the family resides in. This initial creation step in the development of one's cultural identity is itself based on a closed groups system of mating, marriage or its monogamous equivalent, child rearing, and family structure. Even within a uniform politically designated society such family orientations produce regional differences. All our basic assumptions are tethered like a life sustaining umbilical cord to this first level and this exposure tends to act as the anchor of our core values. The saying "it takes a village to bring up a child" is indicative of the surrounding geographical social arena, one's associations with others, that one grows in. It is also made up of one's climatic and physical environment as well as the socioeconomic and political exposure one encounters with a particular sovereign territory. As with family units even the norms and behaviors experienced with a given bordered nation may be further segregated by differences in domestic regional characteristics setting them apart from other citizens of the same nation.

While the nomenclature of culture is normally prescribed to identify the national culture of a particular geographical area of the world there are other influencing factors often denoted as subcultures as they are embedded in a country or regional territory. Two identifiable contributory components are educational/professional and organizational. Some would argue that these additional cultural steps are not a set of values but instead are merely a series of acceptable group practices imposed by the power channels of such institutional subgroups one associates with and hence are not a natural process of cultural assimilation.[7] However, as powerful stimulators of behavior and perceptual development they are part of the cultural building process. One's cultural path in life is further influenced by the structured choice of the formal education afforded them.

From primary or grade school up and through undergraduate university, masters, and perhaps even the doctorate level such scholastic exposures to specific instructional programs and curriculums chosen alter one's thinking matrix and cultural indoctrination. With some degrees culminating in acceptance into the professional ranks or a specialized field of study the endowments provided by one's academic experiences assist in the manifestation of selected cultural inputs.

At the top level is organizational culture. Organizational culture is a relatively new field in the arena of cultural anthropology with research in the area pioneered by studies of commercial institutions and managerial approaches to the internal psychology, attitudes, experiences, beliefs, and values of shared groups of people operating toward a unified goal. It is the goal orientation that defines and separates this category of culture, how things are accomplished, from the normative other levels of cultural development. Organizational culture can be simply stated as *the way things get done around here*.[8] It is reflective of a patterned activity of shared assumptions the group have evolved to solve problems. As such the paradigm created runs the gamut from mission values, the expectation or goal creator, to tangible control systems and structures while also containing influential emotion-based intangible elements such as institutional symbols, rituals, and routines as well as stories and myths, all working together to sustain and perpetuate the culture of an organization.[9] Organization culture is shaped and its character devised from a firm's unique historical roots, its situational development as it has responded to internal and external forces in its growth cycle. It reflects not only on employees but also relationship dealings with customers and suppliers as well as responses to competitors. Organizational culture tends to be forced acceptance as opposed to the more hidden reinforced acculturation occasioned by acquiring culture via birthright, the passive accumulation of geographical influences and the volunteered or sought after educational elements that all result in acquiring one's cultural acquisitions in the tiered building system per Figure 1.2.

The first two layers, birthright and geographical, of cultural development are the deepest felt, the most difficult to change, and vary the most as one moves from one society to another. The top two layers, educational and organizational, may by their broader indoctrination acquisition

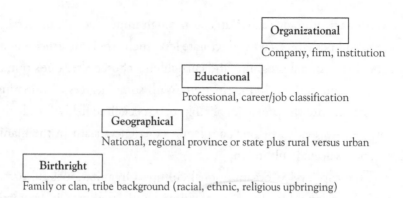

Figure 1.2. Cultural building staircase: levels of group induced affiliations.

surpass the constraints of the more limited originating family/geographical inputs thereby allowing for greater flexibility, alteration, and change. People are more apt to modify the higher educational institutions they attend much less than the subjects they major in and the collateral courses selected. The same occurs over their business careers they tend to adjust their professional associations and certainly move from company to company; a readjustment of organizational culture but continue to perform many of the identical tasks within them.

Examining One's Cultural Self-Identity

An exercise based on the various group affiliations one is exposed to in life, the levels of cultural indoctrination as provided by other associations to induced self-identity is proposed by Taylor Cox, Jr. and Ruby L. Beale in their book on managing diversity.[10] The activity, with the goal of increasing awareness of one's socially induced self-identity, directs one to create a "pie chart" based on two dimensions of diversity related to one's group affiliations in their lives by indicating the approximate importance of membership in groups as represented by the size of the slice of pie assigned to them. An evaluation of one's primary associations (e.g., sex and orientation, race, ethnicity, age, physical and mental abilities) and secondary associations (education, income, marital and parental status, religion, political affiliation, work experience as well as hobbies, grooming and clothing style, music preference) provide the criteria for assessment. This combination of forces, under the control or inducement of others, and self-selected group affiliations examines how people categorize themselves and hence allows for an insight into one's cultural profile as well as indicating the force or influence these associations exert on the individual. While the criteria are much wider than the four cultural levels concept that begins with the family and progresses up to organizations, it can be a valuable tool in assessing one's cultural drivers. The only drawback to the exercise is that the journey to self-discovery is complicated and a number of false positives may be encountered as the integration of associations tends to contaminate one another as opposed to direct linkages specifically affecting behavior and perceptual thinking. A simpler, less complex set of cultural components or determinants might afford a better guide to one's cultural self-identity.

The Cultural Pond

Another way to visualize the cultural development of the individual but with an added component is the undulating pebble in the pond example. As a small stone is dropped in the center of the water, a ripple upon which the individual cultural ship sails is created. The vessel containing one's cultural identity is propelled outward engaging larger and wider cultural experience and assimilation as the ship moves out through ever expanding circles (see Figure 1.3). It first passes through the family unit absorbing both the surface and deep undercurrent characteristics. As the pebble, birth cultural development, sinks at this spot in the pond it more

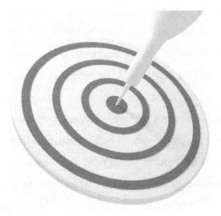

Figure 1.3. Cultural circles.

intensively draws down the cultural affinity, almost anchoring the ship. The cultural ship's journey moves through the three remaining circles encountering the geographical area then passing the educational segment and finally progressing across the organizational area.

The cultural pond is at its deepest at the center, the spot of initial contact of the pebble and the start of the ship's cultural journey. The water depth drops off as the bottom rises as one ventures out and collaterally so does the intensity of the influential conditioning the cultural pond provides. Think in terms of a right-angled triangle lying on its side with the family providing the strongest influence and in descending order geographical, educational, and organizational (see Figure 1.4).

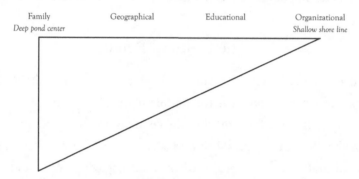

Figure 1.4. *Cultural pond depth: from deep to shallow influence.*

Cultural Push Back: *Culture Shock*

Calm sailing of the cultural ship normally occurs as one progresses outwardly and comes to rest on the eventual shoreline of their own pond. However as one crosses over the land bridge to a new culture the track can be torturous as one's cultural security is threatened. Sometimes the beach terrain is uneven and rocky or ends at an embankment such as natural cliffs or a man-made sea wall. The cultural wave that propelled in their home pond does not gently wash up and over to a new alien cultural pond. The waters upon which one's cultural ship ventures is repelled backwards and may be forced to recede. An upsurge in the surf occurs, disturbing the tranquility of the home or domestic cultural pond affecting one's emotional and rational mind-set. This push back is cultural shock. Cultural shock is theoretically defined as the "psychological reaction to an unfamiliar or alien environment" referred to by Kalervo Oberg as "a generalized trauma one experiences in a new and different culture because of having to learn and cope with a vast array of new cultural cues and expectations, while discovering that your old ones probably do not fit or work."[11]

The more different the shoreline obstruction erected by the alien society is from one's domestic waters the stronger the reverse wave and the cultural ship is tossed around, upsetting the navigational balance and affecting its structural identity. Americans traveling to their northern neighbor Canada would experience minimal culture shock as the two countries share an abundance of similarities making up the radiating circles; and one might be said to be sailing on a conjoined cultural pond feed from related cultural springs. As one "jumps across the pond," a common vernacular expression for crossing the Atlantic Ocean to Europe, a stop in England, a nation that shares a common heritage and basic language with the United States (accent and terminology aside), might not be so shocking but certainly more then a Canadian venture. Moving east onto Europe increased cultural strains might be encountered. As one ventures south and further east, across the Mediterranean onto the African continent, the Middle East and still further east toward the Asian subcontinent and into China the divide between East and West, first mentioned in the Introduction, gets wider and the push back or cultural shock deepens, becoming more acutely felt on all the senses. While initially the disturbing feeling occasioned by entering culturally alien societies tends to be on the surface of the cultural iceberg (see Figure 1.1) the physical observed differences, those below the surface, mind-sets affecting core values and therefore determining beliefs, attitudes, outlooks, and perceptional realities begin to rise, psychologically affecting the cross-cultural engager. One has a natural tendency to retreat to what they feel is normal, deeply desirous of the safety of their ingrained learned cultural attitudes and beliefs, their pond, as they attempt to combat alien cultures.

The push back can be just a mere ripple or a more destructive intensive undulation akin to a rip tide. It is felt most dramatically in descending reverse order as it moves offshore to deeper home cultural waters. Organizational or institutional culture is first affected as it based in shallower waters. Then to a lesser but still strong degree educational culture, then to a minor extent geographical and finally to the least amount family culture as this element is most deeply entrenched in higher waters, anchored in the middle of the pond. Within a business context one may first notice differences in institutional hierarchy structuring, the organizational circle, duties, responsibilities, and decision-making roles; the way things get done within a group vary. Strategic goals may be based on alternative value assessments. Time orientations and meeting models may differ. Parties that share professional backgrounds, the educational circle, with similar sounding titles or positions are not equal in how they apply basic skill sets and interact with other segments of the company. The regulatory and economic environment the alien business operates in, the geographical circle, impacts operational activities. The infrastructure, from communication in marketing programs to affected channels of trade and distribution, may differ. Commercial relationships whose underpinnings stem from one's personal indoctrinations, the family circle, may not be established in the same way. Individual versus collective group objectives are not uniform with one cultural determinant taking precedence over the other.

The process of acculturation, a hopefully gentle immersion into a new society, is not easy and recognizing this is important. It is this backdrop of cultural development, its acquisition and potential disruption, that international managers must first appreciate and understand before their formal education on the subject begins. A cross-cultural education enables one to build a *bridge over troubled water*[12] allowing our individual ships to sail smoothly between one's home harbor ponds and those inhabited by alien societies while minimizing culture shock.

Other Aspects of Culture

Culture as Acquired Knowledge

Culture is a process wherein one acquires the knowledge to deal with accepted social behaviors in a given group or society. The process is characterized by a series of key factors. It is a learning experience (a) passed on from one generation to the next, (b) mutually shared with others resulting in common outlooks and responses of a group, (c) exemplified by interlocking cross-influential patterns that sustain and play off each other, (d) observable via commonly understood symbols and finally part of a (e) fluid state with adaptive changes altering all of the previous contributing factors.

Culture as a Sensory Filter

Culture is the prime motivator of our conscious and unconscious thought. It influences our brain and heart, impacts our rational determinations and emotional intuitions. It is the filter of our senses, what we see, hear, smell, taste, and touch. The inputs from these collectors are interpreted, assigned values and therefore classified as important or not, depending upon our cultural indoctrinations. Culture determines our value system and prejudices our perceptions. While we all see the same things, like peering through the lens of a camera, the imprint process on the film of our brain causes different culturally induced images to appear. The colors and the shades are altered. Some images are sharp while others are grainy or out of focus. The expression "don't you see it" is most appropriate as in fact we don't all see identically. The axiom "beauty is in the eyes of the beholder" is true and exemplifies our cultural induced bias as we unconsciously apply our predetermined socially induced beliefs, values and traditions dispositions.

The Ethnocentric Nature of Culture

One of the dangers of culture is that it creates and supports ethnocentric dispositions. It is natural for one to think that their way is the best or correct way and such presumptive thinking is an impediment to being open to the acceptance of alien cultures. Ferraro defines ethnocentrism as "literally 'culture centered'—the tendency for people to evaluate a foreigner's behavior by the standards of their own culture and believe that their culture is superior to all others."[13] When confronted by difference, instead of re-evaluating our own stance on issues there is a penchant to fail back on what one has first learned and treat such knowledge as sacrosanct; failing to recognize our own biases. This is the trapdoor in the cultural learning process and one must be ever vigilant not to fall through it.

Cultural Stereotyping

We all come equipped with a nuanced picture of the world called cultural stereotyping. It is the product of retained memory and learned patterns of associations. Such dual programming often results in snap judgments about those we meet with preconceptions of expectations. While cultural investigating and the process of providing value determinants to access and qualify the pronounced group characteristics of particular societies is a valuable guidance tool in both understanding and appreciating social interaction and relationship development, it has its dangers. There is a marked tendency to prejudge relative similarities or differences between two cultures based on applied research and quantified historical inspectional criteria. To stereotype people and place them into prelabeled categories so one can know what to expect and hence plan to act and react accordingly seems to be a reasonable and prudent device. It is a very natural consideration, like doing one's homework in advance and being prepared; an axiom we have all heard. In doing so there is a related risk, as all too often caricature-based descriptions of people can contain oversimplifications, biased images and impressions, gossip, and myth related stories resulting in a clichéd profile of a society. Best to resist this temptation and therefore tread lightly between the factual and the fictional.

What the study of culture and the principles used in the examination process should really be intended for is to provide a template for investigation as opposed to generating predisposed dispositions of expected values, behavior, and attitudes. A knowledge of culture is best applied when it is joined by observation and experience. One's cultural education is best used when it allows for the actual input to be correlated with definitive criteria and a meaningful classification system. In other words create a reservoir of information that allows one to be a cultural detective. Besides first appreciating one's own cultural profile, watch, monitor, and examine others before forming cultural opinions, then correlate such familiarity into usable understandable and workable knowledge on how to best engage and form relationships with new parties.

Notes

1. Ferraro (2006), p. 19.
2. Tylor (1871), p. 1.
3. Herskovits (1955), p. 305.
4. Hofstede (1991).
5. Hall (1976).
6. Ferraro (2006), p. 19.
7. Hofstede (1999).
8. Deal (1982).
9. Johnson (1988), pp. 75–91.
10. Cox (1997).
11. Harris (1996), p. 140.
12. Song title and lyric, *Bridge over troubled water* published in 1970 with words and music by Paul Simon, New York, NY, Columbia Records.
13. Ferraro (2006), p. 35.
14. The term has been attributed to those describing the uncanny ability of Apple Computer founder Steve Jobs to motivate others by misleading his audience into believing that the task at hand could be accomplished, in spite of the realities of difficulty surrounding a project. The phrase may have been borrowed from the popular *Star Trek* science fiction TV program and movie series to explain a phenomenon whereby normal observations are altered causing the brain to not to perceive things as they really are.
15. Bellah (2011).
16. Kissinger (2011).
17. Aydon (2007), p. 1.
18. Angier (2011); referencing David Wilson.
19. Delanty (2011).

Discussion Questions: What is Culture? Where Does it Come From?

1. If you are ethnocentric about food, what does that mean?
2. Briefly describe two ways that culture is acquired or learned. When does culture acquisition begin?
3. What is culture shock? How would this be experienced with food?
4. List and describe 4 different sources for the development of your own food culture.

Topic II: On Biology & Nutrition

As is true for all mammals, there are aspects of our biology that can have an impact on the way we eat and process food; hence, *Skin and Sun* provides an example of one such biological trait, skin, that mediates micronutrient synthesis and uptake. One's skin is responsible for generating or regulating the levels of several vitamins critical to human health. This selection goes through the important role played by the largest of our organs in maintaining one's health, detailing the way this adaptation came about and what happens if we disregard our biology. When one understands what this massive organ in the body does, then it becomes clear how biology and culture work together to maximize health.

Malnutrition includes both undernutrition and overnutrition or obesity. The selection *Malnutrition and Obesity*, defines the label or term obesity, based upon world standards. The reader learns about the way in which malnutrition, or bad nutrition, and related sequelae compromise one's nutrition and health status worldwide. One can also consider the differences in the cultural concepts of beauty, patterns of thinness and fatness, and trends such as the 'nutrition transition' that is now in process in many countries around the world.

Anthropometric Characteristics of Underprivileged Adolescents: A Study from the Urban Slums of India describes growth and development, as well as gender, socioeconomic, and age issues that are uncovered during an 'anthropometric' assessment of malnourished adolescents in India. To understand how nutritional intake can affect growth, there is a discussion of differential need in terms of dietary consumption, across the life span, and between males and females. Other factors that affect growth and development patterns during adolescence are included. One can see how the use of basic anthropometry, gathering values for height, weight, and mid-upper arm circumference (MUAC), are part of a critical and non-invasive approach to the study of overall body health and nutritional status.

skin and sun

Nina Jablonski

As we go about our daily lives, our skin is always active, and its complex chemistry is constantly changing. Skin cells are dividing, important molecules are being broken down, others are being repaired, and yet others are being created on the spot. Because the human lineage originated in the tropics and spent most of its six million or so years of existence in tropical areas, part of the skin's activity has involved a series of anatomical and biochemical adaptations to heat and sunlight. Sweating is only part of the story. Our skin has also evolved other ways to mediate vital chemical transactions between the body and the environment, and particularly between the body and sunlight.

The sun emits a wide variety of electromagnetic radiation, ranging from very short-wavelength ionizing radiation such as gamma rays to very long-wavelength infrared radiation and radio waves (figure 17). Ultraviolet radiation (UVR) itself includes a broad spectrum of wavelengths, from very short-wavelength vacuum UV to longer-wavelength UVC, UVB, and UVA. Although it is maligned by most biologists because of its destructive effects on bio-

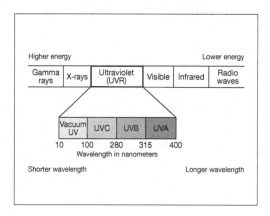

FIGURE 17. Solar radiation comes in a wide range of wavelengths and energy levels. The most harmful types of radiation are those with the shortest wavelengths and the highest energy, such as gamma rays and UVC. Oxygen and ozone in the earth's atmosphere filter out much of the harmful UVR, but overexposure to UVR can damage DNA and destroy folate in the body. (© 2005 Jennifer Kane.)

logical systems, UVR has been one of the most important forces in the evolution of life on earth. From the early days of our planet's history, unicellular and multicellular organisms have been forced to evolve mechanisms to protect their delicate chemical reactions from its disruptive effects.[1]

For living creatures, the most damaging types of radiation are those with the shortest wavelengths and the highest energy, such as gamma rays and UVC. During the long sweep of earth's history, our planet has developed an atmosphere rich in oxygen and ozone, which very effectively screens out the most harmful wavelengths of solar radiation. Longer wavelengths of UVR (specifically UVB and UVA), along with visible light and infrared and radio waves, penetrate the atmosphere much more easily. Scientists and some politicians today are rightly concerned about the health of the earth's atmosphere and, in particular, the state of our protective ozone layer. If this ozone layer becomes thinner or badly perforated, most forms of life on earth would suffer from the destructive effects of high-energy solar radiation, especially excessive UVB.

Using satellite data, we can generate a map showing average UVR levels at the earth's surface (see color map 1).[2] This map reveals some predictable patterns and a few surprises. Levels of UVR are highest in the tropics and especially at the equator. But latitude is not the only determinant; some places near the equator experience much higher levels of UVR than others.

Arid regions like the Sahara Desert receive very high levels of UVR, whereas more humid or cloudy equatorial areas like the Amazon rain forest receive lower levels. Outside the tropics, UVR levels are generally lower, with a few conspicuous exceptions. The Tibetan plateau, for instance, experiences very high levels of UVR because of its high altitude and thin atmosphere.[3]

Different types of UVR penetrate the earth's atmosphere to different extents. As UVR approaches the earth, the most high-energy wavelengths (UVC and about 90 percent of UVB) are absorbed by the oxygen and ozone in the atmosphere. The remaining 10 percent of the UVB and all of the UVA pass through, but the amount that actually makes it to any given spot on the earth depends on the latitude and the angle of the sunlight at that particular place and time. As one moves away from the equator and the angle of the sunlight decreases, the atmosphere becomes thicker and filters out more UVB. Thus, low levels of UVB fall on areas at high latitudes. Very small changes in UVB levels have substantial effects on plants and animals. Organisms living at extremely high northern and southern latitudes, for example, have adapted to receiving only tiny doses of UVB, and only at the peak of summer.[4] The unequal distribution of UVB and UVA on earth has had enormous consequences for the evolution of life at different latitudes, and for the evolution of human skin color, as we will see later.

Most of the chemical reactions that UVR causes in the body are harmful. If you've ever had a sunburn, you know that your skin has been damaged—you can feel and see it. But a sunburn is only the most immediately palpable and visible negative effect of UVR exposure. The most serious destruction wrought by UVR is more sinister because it can go unnoticed for years. At the molecular level, UVR can damage DNA, the most important information-carrying molecule in the body, which is essential to cell division. UVR can affect a DNA molecule directly by changing the molecule's chemical composition when it absorbs the UVR or indirectly through the potentially destructive free radicals generated by UVR.

The worst damage is caused when DNA absorbs shorter-wavelength

UVR (mostly UVB). Specific chemicals, known as "photoproducts" because they are the result of solar radiation, are then produced within the DNA molecule, causing small physical distortions in its structure. These distortions are normally corrected by a process known as nucleotide excision repair, which removes and replaces the damaged DNA strands—a sort of corrective surgery at the molecular level. The evolution of the ability to repair DNA was one of the most important innovations in the history of life on earth. The repair usually proceeds uneventfully, provided that not too much DNA was affected and that the repair mechanism itself is in good shape. But if the repair is inadequate, cells will then reproduce with faulty DNA. Given enough time and continued exposure to UVB, cells with faulty DNA can build up in the skin, eventually leading to skin cancer.[5] UVA also causes considerable harm to DNA, although this damage is somewhat different in its structure, and possibly in its effect, from that caused by UVB. UVA has been implicated as a major culprit in the premature aging of skin caused by sun exposure (known as photoaging), and it has been associated in epidemiological studies with the most dangerous form of skin cancer, malignant melanoma.[6]

DNA is not the only molecule adversely affected by UVR. Folate, for example, is a water-soluble B vitamin that is necessary to produce DNA. The body must constantly manufacture new DNA, because so many of its routine functions require cell division: creating new blood cells; replenishing the skin, hair follicles, and linings of the mouth and gut; and producing sperm cells in men (a process that continues throughout adult life).[7] But a lack of folate will slow or curtail DNA production, and all the processes that require new DNA will suffer, especially those that need the DNA quickly or continually. DNA is especially critical for fueling the rapid cell division that occurs in a developing human embryo or fetus, particularly in the early weeks of pregnancy, when organs are beginning to form and the overall plan of the body is being laid out. Without sufficient folate in a mother's body, not enough DNA will be produced to promote the cell division that allows embryonic tissues to differentiate and grow.[8]

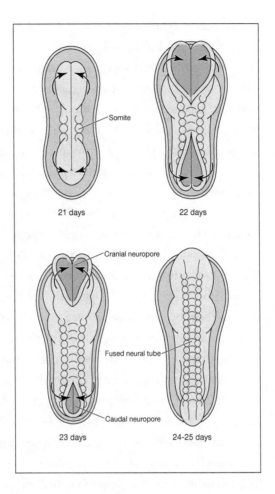

FIGURE 18. The nervous system in a human embryo begins to develop with the formation of the neural tube during the first few weeks of pregnancy. This process involves the precise, zipperlike closing of neural folds on the top of the embryo, as depicted in the sequence here. For this process to succeed, cell division in the neural folds must occur exactly on schedule. If there is not enough folate to fuel DNA production for the rapidly dividing cells of the neural folds, a neural tube defect can develop. The somites, structures flanking the neural tube, are the building blocks for many of the body's future muscles and bones. (Illustration by Jennifer Kane.)

Folate also plays a crucial role in the development of the embryonic nervous system. A shortage of folate at a critical time in early development can lead to birth defects of varying degrees of severity, including some that may be lethal. Folate deficiency is now widely acknowledged as a risk factor for numerous complications of pregnancy as well as for a group of birth defects called neural tube defects (figure 18).[9] The neural tube is the forerunner of the central nervous system in the embryo. It extends from the top of the primordial brain (the cranial neuropore) to the end of the spinal cord (the caudal neuropore).

Few nutrients compare with folate in terms of its impact on health, especially the reproductive health of both men and women. We derive folate mostly from green leafy vegetables, citrus fruits, and whole grains. Because folate is so vital to the body's machinery and to maintaining reproductive health, it has become a focus of public health campaigns in many countries. Folate is now added to many foods (especially breads and cereals) in the form of folic acid to ensure that people sustain adequate levels in their bodies, and women of reproductive age are encouraged to take folate supplements.[10]

UVR and other high-energy radiation can destroy folate in the body. When this occurs suddenly or on a large scale, the consequences are serious because all the chemical processes that depend on folate are affected.[11] Although scientists first documented the adverse effects of UVR on folate in humans nearly thirty years ago,[12] only in the past decade, as the importance of folate became clear, have we begun to understand the implications of this phenomenon. The details of the chemical destruction of folate by UVR have recently been documented in laboratory experiments, which have shown that folate is most susceptible to damage by the longer wavelengths of UVR, UVA.[13] These studies are paving the way for investigations of how naturally occurring UVA affects folate levels in humans during real life. If UVR can destroy folate, a substance essential to human life and reproduction, it is clear that some sort of defensive mechanisms must have evolved through natural selection to help maintain folate levels in the body. This is where the story of skin color comes in, as chapters 5 and 6 explain in greater detail. When the body is suffering from the effects of sun, the evolutionary solution has been to add natural sunscreen to the body's surface, the skin.[14]

Despite the destructive effects of UVR, it is not universally harmful and in fact has some positive biological effects. The most important of these—the production of vitamin D, popularly known as the "sunshine vitamin"—occurs in the skin.[15] Vitamin D exists in several forms: vitamin D_3 is made by vertebrates, and vitamin D_2 is the primary form found in plants. Vitamin D is a unique natural molecule that first appeared on earth as a product of photosynthesis in tiny marine phytoplankton over 750 million years ago.[16] Although its function in the earliest vertebrates (ancient fish) is not well understood, by about 350 million years ago—the time the first tetrapods emerged, the first animals to spend significant amounts of time on dry land—this vitamin had taken on an essential role in vertebrate evolution.

Vitamin D is important to all vertebrates because it allows them to absorb calcium from their diet and build a strong internal skeleton. Fish can easily get enough vitamin D by eating plankton or other fish that contain it. For the earliest land-living vertebrates, however, these sources of vitamin D were not available, even though their need for calcium in order to maintain a rigid skeleton was great. At this stage in evolution, with natural selection operating full force, vertebrates developed the ability to make their own vitamin D. Because vitamin D is manufactured by a photochemical, or sunlight-induced, process, early tetrapods could help to satisfy their body's requirements for the substance by exposing themselves to sunlight. In this way, they could potentially get vitamin D both from their diet and from the vitamin factory in their skin.

UVR in the UVB range stimulates the production of vitamin D_3 in the skin. High-energy UVB photons first penetrate the skin and are absorbed by a cholesterol-like molecule residing in the cells of the epidermis and dermis, which catalyzes the formation of a molecule called previtamin D_3. This precursor molecule is then transformed in the skin at body temperature to vitamin D_3, which undergoes further chemical conversion in the liver and kidney to become the biologically active form of the vitamin. This reaction is self-limiting: if the body's circulation already contains enough of the active form of vitamin D, the process of making more is discontinued, and the chemical precursors are broken down into various inert by-products. In this way, the body averts "vitamin D intoxication," or vitamin D poisoning, the overproduction of the active form.[17]

The active form of vitamin D is used throughout the body for a variety of purposes. It regulates calcium and phosphorus metabolism, the basis of making a strong skeleton. It also facilitates calcium absorption from the

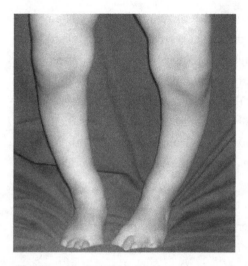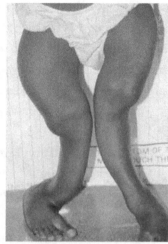

FIGURE 19. The soft, poorly calcified bones of children afflicted with nutritional rickets are bent under the weight of the body. This condition is caused by a serious vitamin D deficiency, which prevents absorption of calcium from the diet. Historically, rickets afflicted mostly children living in far northern latitudes with little UVB, but it is becoming increasingly common in children with dark skin at all latitudes who lack calcium in their diet or who are not exposed to sunlight. (Left, © NMSB/Custom Medical Stock Photo; right, courtesy of Tom D. Thacher, MD.)

gut and has a direct effect on bone-forming cells. We have long known that vitamin D is necessary for the growth of bones because it allows the body to absorb calcium from food.

A shortage or lack of vitamin D has negative effects on the body throughout the human lifespan. A vitamin D deficiency during childhood or adolescence can reduce a person's reproductive ability later on. The most serious and infamous condition caused by vitamin D deficiency is nutritional rickets, a childhood disease in which the long bones of the legs bow under the body's weight (figure 19). In children with rickets, the cartilage in developing bones fails to mineralize properly because the body is not absorbing calcium and phosphate. Serious cases of rickets in girls also prevent the pelvis from forming normally, which can cause later problems with pregnancy, including obstructed labor and a high incidence of infant and maternal health problems and mortality. Abnormally low levels of vitamin D can also interfere with normal ovarian function. Among pregnant women, vitamin D deficiency contributes to pathologically low calcium levels in their blood and later to rickets in their babies. Among all adults, it can produce osteomalacia, a painful softening of the bone's structural framework, and can also affect the functioning of the immune system.[18]

Less widely known than vitamin D's importance to a healthy skeleton is its role in regulating normal cell growth and inhibiting cancer cell growth.[19] Insufficient vitamin D has recently been related to an increased risk of several types of cancer that commonly afflict people in industrialized countries, namely, colon, breast, prostate, and ovarian cancer.[20] These cancers appear to be particularly prevalent among people with chronic, low-level vitamin D deficiencies who live in high latitudes—a finding whose evolutionary significance will become evident in the following two chapters.

Ultraviolet radiation has been a relentless force in the evolution of life on earth. Because of its destructive power, organisms have had to evolve sophisticated means to protect their most basic reproductive machinery—DNA and its folate precursors—from annihilation. Like most villains, however, UVR has a good side that isn't often taken into account. Its ability to transform molecules in the skin into the precursors of vitamin D has been of paramount importance to all vertebrate organisms living on land, including people. The real trick in evolution has been to figure out a way to control the amount of UVR entering the skin, and that is the skin's dark secret.

Discussion Questions: Skin and Sun

1. How is one's skin linked to nutrition? How does skin mediate nutrition and which nutrients are affected or involved?
2. What is UVR and what happens if one has too much UVR?
3. What is rickets and how does it develop?
4. Ultimately, why does skin color vary throughout the world?

Malnutrition and Obesity

Thomas J Bassett and Alex Winter-Nelson

Malnutrition takes many forms. Previous maps focused on inadequate consumption of nutritious food among populations. The consumption of too much of certain foods can also result in malnutrition, but not hunger. When people do little physical activity and their diets include excessive amounts of saturated fats, starches, and carbohydrates, they become overweight or even obese. Nutritionists and health policy experts are increasingly concerned about this form of overnutrition because of its public health implications. Overweight and obese people are more prone to chronic diseases such as diabetes, hypertension, heart disease, osteoarthritis, and some cancers. Although the WHO and FAO focus their activities on ending hunger in the world, obesity is a growing concern (box 5.1).

The prevalence of obesity in a population is measured through body mass index (BMI) classifications developed by The National Center for Health Statistics (NCHS). A person's BMI score is his or her weight (in kilograms) divided by his or her height in meters squared. For example, a young woman who weighs 58 kilograms (128 lbs) and is 1.7 meters tall (5 feet 7 inches) has a BMI score of 20 $(58/(1.7)^2)$. This number can be compared to the ranges developed by NCHS that classify subjects as underweight, normal weight, overweight, and obese (table 5.1). The ranges are indicative only of the frequency of these conditions in a population. Whether or not a specific individual's weight is a health concern should be determined in consultation with a physician.

Table 5.1 shows BMI cutoff levels that determine the NCHS classifications and presents the share of women in selected countries whose BMI scores fall into each of these ranges. NCHS nutritionists believe that people are at risk for diseases associated with undernutrition if their BMI is less than 18.5 and at risk of problems from overnutrition if their BMI is greater than 25. The use of a low BMI to indicate risks associated with undernutrition is described in box 5.2. With a BMI of 20, the young woman in our example would be consid-

ered to have a normal weight for her height. In contrast to this hypothetical woman, 52.2% of women in Turkey are classified as overweight with a BMI above 25. Almost 20% of the Turkish women surveyed were considered obese (BMI > 30). In Brazil, about 10% of women were obese, while 6% were underweight.

Like other indicators used in this atlas, the BMI measure has its strengths and weaknesses. First, the data are deficient in terms of the number of countries reporting. When data exist for a country, they are often for just one or two years. Poor geographical coverage and shallow time series make it difficult to chart global trends in obesity and related chronic diseases. Second, the cutoff points fixed by NCHS were developed for US citizens at high risk of disease above a BMI of 25 and below a BMI of 18.5. These standards and risks may not equally apply to other populations. When they are applicable, their relevance is limited to indicating tendencies in a population. The ranges and associated risks are not reliable diagnostics for individuals. We can think of examples that point to the limitations of BMI as a health indicator (e.g., a 6-foot-6-inch, 235-pound athlete with a BMI score of 27). There is consensus, however, that an adult BMI of greater than 30 kg/m^2 places individuals at considerable disease risk (WHO 2006a).

Table 5.1. Women's body mass index percentiles for selected countries

	BMI < 18.5 Underweight	18.5 < BMI < 25.0 Normal	BMI > 25 Overweight	BMI > 30 Obese
Bangladesh	45.4	50.1	4.4	0.7
Brazil	6.2	58.9	34.8	9.7
Burkina Faso	13.2	81.0	5.7	0.9
Egypt	0.6	28.2	71.2	32.4
Ethiopia	26.0	71.6	2.3	0.2
Guatemala	2.0	54.1	43.8	12.1
India	26.6	69.7	3.7	1.0
Kazakhstan	9.8	67.5	22.8	8.4
Turkey	2.6	45.2	52.2	18.8
Uzbekistan	9.8	71.6	18.5	4.1

Source: WHO 2004a, Annex 11.

Box 5.1. The Nutrition Transition and the Double Burden of Malnutrition

Nutrition and health experts note that diets change significantly as a population becomes more urban and incomes rise. The "nutrition transition" refers to a shift from a predominately plant-based diet high in complex carbohydrates, fiber, and vegetables to an energy-dense (high calorie) diet in which a higher percentage of calories come from sugar, fat, and processed foods. For example, soft drink consumption has increased by 400% in Brazil since the mid-1970s and is believed to be a major contributor to obesity (Rohter 2005). Over the same period the population has shifted from 80% rural to 80% urban. The relatively lower cost of energy-dense foods versus vegetables, fruits, and lean meats partly explains the phenomenon of obesity among the urban poor (Drewnowski and Spencer 2004). Research shows that the income required to purchase fatty foods has decreased over the past 30 years (FAO 2006a).

The coexistence of underweight and overweight people in a population is not uncommon (Barquera et al. 2006). In Brazil, there are four million undernourished people but ten million who are obese. There is even evidence of malnutrition of both types within the same family. In one poor urban community in the Philippines, 8.2% of the households had an underweight child and an overweight mother. The percentage increased to nearly 20% in a more affluent urban community (Pedro and Benavides 2006). The "double burden of malnutrition" refers to the coexistence of undernutrition and overnutrition and their related infectious and chronic diseases. Government health programs must be versatile and well financed to prevent and control these twin nutritional problems.

Box 5.2. Low BMI

Just as a high BMI can indicate overnutrition, a low BMI suggests undernutrition. If a person has a BMI of less than 18.5, then he or she is considered underweight. Unfortunately, the data for low BMI are very limited and focus on adult women. Another problem with the data is that the BMI cutoff point of 18.5 may be too low for individuals whose weight fluctuates with food availability, work, illness, and income. A BMI of 20 would provide some additional weight as a buffer for these lean periods (Svedberg 1999, 2087). Despite these data limitations, table 5.3 shows those countries with the highest levels of underweight women based on the low BMI measure. If we use this indicator alone, South Asia and Sub-Saharan Africa stand out as containing the highest percentages of malnourished women.

Data limitations make mapping the geography of obesity particularly challenging. The data that do exist are collected for children under the age of five and for women during their childbearing years. Map 5.1 shows obesity rates for children ages 0–5 based on the WHO's international child growth standards. The reference population for these standards is derived from surveys undertaken between 1997 and 2003 in six countries (Brazil, Ghana, India, Norway, Oman, and the United States). Obesity rates are lowest in Sub-Saharan Africa and South Asia and highest in East-Central Europe, the Middle East and North Africa. The countries with the highest rates of overweight and obese children are listed in table 5.2.

The United States has one of the highest adult obesity rates in the world (map 5.2). The Centers for Disease Control and Prevention estimate that 30% of adults in the United States are obese (CDC 2008). This represents 60 million people or one-fifth of the world's 300 million obese adults. The prevalence of obesity is on the rise in the United States. In 1995 obesity rates were less than 20% in all 50 states. By 2005 there were just four states (Hawaii, Kansas, Connecticut, and Vermont) with prevalence rates less than 20%. Seventeen states recorded obesity levels greater than 25%, with three of them greater than 30% (Louisiana, Mississippi, and West Virginia). The obesity epidemic in the United States is associated with unbalanced diets and limited physical activity. The stereotype "couch potato" who sits in front of a video screen eating packaged snacks contains an element of truth about the reason for obesity in the United States. Obesity is also strongly associated with

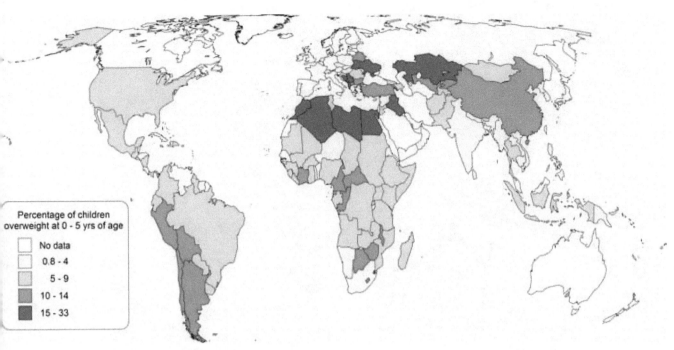

Map 5.1. Overweight and obese children 0–5 years of age.

Table 5.2. Countries with the highest rates of overweight and obese children (BMI = +2SD)

Country	BMI
Albania	33.0
Ukraine	27.6
Bosnia and Herzegovina	26.0
Comoros	25.3
Serbia	19.5
Kazakhstan	18.9
Swaziland	18.2
Iraq	17.1
Algeria	16.8
Libya	16.2
Morocco	15.5
Egypt	15.1

Source: WHO 2008c, most recent years.

Table 5.3. Percentage of adult women underweight (BMI < 18.5)

Country	Rate (%)
Bangladesh	45
India	41
Eritrea	41
Nepal	27
Ethiopia	26
Yemen	25
Kampuchea	21
Chad	21
Niger	21
Madagascar	21

Source: United Nations System, Standing Committee on Nutrition, 2004.

low income and low educational levels (Drewnowski and Spencer 2004). In many poor neighborhoods in US cities minimarts readily provide low-fiber, high-fat processed foods, but fresh produce and whole grain products are scarce and expensive.

The profile of obesity in the developing world is complex. In some countries, being overweight is a sign of wealth and high status. This is the case in urban Africa among the upper classes, and among "big men" in many rural African communities. In countries like Brazil and Mexico, it used to be prestigious to be over-

weight. While the elites of these countries are today adopting a slimmer look, obesity afflicts all socioeconomic groups (Rohter 2005).

In general, obesity tends to be higher in urban areas and is correlated with recent increases in a country's income (Martorell 2006). Urban populations in Latin America, Africa, and Asia are growing rapidly. As people move to cities, they encounter food that is high in sugar and fat and that is cheaper than more nutritious foods (Drewnowski and Spencer 2004; FAO 2006a) (figure 5.1). Poor people's access to nutritious

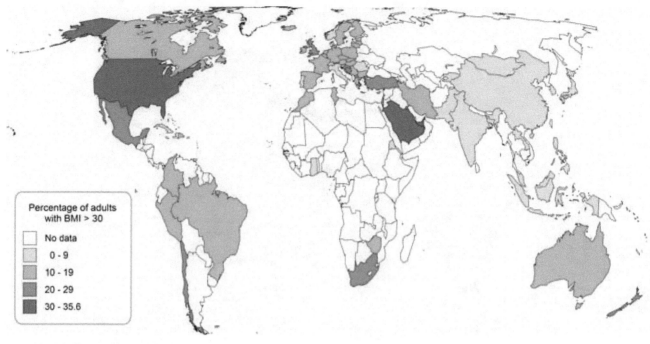

Map 5.2. Obese adults in the world.

Percentage of adults with BMI > 30

- No data
- 0 - 9
- 10 - 19
- 20 - 29
- 30 - 35.6

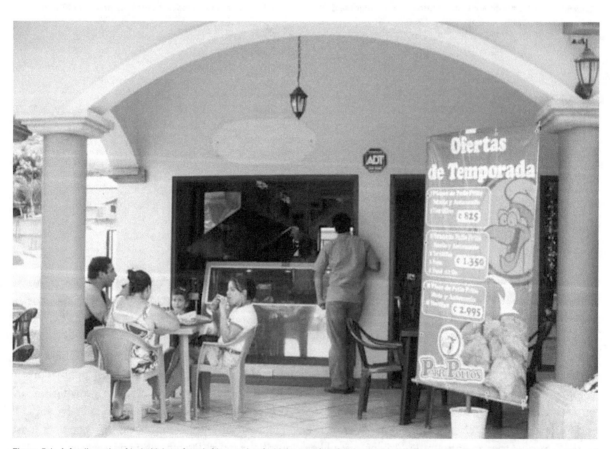

Figure 5.1. A family eating fried chicken, french fries, and soft drinks at a fast-food restaurant in Tamarindo, Costa Rica. The consumption of high-fat foods and soft drinks combined with little physical exercise leads to weight gain and the onset of chronic diseases like diabetes.

food often becomes restricted if a limited number of stores sell a variety of fresh produce within walking distance of their homes (Algert, Agrawal, and Lewis 2006). Although people may know that eating more healthy foods is better for them, they cannot always afford to buy foods like fruits and vegetables (Drewnowski and Spencer 2004).

The relatively high prevalence of obesity in Latin America means that overnutrition commonly coexists with undernutrition (box 5.2 describes this phenomenon in Brazil). The combination of limited incomes, reduced physical activity, and an unbalanced diet increases the likelihood that poor children and adults alike will become obese and therefore be at risk for type-2 diabetes and hypertension, breast, colon, and prostate cancer, and heart disease (WHO 2006a). To counter the worldwide upsurge in obesity-related diseases, public policies need to promote the availability of low-fat, high-fiber foods among the poor, increase educational outreach and the opportunities for physical exercise, and support programs that address the links between income inequality, poor diets, and poor health.

Discussion Questions: Malnutrition and Obesity

1. What does malnutrition mean? How should you define the term?
2. What is BMI and what does it indicate?
3. What does the double burden of malnutrition mean?
4. What is the nutrition transition?

Research Article

Anthropometric Characteristics of Underprivileged Adolescents: A Study from Urban Slums of India

Sushama A. Khopkar,[1] Suvi M. Virtanen,[2,3,4] and Sangita Kulathinal[5]

[1]Department of Statistics, H. P. T. Arts and R. Y. K. Sc. College, Nashik 422 005, India
[2]Unit of Nutrition, Department of Lifestyle and Participation, National Institute for Health and Welfare, Helsinki, Finland
[3]School of Health Sciences, University of Tampere, Tampere, Finland
[4]Research Center for Child Health, Tampere University and University Hospital and the Science Center of Pirkanmaa Hospital District, Tampere, Finland
[5]Department of Food and Environmental Sciences, Division of Nutrition, University of Helsinki, 00014 Helsinki, Finland

Correspondence should be addressed to Sushama A. Khopkar; sakhopkar@gmail.com

Received 2 October 2014; Revised 29 November 2014; Accepted 30 November 2014; Published 24 December 2014

Academic Editor: Kaushik Bose

Purpose. The anthropometric status and growth of adolescents living in challenging conditions such as slums are insufficiently studied. The purpose here was to describe anthropometric characteristics and nutritional status of adolescents from urban slums of India and to study the factors affecting it. *Methods.* Anthropometric, socioeconomic and dietary habit data were collected using structured questionnaires of six hundred adolescents aged 10–19 years by house-to-house survey conducted in two randomly selected slums of Nashik, Western India. The growth of adolescents was compared using WHO and Indian reference populations. Mixed effects logistic regression models were used to examine associations between anthropometric measures and income, mother's education, household size, and dietary intake. *Results.* Prevalences of stunting and thinness were lower using the Indian reference population compared to that of WHO. Stunting was more prevalent than thinness in the study subjects, and boys suffered more than girls. The effect of age on stunting was different among boys than girls. A mother's education was highly significantly associated with both stunting and thinness in both sexes. Household size and income were significantly associated with the nutritional status of girls. *Conclusions.* Educating mothers about the nutritional needs of adolescents may help to improve adolescents' anthropometric profile and future health.

1. Introduction

Adolescence is a transitional phase between childhood and adulthood characterized by marked acceleration in growth [1, 2]. It is a second chance for growth or catch-up growth for those children who have experienced nutritional deficiencies in early childhood [3, 4]. A large number of adolescents from South and South-east Asian countries suffer from chronic malnutrition and anaemia which affect their development [1]. The high rate of malnutrition in girls contributes to the intergenerational cycle of malnutrition, and in most developing countries nutrition initiatives have focused on children and women, essentially neglecting adolescents, especially boys [1].

Anthropometry helps in assessing nutritional status and health risks among adolescents [5, 6]. Recommended measures for assessing nutritional status in school-aged children and adolescents are BMI-for-age and height-for-age [7]. Low BMI-for-age is classified as thinness and high BMI-for-age as overweight and obesity, and low height-for-age as stunting [7]. Stunting is a primary manifestation of malnutrition in early childhood and is an indicator of chronic undernutrition, while thinness indicates current malnutrition. Stunting increases the risk of morbidity, impairs cognitive development, and reduces work productivity in later life [8]. The consequences of undernutrition extend not only to later life, but also to future generations [9]. Both childhood obesity and thinness are linked to underachievement in school and lower self-esteem [10]. Assessment of stunting and thinness is crucial for adolescents and a reference population is central to it. One of the objectives of the present paper is to compare estimates of malnutrition observed in this study population based on the growth reference curves developed for India [11] and the WHO Multicentre Growth Reference Study [12]. Several factors affect the nutritional status of adolescents. Among these, socioeconomic and demographic factors are associated with worldwide patterns of stunting and thinness [13].

India has a large population of adolescents (10–19 years of age, 21%) and also of slum dwellers in urban areas (15% of total urban population of India, [14, 15]). Although a number of studies from India have been published on adolescents' anthropometry among school children from urban and rural areas reporting prevalence of undernutrition ranging from 17% to 65% [16], there are only a few studies conducted on the growth of adolescents from urban slums covering adolescents not attending school (e.g., [17]). Addressing the growth issues of this underprivileged group could be an important step towards breaking the vicious cycle of intergenerational malnutrition, chronic diseases, and poverty. Such assessments need special consideration since they constitute a large proportion of the urban population and suffer from adverse living conditions such as unsafe water, poor housing, overcrowding, and limited health facilities, especially when compared to school-going urban adolescents not living in slums. The purpose here is to describe anthropometric characteristics and nutritional status of adolescents from urban slums of India and study the factors affecting it. In the current study, nutritional status as determined by height-for-age and BMI-for-age of a sample of adolescents from urban slums of Maharashtra with low per capita income is examined. Their status is also compared with the WHO and Indian reference populations by age and sex. Note that Maharashtra has the highest slum population as a proportion of urban population (27.3%) in India [15]. Further, factors such as mother's education, family income, and diet, known to affect the nutritional status (stunting and thinness) of school children, are examined for these adolescents. Girls have been the focus of nutritional research and growth-related issues stemming from a lack of proper nutrition. The novelty of the present work lies in examining whether the situation among boys differs from that of girls.

2. Methods

The study was undertaken over a six-month period from November 2010 to April 2011 in two urban slums in Nashik city in the state of Maharashtra, Western India. Out of the 32 notified slums by the Nashik Municipal Corporation (NMC) within the city limits, one slum was selected randomly. The slums were enumerated and a number between 1 and 32 was selected randomly. The slum with the selected number was chosen for the study. Similarly, out of 27 slums notified by the NMC on the outskirts of the city, one was selected by randomly choosing a number between 1 and 27.

After the selection of slums, a survey was carried out to gather background information on households, number of family members, and number of boys and girls between the age of 10–19 years from 539 (241 + 298) households. Written consent was also sought, at the same time. One of the selected slums had 1384 households (reported by the NMC) and the first 241 households interviewed, which gave the required number of adolescents for the study, were included. All 298 households from the other slum were included. All the households with at least one adolescent (200 out of 241 and 150 out of 298 households) and which gave consent to participate in the study were selected. This gave 156 (out of 200) and 120 (out of 150) households and 545 adolescents for the present study.

Data on household characteristics, socioeconomic indicators, and eating habits were collected using structured questionnaires by house-to-house survey. The adolescents whose parents gave consent were interviewed to collect data on their demographic and life style factors, habits, physical activity, diet, and so forth. The questionnaires were administered by two teams consisting of three trained surveyors each. Another team of five members carried out measurements. One member of the team collected data on weight, one on height, and the other three on blood pressure. The field study was approved by the Institutional Review Board of Tampere School of Health Sciences in 2010. The study was conducted in accordance with the ethical guidelines in the Helsinki Declaration of 1975, as revised in 2000.

In the present paper, the analysis of anthropometric data is restricted to the age group 10–18 years (boys = 257, girls = 261, total = 518) since the growth curves from India are available up to the age of 18 years.

2.1. Anthropometric Measurements. Data on height and weight were collected in the present study. The participants were invited to camps at scheduled times with their parent or guardian for the recording of anthropometric measurements. Height (in cm) was measured using a simple nonelastic measurement tape to the nearest integer. Weight (in kg) was recorded using a new bathroom scale (brand Libra, Model no. 770) to the nearest integer. Two readings each were taken for height and weight and the average was used for analyses here. Body mass index (BMI) was defined as the ratio of weight (in kg) to the square of height (in m).

2.2. Stunting and Thinness. Height-for-age and BMI-for-age Z-scores were derived using WHO as well as Indian reference populations [11, 12]. A subject was classified as stunted if the height-for-age score was below −2, as thin if BMI-for-age score was below −2, and overweight if BMI-for-age score was above 1 [18].

2.3. Independent Variables. In this study, it was examined whether differences in household per capita income, mother's education, household size, and dietary intake of protein/fat within the slum population were associated with variation in anthropometric status. The level of economic wellbeing is one of the basic factors of the household that is reflected in child undernutrition. The poverty that children experience is associated with inadequate food, poor sanitation, and poor hygiene, which lead to increased infections, and is also associated with low maternal education, increased maternal stress, and depression [19–21]. Household characteristics such as mother's education, poverty, and household size are closely linked to aggregate anthropometric failure in India [22, 23]. Interestingly, a larger number of over-5-year-old children in a household have been found to be associated with *less* child anthropometric failure than if there were fewer children [23]. The role of household size in determining the nutritional status of children remains unclear. It is known that the mother's education is generally reflected in a child's wellbeing. Educated mothers could be more aware of health issues, with more means to get information than uneducated mothers [22]. Children of mothers with higher education tend to have better nutritional status [19, 23]. The mother's education level here was grouped into two categories for analysis: (i) primary or no education and (ii) secondary or higher education. Per capita income was obtained by dividing the total household income by the household size.

Fat and protein are important macronutrients for the growth of children. The main sources of fat and protein in the diet of the present study population were oil, dal/pulses, and meat/egg/fish among other foods. Information about per capita weekly consumption of oil, dal/pulses, and meat/egg/fish was derived from the household questionnaire where the adult respondent (in most cases the mother) was asked how often various items were consumed weekly in the household and the quantity of each item bought per week. Per capita weekly consumption of a specific item was derived by dividing the weekly purchase of that item by the number of family members. Specifically, weekly consumption of meat/egg/fish was derived by combining consumption of meat (in kg), eggs (1 egg ≈ 50 g), and fish (in kg).

2.4. Data Analysis. Basic characteristics of households and adolescents were described. Overall mean and standard deviation were obtained for height, weight, and BMI. We first compared the observed percentiles of height, weight, and BMI for the study population to the WHO and Indian reference populations. Percentages of stunting and thinness using the WHO and Indian reference populations were presented in bar charts. Not much is known about the correlation between height, weight, and BMI among adolescents of low-income and middle-income countries. We also computed Pearson correlation coefficients between these three measures separately for boys and girls. Descriptive statistics of independent variables are also presented.

The study subjects were recruited from 276 households and that resulted in more than one adolescent per household (171 households, 65%). The data on adolescents from the same household might be correlated and, hence, regression models used for the analysis included a household-specific random effect. The analysis was carried out using a generalized linear mixed model [24]. Age-adjusted means were obtained using linear regression of each (denoted by y) height, weight, and BMI over age (denoted by x) using

$$y_{ih} = b_0 + b_1 x_i + \epsilon_{ih} + u_h, \quad i = 1, \ldots, n_h, \ h = 1, \ldots, H, \quad (1)$$

where b_0 and b_1 are the fixed effects, x is the age, ϵ is the random error due to the model, and u is the household-specific random effect. Both ϵ and u are assumed to be independent and normally distributed.

For the analysis of stunting and thinness, mixed effects logistic regression models were used. Regression analyses were carried out with age as an independent variable, and the other variables added to the model one by one. Multivariate analyses with age and consumption data were carried out in model 1, and in model 2, family information was added. The mixed effects logistic regression model specified in terms of the log odds is given as follows:

$$\log \left(\frac{p\left(y_{ih} = 1 \mid x_{ih}, b, h\right)}{p\left(y_{ih} = 0 \mid x_{ih}, b, h\right)} \right)$$
$$= b_0 + b_1 x_{1i} + b_2 x_{2i} + \cdots + b_p x_{pi} + u_h, \quad (2)$$
$$i = 1, \ldots, n_h, \quad h = 1, \ldots, H,$$

where y is a response variable (stunting or thinness), $x = (x_1, x_2, \ldots, x_p)$ is a vector of p independent variables, $b = (b_0, b_1, \ldots, b_p)$ is a vector of fixed effects, and u is the household-specific random effect.

All analyses were performed using the statistical computing environment R and the regression analyses were implemented using the glmer function from the package lme4 of R [25–27].

3. Results

3.1. Descriptive Statistics. The slum population was rather homogeneous with regard to native place (Maharashtra), mother tongue (Marathi), and eating habits. The major religion was Hindu (87%), followed by Muslim (10%), Buddhism (2%), and other (1%). Forty percent of the population belonged to scheduled caste (SC), 32% scheduled tribe (ST), 10% open, 9% other backward class (OBC), and 9% other caste. 51% houses were of type kaccha, 45% were of type pucca, and the rest 3% were semipucca.

The median ages (14 years) of boys and girls were the same (Table 1). 79% of boys and 82% of girls were currently studying and 52% (45%) of boys and 56% (41%) of girls described their general health as very good (good). 42% of the adolescents were in class 5–7 and 38% were in class 8–10, and 30% boys and 24% girls were engaged in earning money. 25% boys were smokers and 24% and 35% either chewed tobacco or used gutka. Among girls these percentages were the same (7%) but smaller compared to that of boys. 64% of mothers were at home while 18% worked as household helpers. The maximum percentage (44%) of fathers was labourers, 22% had small businesses, and 10% were in the service sector. Comparison of mean values showed that boys were taller than girls but there was no difference in the mean weight (Table 1). The 75th and 90th percentiles of height were higher by 7–9 cm among

TABLE 1: Means, standard deviation (SD), and percentiles of height, weight, and BMI for adolescents (combining 10–18 years) by sex.

	Boys (N = 257)						Girls (N = 261)					
	Mean (SD)	Percentiles					Mean (SD)	Percentiles				
		10	25	50	75	90		10	25	50	75	90
Age (years)	14 (2.5)	10	12	14	16	17	14 (2.3)	11	12	14	15	17
Height (cm)	150 (14)	131	139	149	162	169	147 (10)	131	140	148	155	158
Weight (kg)	37 (11)	23	29	36	45	50	37 (9)	25	30	38	43	48
BMI (kg/m^2)	16 (2)	13	15	16	18	19	17 (3)	14	15	17	19	21

TABLE 2: Means of height, weight, and BMI for adolescents by age and sex.

Age (years)	Boys				Girls			
	N	Height (cm)	Weight (kg)	BMI (kg/m^2)	N	Height (cm)	Weight (kg)	BMI (kg/m^2)
10	27	134	25	14	16	136	28	14
11	30	138	29	15	36	139	30	15
12	40	142	32	15	40	142	33	15
13	31	146	35	16	31	144	35	16
14	25	151	38	16	33	147	38	16
15	21	155	41	17	40	150	40	17
16	32	159	44	17	26	153	43	17
17	29	163	47	18	22	156	45	18
18	22	167	50	18	17	158	48	18

boys compared to girls. The 10th, 25th, and 50th percentiles of weight were higher by about 2 kg among girls but the 75th and 90th percentiles were lower among girls compared to boys. The average BMI as well as percentiles were higher among girls than boys by 1-2 kg/m^2 (Table 1).

An age-wise summary of height and weight showed that height and weight increased with the increase in age in both sexes (Table 2). An average yearly increment in the mean height of boys was 3.6 cm, while that of girls was 2.4 cm, and an average yearly increment in the mean weight of boys was 2.7 kg, while that of girls was 2.2 kg. Girls were at least as tall as boys to the age of 12 years and the mean weight of girls showed a similar pattern to the age of 14 years. Boys tended to be taller than girls from the age of 13 years and heavier from the age of 15 years. The mean BMI for boys and girls was the same at all ages but showed increasing trend with age.

For boys, the Pearson's correlation coefficient between height and weight was 0.89, height and BMI was 0.50, and weight and BMI was 0.83, while for girls the same between height and weight was 0.76, height and BMI was 0.35, and weight and BMI was 0.87. For all adolescents combined, the Pearson's correlation coefficient between height and weight and between weight and BMI was 0.83, while it was lower between height and BMI (0.38), as observed in other studies.

3.2. Stunting and Thinness. The study population had lower median values (about 10 cm for height and 3 kg/m^2 for BMI) for all ages compared to both reference populations (Figure 1). The difference in median height narrowed after the age of 15 years but that of BMI remained the same. This was seen among boys as well as girls. It should be noted that the Indian reference population (of affluent urban adolescents)

had similar median values of BMI but slightly lower median heights compared to the WHO reference population. In the sequel, WHO and IND refer to the classifications based on the WHO and Indian reference populations, respectively. The percentages of stunting among boys (range WHO 13%–59% and IND 13%–41%) were similar using both the reference populations to the age of 12 years and after that the proportion was higher when the WHO reference population was used (except for the age 17 years, Figure 2). Among girls (range WHO 14%–44% and IND 4%–31%) the two classifications differed at all ages. Stunting showed an increasing trend with age among boys and a decreasing trend among girls. It was interesting to note that the proportion of stunted boys was lower compared to girls at ages 10 and 11 years, after which the trend was reversed.

The differences in the two classifications for thinness were much larger compared to stunting (Figure 3). The proportion of thinness, both among boys (range WHO 23%–52% and IND 0%–18%) and girls (range WHO 15%–38% and IND 4%–19%), first increased with age and then tapered off. Small proportions of overweight adolescent boys (range WHO 0%–8% and IND 0%–8%) were observed at ages 11, 15, and 16 years under the WHO but at the age of 14 years under both the classifications. Among girls (range WHO 0%–13% and IND 0%–10%) overweight was observed at ages 11, 12, 13, and 16 years under both classifications. For further analysis, stunting and thinness as defined by the Indian reference population were used.

3.3. Summary of Independent Variables (Table 3). The mean per capita income per month was INR 960 and INR 843 for boys and girls, respectively, which puts 60% boys and 68%

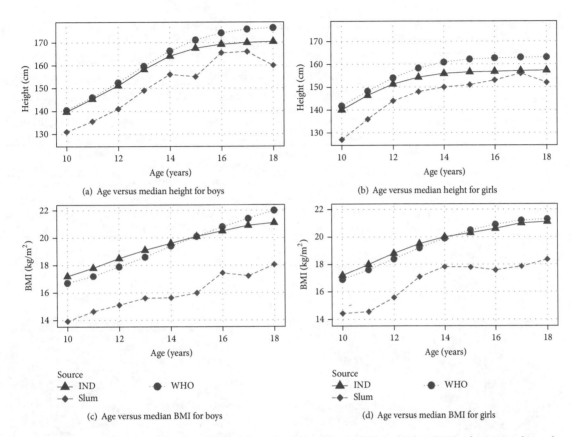

(a) Age versus median height for boys

(b) Age versus median height for girls

(c) Age versus median BMI for boys

(d) Age versus median BMI for girls

FIGURE 1: Age versus median values of height and BMI of the study subjects (Slum), WHO, and Indian (IND) reference populations by sex.

TABLE 3: Mean, standard deviation (SD), and range (minimum, maximum) for dietary consumption data, income, household size, and percentage of mother's education by sex.

	Income* (INR)		Consumption of		Household size (%)			Mother's education (%)
		Oil* (kg)	Egg/meat/fish* (kg)	Dal/pulses* (kg)				
	Mean (SD)	Mean (SD) range	Mean (SD) range	Mean (SD) range	4 or less	5	More than 5	Primary or no
Boys (N = 257)	221 (140) (28, 1073)	0.23 (0.11) (0.02, 0.75)	0.13 (0.10) (0.00, 0.45)	0.08 (0.04) (0.00, 0.25)	35	30	35	49
Girls (N = 261)	194 (101) (29, 1035)	0.21 (0.10) (0.00, 0.75)	0.12 (0.09) (0.00, 0.45)	0.08 (0.05) (0.00, 0.40)	23	27	50	49

*Per capita weekly.

girls below the poverty line (below INR 961.1 per person per month for urban Maharashtra, [28]). 49% of mothers of the adolescents had primary or no education. The per capita weekly overall consumption of animal protein (meat, fish, and eggs, 120–130 g with SD of 100 g) as well as vegetable protein (dal/pulses, 80 g with SD of 40 g) was very low and similar in households with boys and girls. Intake of a source of energy, which was mainly oil (peanut oil in the study area), varied between negligible and 750 g per person per week. The distribution of household size differed between boys and girls with 50% girls having a household size of

more than 5 members while only 35% boys had more than 5 members. Except for consumption data on meat, egg, or fish (4% missing data), the proportion of missing data was less than 1% (Table 3).

3.4. Regression Analysis. A univariate regression analysis where log odds of stunting versus no stunting were modelled with age as an independent variable showed a significant effect in both boys and girls, but positive in boys and negative in girls (Table 4). An increase in age by one year increased the

TABLE 4: Stunting-regression coefficients (β) and 90% confidence intervals under the mixed effects logistic regression model for stunting by sex. Log odds of stunting versus no stunting were modeled. Each model included age and an additional covariate.

		Boys		Girls	
		β (CI)	$\exp(\beta)$ (CI)	β (CI)	$\exp(\beta)$ (CI)
Age		0.12* (0.01, 0.24)	1.13 (1.01, 1.27)	−0.18* (−0.35, −0.02)	0.83 (0.70, 0.98)
Household size	4 or less	Reference		Reference	
	5	0.28 (−0.41, 0.99)	1.33 (0.66, 2.69)	−0.88 (−1.87, 0.11)	0.41 (0.15, 1.12)
	More than 5	0.42 (−0.26, 1.11)	1.53 (0.77, 3.03)	−0.76 (−1.56, 0.03)	0.47 (0.21, 1.03)
Mother's education	Primary or no	Reference		Reference	
	Secondary or higher	−0.89* (−1.46, −0.33)[1]	0.41 (0.23, 0.72)	−1.42* (−2.32, −0.52)[3]	0.24 (0.10, 0.59)
Income	Standardized	0.11 (−0.15, 0.38)	1.12 (0.86, 1.46)	−1.02** (−1.64, −0.41)	0.36 (0.19, 0.66)
Consumption of	Oil	−0.89 (−3.62, 1.85)	0.41 (0.03, 6.36)	1.41 (−1.88, 4.69)	4.08 (0.15, 108.85)
	Dal/pulses	−0.90 (−7.68, 5.88)	0.41 (0.0005, 357.81)	3.84 (−2.78, 10.46)	46.53 (0.06, 34891.55)
	Egg/meat/fish	−2.93 (−6.23, 0.36)[2]	0.05 (0.002, 1.43)	0.49 (−3.53, 4.52)[4]	1.64 (0.03, 91.84)

[1] Age effect did not remain significant.
[2] Age effect became stronger, regression coefficient and CI were 0.14 (0.03, 0.27), P value = 0.05.
[3] Age effect became stronger, regression coefficient and CI were −0.22 (−0.40, −0.05), P value = 0.04.
[4] Age effect did not remain significant.
* $0.01 \leq P$-value ≤ 0.10, and ** P-value < 0.01.

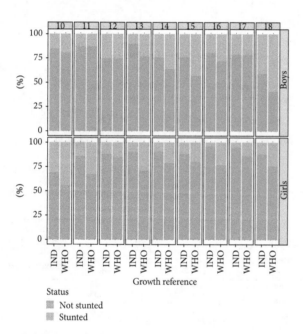

FIGURE 2: Percentages of stunted and not stunted study subjects by age and sex using WHO and Indian (IND) reference populations.

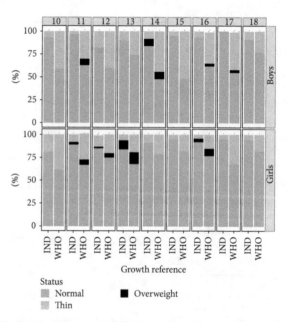

FIGURE 3: Percentages of thin, normal, and overweight study subjects by age and sex using WHO and Indian (IND) reference populations.

odds of stunting among boys by 13%, whereas it reduced the odds by 17% among girls.

Further, bivariate regression analyses were carried out by adding the independent variables, namely, household size, mother's education, income, and dietary data on consumption of oil, egg/meat/fish and dal/pulses, one by one to the model in addition to age. Mother's education was significantly associated with stunting (Table 4). When moving from primary or no education to secondary or higher education of

the mother, the odds of stunting reduced by 59% among boys and 76% among girls. Income was significantly associated with stunting among girls, with a ten standard deviation unit increase in income reducing the odds of stunting by 20% among girls. There was no significant effect of dietary data observed in this study.

The multivariate analysis under model 1 which included age and dietary data did not alter the age effect. The second model which in addition included mother's education,

TABLE 5: Thinness-regression coefficients (β) and 90% confidence intervals under the mixed effects logistic regression model for thinness by sex. Log odds of thinness versus normal BMI were modeled. Each model included age and an additional covariate.

		Boys		Girls	
		β (CI)	$\exp(\beta)$ (CI)	β (CI)	$\exp(\beta)$ (CI)
Age		−0.10 (−0.26, 0.06)	0.91 (0.77, 1.06)	−0.18* (−0.35, −0.02)	0.83 (0.70, 0.98)
Household size	4 or less	Reference		Reference	
	5	0.17 (−0.89, 1.23)	1.18	−0.88 (−1.87, 0.11)	0.41 (0.15, 3.42)
	More than 5	0.36 (−0.68, 1.41)	1.44 (0.51, 4.10)	−0.76 (−1.56, 0.03)	0.47 (0.21, 1.03)
Mother's education	Primary or no	Reference		Reference	
	Secondary or higher	0.12 (−0.71, 0.96)	1.13 (0.49, 2.61)	−1.42** (−2.32, −0.52)	0.24 (0.10, 0.59)
Income	Standardised	0.04 (−0.34, 0.43)	1.04 (0.71, 1.54)	−1.02** (−1.64, −0.41)	0.34 (0.19, 0.66)
Consumption of	Oil	1.13 (−2.62, 4.87)	3.08 (0.07, 130.32)	1.40 (−1.88, 4.69)	4.08 (0.15, 108.85)
	Dal/pulses	−7.44 (−19.26, 4.38)	$0.0006 (0.43 \times 10^{-8}, 79.83)$	3.84 (−2.78, 10.46)	46.36 (0.06, 34891.55)
	Meat/egg/fish	−2.06 (−6.47, 2.35)	0.13 (0.002, 10.49)	0.49 (−3.53, 4.52)[1]	1.64 (0.03, 91.84)

[1] Age effect was not significant.
*$0.01 \leq P$-value ≤ 0.10, and **P-value < 0.01.

household size and income did not change the results of univariate analysis of each of these variables (adjusted for age). For boys, age did not remain significant in the second model but mother's education remained significant and had a similar effect as described earlier. For girls, age, mother's education, and income remained significant and in addition household size was also significantly associated with stunting. When moving from a household size of 4 or less to more than 5, the odds of stunting among girls were reduced by 70% (*data not shown*).

Similarly, odds of thinness versus normal BMI were analysed under the regression models with age as an independent variable and then each of the other variables was added to the model. None of the independent variables showed significant association with thinness among boys (Table 5). However, for girls, age, mother's education, and income were significantly associated with thinness. When mother's education increased from primary or no education to secondary or higher education, the odds of thinness versus normal BMI were reduced by 76%. One unit increase in a girl's age reduced the odds by 17% while a ten-standard-deviation-unit increase in income reduced the odds by 66%. Once again, dietary data did not show any significant effect. Multivariate analysis including all the independent variables did not change the results of univariate analysis, and age, mother's education, and income remained significant for girls with similar effects as described above (*data not shown*).

4. Discussion

This study examined the nutritional status and possible associated factors, of adolescents from an economically deprived slum population which constitutes a sizeable proportion of the overall Indian urban population. With increasing urbanization, this population is likely to grow. The adolescents of the present study had lower mean height and weight but comparable BMI-for-age compared to those reported in other studies on school children from Indian cities [13, 16, 29, 30]

but higher height and weight but lower BMI compared to school children (10–17 years) from the rural area of Wardha, Maharashtra, and rural area of northern Karnataka [30, 31].

Adolescent growth spurt is a universal phenomenon and occurs in all children during adolescence, though it varies in intensity and duration from one child to another. Growth spurt among girls was observed around the age of 13 years and it was around this age when menarche was attained (median age at menarche of the study girls was 13.7 years, data not shown) after that the BMI tapered off and so did height. For boys it happened about 2 years later that was around 15 years of age. During the growth spurt, boys gained about 20 cm (range 10–30 cm) in height accompanied by a gain in weight of about 20 kg (range 7–30 kg). The peak velocity of height growth averaged about 10 cm per year. In girls the spurt was somewhat narrower in magnitude, and the peak height velocity was averaging about 8 cm per year. Similar observations were also made in other studies [29, 32]. The difference in size between adult men and women is to a large extent the result of the differences in adolescent growth spurt occurrence. In boys the spurt occurs later, allowing an extra period for growth, even at the slow prepubertal velocity and partly because of the greater intensity of the spurt itself; prior to it, boys and girls are practically of the same height [29].

The growth reference curves for India were derived using apparently healthy affluent Indian children [11] and the present slum population seemed to have lower anthropometric profile in comparison. The prevalence of stunting was higher than the prevalence of thinness among boys and girls. The phenomenon of the higher proportion of stunting may indicate that consumption of foods rich in protein responsible for height was far below the required level. We make an observation that the Indian reference population had a higher median BMI-for-age than the WHO reference population which was derived from several countries including India (Figure 1). The prevalence of stunting and thinness was reduced when using the Indian reference population compared to the WHO reference population and similar observations were also made in other studies [33].

The prevalence of stunting was higher among boys than girls after the age of 11 years and also the prevalence of thinness was higher among boys at all ages, though not showing such trend systematically (Figures 2 and 3). This could be because girls were nutritionally better off than boys [34]. The total proportion of stunting was higher among boys (21%) compared to girls (11%) in this study. This highlights a less researched question about boys suffering growth related issues and possibly nutritional deficiency as the focus of such research has been mostly on girls and women.

With regard to BMI-for-age, a high proportion (90%) of the study population had normal nutritional status. The overall prevalence of being overweight (1% boys and 2% girls) and thinness (8%) were low compared to other studies on urban children. In this paper, no association was observed between dietary data and nutritional status. One reason for this could be that the study population was rather homogeneous with regard to the food habits and to some extent, life style.

A study from rural Wardha observed a significantly higher prevalence of stunting among adolescents from the lower family income group [35]. Surprisingly, one study found that a larger number of over-5-year-old children in a household was associated with less child anthropometric failure than if there were fewer children [23].

The association between stunting and thinness with higher income and more family members among girls is in line with the rural Wardha study [35] and Gaiha's study [23]. The mother's education was found to be an important factor affecting stunting as well as thinness among boys and girls in accordance with other studies [35–37].

In summary, boys with a higher prevalence of stunting compared to girls might have suffered from high levels of chronic undernutrition, a consistent lack of consumption of required nutrients both in quantity and quality, and partly from untreated infections. Proper care is needed for growing boys to meet their nutritional requirement according to age. Mother's education was highly significant in reducing stunting among both sexes, and hence, educating the mothers of adolescents about their nutritional needs may help in improving adolescents' anthropometric profile and future health. A longitudinal study looking at anthropometry and dietary intake data would be needed for planning of a proper nutritional intervention for urban slum populations to overcome the problem of stunting.

Conflict of Interests

The authors declare that there is no conflict of interests regarding the publication of this paper.

Acknowledgments

The study was supported by a scholarship of The International Postgraduate Program in Epidemiology and Public Health (IPPE) at the School of Health Sciences, University of Tampere, Finland. Sangita Kulathinal's work was supported by a research grant from the Academy of Finland (no. 269053). The authors would like to thank Minna Säävälä, Väestöliitto, Helsinki, Finland, for helpful discussion and comments on the paper. Dr. V. V. Khadilkar kindly provided the LMS values to calculate Z-scores on request.

References

[1] "Adolescents Nutrition: a review of the situation in selected South East Asian countries," World Health Organization, Regional office of South East Asia, Executive Summary, 2005, http://apps.searo.who.int/PDS_DOCS/B0239.pdf?ua=1.

[2] K. Anand, S. Kant, and S. K. Kapoor, "Nutritional status of adolescent school children in Rural North India," Indian Pediatrics, vol. 36, no. 8, pp. 810–815, 1999.

[3] S. Rao, "Nutritional status of the Indian population," Journal of Biosciences, vol. 26, no. 4, pp. 481–489, 2001.

[4] H. Delisle, V. C. Mauli, and B. De Benoist, "Should adolescents be specifically targeted for nutrition in developing countries? To address which problems and how?" http://www.idpas.org/pdf/1803ShouldAdolescentsBeTargeted.pdf.

[5] World Health Organization, "Physical status: the use and interpretation of anthropometry," Tech. Rep. 854, World Health Organization, Geneva, Switzerland, 1995.

[6] H. G. Thakor, P. Kumar, V. K. Desai, and R. K. Srivastava, "Physical growth standards of Urban Adolescents (10–15 years) from south Gujarat," Indian Journal of Community Medicine, vol. 25, no. 2, pp. 86–92, 2000.

[7] M. de Onis, A. W. Onyango, E. Borghi, A. Siyam, C. Nishida, and J. Siekmann, "Development of a WHO growth reference for school-aged children and adolescents," Bulletin of the World Health Organization, vol. 85, no. 9, pp. 660–667, 2007.

[8] D. Basu, G. Islam, R. Gogoi, S. Dey, and J. Deori, "Child's growth and nutritional status in two communities—Mishing tribe and Kaibarta caste of Assam," International Journal of Sociology and Anthropology, vol. 62, pp. 59–69, 2014.

[9] Fact sheet EURO/06/05, The Health of Children and Adolescents in Europe, World Health Organization, Copenhagen, Bucharest, 2005.

[10] M. S. Kramer, "Determinants of low birth weight: methodological assessment and meta-analysis," Bulletin of the World Health Organization, vol. 65, no. 5, pp. 663–737, 1987.

[11] V. V. Khadilkar, A. V. Khadilkar, T. J. Cole, and M. G. Sayyad, "Cross-sectional growth curves for height, weight and body mass index for affluent Indian children," Indian Pediatrics, vol. 46, no. 6, pp. 477–489, 2009.

[12] M. De Onis, "Assessment of differences in linear growth among populations in the WHO Multicentre Growth Reference Study," Acta Paediatrica, International Journal of Paediatrics, vol. 95, no. 450, pp. 56–65, 2006.

[13] G. J. Haboubi and R. B. Shaikh, "A comparison of the nutritional status of adolescents from selected schools of South India and UAE: a cross-sectional study," Indian Journal of Community Medicine, vol. 34, no. 2, pp. 108–111, 2009.

[14] Census of India, Single Year Age Data Table C13, 2011, http://www.censusindia.gov.in/2011census/Age_level_data/Age_level_data.html.

[15] S. Upinder, "Slum population in India: extent and policy response," International Journal of Research in Business and Social Science, vol. 2, no. 1, pp. 2147–4478, 2013.

[16] V. Kumaravel, V. Shriraam, M. Anitharani, S. Mahadevan, A. N. Balamurugan, and B. W. C. Sathiyasekaran, "Are the current

Indian growth charts really representative? Analysis of anthropometric assessment of school children in a South Indian district," *Indian Journal of Endocrinology and Metabolism*, vol. 18, no. 1, pp. 56–62, 2014.

[17] S. Mandal, V. R. Prabhakar, J. Pal, R. Parthasarathi, and R. Biswas, "An assessment of nutritional status of children aged 0–14 years in a slum area of Kolkata," *International Journal of Medicine and Public Health*, vol. 4, pp. 159–162, 2014.

[18] V. V. Khadilkar and A. V. Khadilkar, "Growth charts: a diagnostic tool," *Indian Journal of Endocrinology and Metabolism*, vol. 15, supplement 3, pp. S166–S171, 2011.

[19] R. H. Bradley and R. F. Corwyn, "Socioeconomic status and child development," *Annual Review of Psychology*, vol. 53, pp. 371–399, 2002.

[20] C. Paxson and N. Schady, *Cognitive Development Among Young Children in Ecuador: The Roles of Health, Wealth and Parenting*, World Bank, 2005, http://wws-roxen.princeton.edu/chwpapers/papers/paxson_schady_childrenecuador.pdf.

[21] A. Deaton and J. Drèze, "Food and nutrition in India: facts and interpretations," *Economic and Political Weekly*, vol. 44, no. 7, pp. 42–65, 2009.

[22] F. Arnold, S. Parasuraman, P. Arokiasamy, and M. Kothari, "Nutrition in India," National Family Health Survey (NFHS-3) 2005-06, International Institute for Population Sciences, Mumbai, India, ICF Macro, Calverton, Md, USA.

[23] R. Gaiha, R. Jha, and V. S. Kulkarni, "Child Under nutrition in India," http://ssrn.com/abstract=1734591.

[24] C. E. McCulloch, S. R. Searle, and J. M. Neuhaus, *Generalized, Linear, and Mixed Models*, Wiley Series in Probability and Statistics, John Wiley & Sons, Hoboken, NJ, USA, 2nd edition, 2008.

[25] R Core Team, *R: A Language and Environment for Statistical Computing*, R Foundation for Statistical Computing, Vienna, Austria, 2013, http://www.r-project.org/.

[26] D. Bates, M. Maechler, B. Bolker, and S. Walker, "lme4: linear mixed-effects models using Eigen and S4," R Package Version 1.1-7, 2014, http://cran.r-project.org/web/packages/lme4/.

[27] D. Bates, M. Maechler, B. M. Bolker, and S. Walker, "lme4: linear mixed-effects models using Eigen and S4," Submitted to *Journal of Statistical Software*.

[28] *Press Note on Poverty Estimates, 2009–10*, Government of India, Planning Commission, 2012, http://planningcommission.nic.in/news/press_pov1903.pdf.

[29] S. S. Patil, S. R. Patil, P. M. Durgawale, S. V. Kakade, and K. Abhishek, "Study of physical growth standards of adolescents (10–15 years) from Karad, Maharashtra," *International Journal of Collaborative Research on Internal Medicine & Public Health*, vol. 5, no. 1, pp. 10–18, 2013.

[30] T. Rajaretnam and J. S. Hallad, "Nutritional status of adolescents in northern Karnataka, India," *Journal of Family Welfare*, vol. 58, no. 1, pp. 55–67, 2012.

[31] A. Taksande, P. Chaturvedi, K. Vilhekar, and M. Jain, "Distribution of blood pressure in school going children in rural area of Wardha district, Maharashatra, India," *Annals of Pediatric Cardiology*, vol. 1, no. 2, pp. 101–106, 2008.

[32] T. Bano, *A comparative study of health nutrition and socio-psycho behaviour of adolescent boys and girls [Ph.D. thesis]*, University of Kashmir, 2012.

[33] S. Maiti, D. De, K. Chatterjee, K. Jana, D. Ghosh, and S. Paul, "Prevalence of stunting and thinness among early adolescent school girls of Paschim Medinipur district, West Bengal," *International Journal of Biological and Medical Research*, vol. 2, no. 3, pp. 781–783, 2011.

[34] K. Venkaiah, K. Damayanti, M. U. Nayak, and K. Vijayaraghavan, "Diet and nutritional status of rural adolescents in India," *European Journal of Clinical Nutrition*, vol. 56, no. 11, pp. 1119–1125, 2002.

[35] P. R. Deshmukh, S. S. Gupta, M. S. Bharambe et al., "Nutritional status of adolescents in rural Wardha," *Indian Journal of Pediatrics*, vol. 73, no. 2, pp. 139–141, 2006.

[36] D. K. Das and R. Biswas, "Nutritional status of adolescent girls in a rural area of North 24 Parganas district, West Bengal," *Indian Journal of Public Health*, vol. 49, no. 1, pp. 18–21, 2005.

[37] A. Abudayya, M. Thoresen, Y. Abed, and G. Holmboe-Ottesen, "Overweight, stunting, and anemia are public health problems among low socioeconomic groups in school adolescents (12–15 years) in the North Gaza Strip," *Nutrition Research*, vol. 27, no. 12, pp. 762–771, 2007.

Discussion Questions: Anthropometric Characteristics of Underprivileged Adolescents: A Study from the Urban Slums of India

1. What is anthropometry, what is done during an anthropometric assessment, and how is it used?
2. What is stunting and what does it tell you about an individual?
3. What characteristics of a mother are correlated with healthier children?
4. Which macronutrients are often limited in the diets of malnourished children?

Topic III: Social and Cultural Aspects of Food and Nutrition

Archaeology provides clues about the way in which human populations have lived through time. In *Food Preparation, Social Context, and Ethnicity in a Prehistoric Mesopotamian Context*, the reader is provided evidence for food preparation, including food types, butchering techniques, and cooking patterns, to examine gender and the associated division of labor, but also the interactions between ethnic groups, of those living in early Mesopotamian state societies. The remnants of this past life, one that unfolded along an important trade route, help the past come alive as the gendered tasks are described, allowing comparisons with contemporary life. There are also outlines of the way in which different ethnicities co-existed in the same space through time.

Most of us have clear and established social meanings that we attach to food and drink. If prompted, we can name items that we ingest or drink on a particular social occasion or at a time we wish to convey a specific social meaning. In *Theories of Food and the Social Meanings of Coffee*, one of the world's most beloved beverages is described in terms of its social meaning or value to peoples around the world. Although coffee is native to Ethiopia, coffee consumption occurs on a daily basis in households and restaurants on every continent. However, the social message connected to this caffeine-rich drink varies, within and between countries, and world regions. In providing a general description of the social context for food and discussing categorization as a means of understanding the social value of a food item in the hierarchy, one can begin to see how 'culture' colors the view one has of all things food.

One significant element of food culture around the world is religion. Thus, in *"I'll Have Whatever She's Having": Jews, Food, and Film*, Jewish dietary laws are explored, as are the foods that are often associated with being Jewish in the United States. Specific food items are included based upon their consumption within Jewish communities and the connection to Jewish characters in a variety of U.S. films. Whether or not you are Jewish, you will recognize many of the food items; they are now part of mainstream U.S. consumption patterns and no longer associated with their original context(s). Most of the foods and recipes that are described as being "Jewish" foods, arrived in the United States with Jewish populations who were emigrating from varied parts of Europe. Jewish dietary laws are discussed so that the origin of particular food restrictions becomes clear. But one also learns the reasoning behind some of the food preparation and consumption patterns that are part of Jewish households throughout the world.

Food Preparation, Social Context, and Ethnicity in a Prehistoric Mesopotamian Colony

Gil J. Stein
ORIENTAL INSTITUTE, UNIVERSITY OF CHICAGO

Food provides a uniquely valuable source of insight into the dynamics of culture. Cooking and consumption often occur in different social contexts, corresponding to the contrast between domestic and more public spheres. For this reason, food preparation and consumption can reflect different context-dependent assertions of social identity such as gender or ethnicity (Crabtree 1990; Gumerman 1997). As recent analyses by Kent Lightfoot (Lightfoot, Martinez, and Schiff 1998) and Kathleen Deagan (1996, 2003) have shown, these contrasts can be especially important analytical dimensions in understanding the dynamics of multiethnic culture contact situations, especially those involving marriage between groups and the establishment of households in colonial encounters.

In this paper I compare the social contexts of food preparation and consumption as a way to investigate the world's earliest known colonial network, established by south Mesopotamian city-states in the Uruk period, ca. 3700–3100 BC. Excavations at Hacınebi in southeast Turkey indicate that south Mesopotamian Uruk merchants established a trading enclave in the midst of this local Anatolian settlement ca. 3700 BC. Evidence for long term peaceful coexistence of Mesopotamians and Anatolians at Hacınebi suggests that social and economic relations were based on strategies of alliance rather than colonialist domination.

I examine several aspects of food preparation (food choice, butchery, and cooking) in relation to gender and ethnicity. Artifacts from the more domestic social context of food preparation are strongly Anatolian in style, while those from more public contexts of consumption are predominantly of Uruk Mesopotamian styles. Significantly, the available data indicate that local Anatolian cooking pot styles predominate even in archaeological contexts that are otherwise overwhelmingly Uruk Mesopotamian in character. The evidence is consistent with the interpretation of gendered ethnic differences between the social arenas of food preparation and consumption. I suggest that the Mesopotamian colonists at Hacınebi were able to maintain a long-term presence as a diasporic community by forging marriage alliances with local elites through the formation of multicultural households composed of Uruk males and Anatolian females.

THE FOURTH-MILLENNIUM COLONIAL EXPANSION OF URUK MESOPOTAMIA

The first state societies of Mesopotamia in the fourth millennium BC Uruk period established a series of trading outposts along the key routes linking the southern alluvium with the highland resource zones of the Taurus Mountains in Anatolia and the Zagros Mountains of Iran (figure 2.1) in order to obtain resources such as copper, lumber, and semiprecious stones (Algaze 1993; Rothman 2002; Stein 1999b; Sürenhagen 1986). A number of Uruk colonies have been excavated in Syria at sites such as Habuba Kabira (Strommenger 1980; Kohlmeyer 1996) and Sheikh Hassan (Boese 1995); in Iran at Godin (Weiss and Young 1975; Young 1986); and in Turkey at sites such as Hassek Höyük (Behm-Blancke 1992; Helwing 2002) and Hacınebi (Stein 1999a, 2002). Uruk colonies and way stations are distributed over a vast area, ca. 1,200 kilometers (east-west) by 1,000 kilometers (north-south). The colonies are distinguishable from the indigenous settlements around them by a complex of material culture, including ceramics, chipped stone, public and domestic architecture, ornaments, and administrative technology (e.g., Sürenhagen 1986, Stein 1999a). The political economy of this colonial network remains the subject of lively debate (e.g., Algaze 2001; Rothman 2001; Stein 1999b).

We are only now beginning to understand the organization of this network and the nature of relations between these Mesopotamian outposts and the local polities with whom they traded. Excavations at Hacınebi in the Euphrates Valley in Turkey indicate that during phase B2, a small Uruk trading enclave was established in the midst of a long-standing local Anatolian settlement (Stein 1999b). Hacınebi is a 3.3 ha village or small town located on the limestone bluffs over-

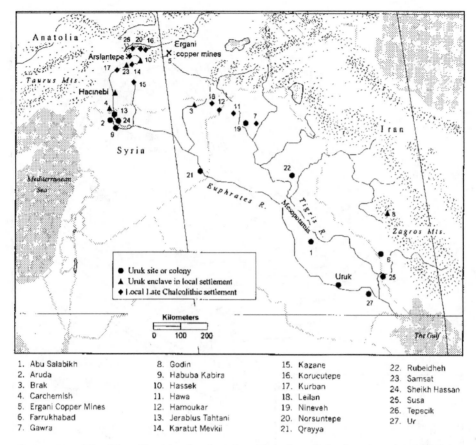

1. Abu Salabikh	8. Godin	15. Kazane	22. Rubeidheh
2. Aruda	9. Habuba Kabira	16. Korucutepe	23. Samsat
3. Brak	10. Hassek	17. Kurban	24. Sheikh Hassan
4. Carchemish	11. Hawa	18. Leilan	25. Susa
5. Ergani Copper Mines	12. Hamoukar	19. Nineveh	26. Tepecik
6. Farrukhabad	13. Jerablus Tahtani	20. Norsuntepe	27. Ur
7. Gawra	14. Karatut Mevkii	21. Qrayya	

Figure 2.1. The Near East in the fourth millennium BC, showing the main sites associated with the Uruk expansion and its colonial network.

looking a ford on the Euphrates River, five kilometers north of the modern town of Birecik. The site's strategic importance derives from its location at the juncture of two of the most important arteries of trade and communication in the central Near East—the north-south riverine route that linked Anatolia, north Syria, and Mesopotamia and the east-west land route that skirted the margins of the eastern Taurus and Western Zagros Mountains.

The available evidence suggests that the preexisting Anatolian Local Late Chalcolithic settlement at Hacınebi in the earlier phases A and B1 had monumental architecture, inherited social ranking, advanced metallurgy, and a complex administrative technology (Stein 2001). Thus, when Mesopotamians established a trading enclave at Hacınebi in phase B2, they were dealing with a society that was already complex. In phase B2 a full range of Uruk material culture is present, from virtually every functional class (Stein 1999a); this gives good evidence for the presence of an actual foreign enclave, rather than simply reflecting

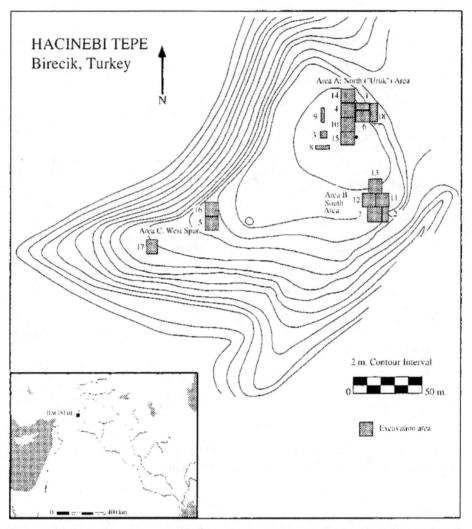

Figure 2.2. Topographic map of Hacınebi showing trenches in Areas A (north), B (south) , and C (west).

emulation by local elites. Stylistically Mesopotamian materials are concentrated in Areas A and B, in the northeast and southeast parts of the site respectively (figure 2.2). A few Uruk deposits are in situ; however, most derive from secondary trash deposits, as do the vast majority of contexts with Local Late Chalcolithic materials. As a result, we cannot really estimate the number of individual Uruk or contemporaneous local Anatolian households in other parts of the phase B2 settlement at Hacınebi. These are contemporaneous with phase B2 Local Late Chalcolithic deposits at Hacınebi. Comparisons between Uruk and local contexts allow us to examine the dynamics of interaction in this prehistoric colonial situation. We need to emphasize three aspects of this encounter:

1. Radiocarbon dates and ceramic styles both suggest an extended period of interaction with Uruk Mesopotamia lasting for 300 to 400 years.

2. Interaction was peaceful—with no evidence for violence or coercion. No weapons, fortifications, skeletons with traumas, or evidence for violent destruction were found anywhere in phase B2 deposits at Hacınebi.

3. Uruk-Anatolian interaction seems to have been in the form of symmetric economic and political relations rather than colonialist dominance (Stein 2002).

Given the lack of evidence for Uruk military or economic control, it is clear that this small trading diaspora was there at the sufferance of the local Anatolian polity. If this was the case, then how were the colonists able to peacefully coexist with the local people for a period of three to four centuries? It is here that gender emerges as a crucial element for any understanding of Uruk-Anatolian interaction in this colonial context.

GENDER IN COLONIAL ENCOUNTERS

Gender imbalances are a common characteristic of colonial encounters. Textual accounts of ancient Greek colonies, the Spanish colonies in Florida and the Caribbean, and the Anglo-French fur-trading frontier in North America suggest a widespread pattern in which the colonizing males often vastly outnumbered the colonizing females. In New Spain, for example, at the city of St. Augustine in what is now Florida, in records from the year 1565, Spanish men outnumbered Spanish women by a ratio of 12:1 (Deagan 1973:57). "The chronic shortage of preferred marriage partners resulted in a regular pattern of intermarriage between Spanish men and Native American women from the earliest years of colonization" (Deagan 1985:304). This was not only sanctioned but encouraged by the Spanish government (McEwan 1991:36). The early French colonial populations in Canada (Faragher 1988:203) and the Iron Age Greek colonies in the eastern Mediterranean showed a similar preponderance of foreign males who formed household with local women in the early stages of colonization at Pithecoussai and in the Greek colonization of Caria (e.g., Coldstream 1993).

Under these conditions of colonial gender imbalance, colonial encounters have historically documented high levels of intermarriage between the foreign men and indigenous women. These marriages took place not only for sexual companionship and colonial access to women's labor but for explicitly political purposes as well. Indigenous women in these situations were cross-cultural brokers, playing a key role in alliance formation between the colonists and the host community. These alliances were essential for colonial attempts to maintain peaceful relations with the host community, while gaining access to land, resources such as furs, or trading privileges. In those cases where the colonists were able to dominate the local peoples militarily or economically, the role of intermarriage in alliance formation was less visible but still present. However, when power relations were more balanced, then cross-cultural marriage alliances played an increasingly important political and economic role. In intercultural households the ability to emphasize one ethnic identity or another, as context demanded, would have been crucial for establishing and maintaining good relations between the colonial and indigenous groups.

If gender imbalances and cross-cultural marriages are such widespread aspects of colonial systems, then they should be detectable in the archaeological record. Kathleen Deagan has explored the phenomenon of Mestizaje or the composite cultural identity that arose through intermarriage between Spanish men and Native American women at eighteenth-century St. Augustine, Florida (Deagan 1973, 1983, 1985). She suggests that this marriage practice can be detected archaeologically through the differential patterning of colonial and local styles of material culture in male- versus female-gendered activities. Female activities with low social visibility such as food preparation would have primarily aboriginal material culture, while socially visible male activities would be mainly associated with colonial styles of artifacts.

It would be naïve to expect that there is any one single gendered model that explains all instances of colonial-indigenous interaction. Other studies grounded in historical archaeology (e.g., Jamieson 2000; Rodríguez-Alegría 2005a, 2005b; Van Buren 1999; Voss 2008) suggest that there was significant variability in both the dynamics of gender relations in intercultural households of colonial Latin America and in their material correlates.

However, Deagan's model provides a particularly useful and archaeologically testable model to examine the role of gender in the interaction of Mesopotamians and Anatolians at Hacınebi. If the Uruk enclave was characterized by a colonial gender imbalance and a pattern of systematic marriage alliances with local Anatolian women, then we would expect to see socially visible male activities associated with Uruk styles of material culture. We would also expect to see clear differences in these activities between the Mesopotamian and Anatolian parts of the site. By contrast, female activities should be associated with local Anatolian material culture. Since Anatolian women would be present in all parts of the site, we would expect to see no differences between Mesopotamian and Anatolian deposits in the artifacts associated with female activities.

The main challenge is the problem of gender attribution. Which activities are predominantly male-gendered domains, and which are predominantly female-gendered? Gender attribution is a controversial topic, not least because of the methodological problems it presents and anthropologists' legitimate reluctance to reify or fix gendered distinctions as if they were immutable social facts.

Table 2.1. Gendered Division of Labor for Selected Household Activities in the 185 Societies—HRAF Files (Murdock and Provost 1973, table 1)

Task	Butchering	Cooking
Exclusively male	122	0
Predominantly male	9	2
Male and female in equal proportions	4	2
Predominantly female	4	63
Exclusively female	4	117

Anthropologists in general have rightly become wary of cross-cultural generalizations about gender (or any other aspect of social and economic behavior), especially when presented out of their culture-specific context. However, certain anthropological questions require that one be able to make reliable gender attributions for classes of activities because, as Costin notes, "there are no known cases of complex society—modern or historic—in which a gendered division of labor is not a critical factor in the domestic and political economies and because gendered relations of production are tied into other complex social and political relations" (Costin 1996:112). Costin suggests that ethnographic analogy, textual data, and figurative representations can all provide useful bases for gender attribution in archaeological analyses (117).

Murdock and Provost's (1973) cross-cultural study of the gendered division of labor in 185 societies showed that stone working and butchering were mainly male activities, while cooking was strongly associated with women (table 2.1). Textual and artistic data from Mesopotamia in the third millennium BC support the identification of cooking as a female-gendered task in households, although large-scale cooking in major institutions such as temples and palaces was often a male-gendered task (Bottero 2001:63). Although far from perfect, these gender attributions for butchery and cooking can serve as useful starting points for investigating the role of gender in the earlier colonial encounters of the fourth-millennium BC Uruk period at Hacınebi.

"INTERCULTURAL" HOUSEHOLDS AND GENDERED PRAXIS AT HACINEBI

The evidence for long-term peaceful coexistence of Mesopotamians and Anatolians at Hacınebi suggests that social and economic relations may have been based on strategies of alliance rather than domination. I suggest that marriage alliances played a key role in cementing good relations between the Uruk enclave and local Anatolian elites and would have formed the basis for symmetric, stable trading conditions. These links would have guaranteed Uruk access to trade goods while building up local elites through their preferential access to foreign exchange networks. As noted above, alliance strategies of this type are well known from historical colonial encounters, such as the French fur trade in Canada.

If this was the case in the fourth-millennium BC Near East as well, then sites such as Hacınebi should have what we can call "intercultural households," in which foreign males cohabitate with local females. This has two important implications: First, the existence of intercultural households requires that we focus on the intersection of gender and ethnicity as a crucial aspect of ancient colonial encounters. Second, it means that we must study the social context of a gendered division of labor in order to understand the ways in which these households actually functioned. We would expect to see at least three gendered ethnic patterns in food processing, cooking, and consumption:

1. Male-gendered food-processing activities, such as butchery, will differ between intercultural and local households.

2. Female-gendered activities, such as cooking, will be similar for "intercultural" and local households.

3. In intercultural households public contexts of consumption will be mainly male-gendered and will emphasize foreign styles.

The key principle here is that *male*-gendered activities would vary, while *female* activities should be fairly constant across the site, in both Uruk and local contexts. It is clearly risky to make specific gender attributions for prehistoric tasks. However, the best way to deal with this problem is to construct explicit hypotheses and see whether the data on food processing, cooking, and consumption are consistent with our expected archaeological correlates.

Evidence for food preferences is provided by a comparative analysis of the faunal data from Uruk and local Anatolian contexts in phase B2 (table 2.2). Animal bone remains from Uruk contexts show a preference for sheep and goats, while fauna from local contexts show a more balanced spread of sheep, goats, cattle, and pigs. Uruk food preferences at Hacınebi match the food preferences found at sites in south Mesopotamia, while the local contexts mirror the preferences at other nearby local sites.

BUTCHERY

Marking a turn from food preferences to food preparation, butchery patterns can provide useful insights about both ethnicity and gender. The tools used to dismember an animal, the specific techniques used (e.g., cutting versus chopping or sawing), and the physical locations of the cut marks can all reflect aspects of daily practice that are consciously or unconsciously indicative of ethnic identity (e.g.,

Table 2.2. Comparison of Fauna Identified to Genus in Uruk vs. Local Contexts at Hacınebi (*N*=1010): Number of Identified Specimens (NISP) and Percentages

Taxon	Local Contexts, NISP	Local Contexts, %	Uruk Contexts, NISP	Uruk Contexts, %
Bos	43	10.8	46	7.5
Cervus	0	0	8	1.3
Canis	2	0.5	0	0
Capra	15	3.8	36	5.9
Dama	13	3.3	10	1.6
Equus hemionus	1	0.3	6	1.0
Gazella	1	0.3	14	2.3
Mus	0	0	1	0.2
Ovis	24	6.0	51	8.3
Ovis/Capra	167	41.9	334	54.6
Ovis/Capra/Gazella	6	1.5	41	6.7
Sus	127	31.8	64	10.5
Total	399	100.0	611	100.0

Langenwalter 1980; Ijzereef 1988). As noted above, butchery is generally a male-gendered activity, so even for the same kind of animal we would expect to see differences between the Uruk and local households. For sheep and goats, the Uruk and local contexts differ strikingly in the locations of the butchery cut marks (figure 2.3). Uruk cut marks cluster on the vertebrae, while the local deposits focus instead on the ribs and the head. The cut marks in the local contexts are wider than those in the Uruk deposits (figure 2.4), perhaps reflecting the use by local butchers of the larger Canaanean blades, while Uruk butchers might have preferred the narrower, smaller simple blades. These differences in cut locations and tool preferences are consistent with the presence of Mesopotamian males in the intercultural households of the Uruk contexts contemporaneous with Anatolian males in the local contexts.

CERAMIC EVIDENCE FOR GENDER-RELATED PATTERNING IN FOOD PREPARATION AND CONSUMPTION

However, the evidence for cooking and serving shows an entirely different pattern. Here our inferences about gender and ethnicity have to rely on the evidence of ceramic vessel function within and between Uruk and local contexts. Local contexts show complete continuity in the relative proportions of ceramic vessel functions between phases B1 and B2. But when we focus on the later phase

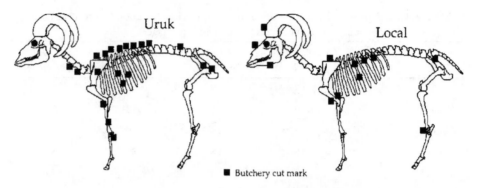

Figure 2.3. Locations of butchery cut marks on sheep/goat skeletons compared for Local Late Chalcolithic vs. Uruk contexts at Hacınebi.

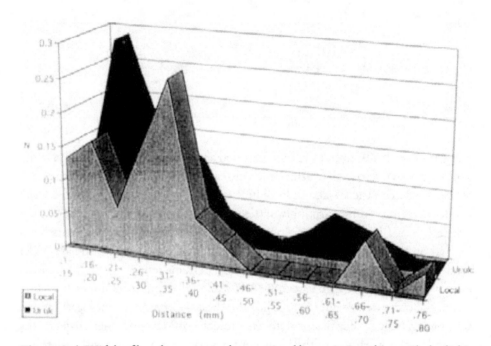

Figure 2.4. Width of butchery cut marks on animal bones in Local Late Chalcolithic vs. Uruk contexts.

B2, we can see clear differences in the functional profiles of Uruk versus local contexts. These differences become even more marked when we look at each vessel class. We have to remember that even in predominantly local contexts, some Uruk ceramics can be found, and vice versa. The question is whether we can observe any patterning in these "crossover" forms.

When we look at storage vessels (table 2.3 and figure 2.5), as we might expect, local forms are most common (81.6 percent) in predominantly local contexts,

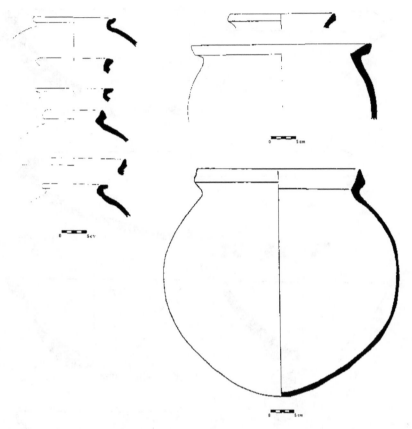

Figure 2.5. Local Late Chalcolithic (*right*) and Uruk (*left*) storage vessels.

Table 2.3. Hacınebi Phase B2 Storage Jars—Style Compared for Uruk and Local Contexts (*N*=565)

| | Ceramic Style | | |
Context	Local	Uruk	Indeterminate
Local	81.6 %	4.6%	13.8%
Uruk	24.7%	47.5%	27.8%

while Uruk forms are the most common class (47.5 percent) in predominantly Uruk contexts. Similarly, local-style serving vessels (table 2.4 and figure 2.6) are the most frequent form (83.2 percent) in local contexts, while Uruk-style serving vessels are the most common (97 percent) in Uruk contexts. This is consistent with our expectation that in intercultural households public food consumption events would reflect the Uruk ethnicity of males.

The only exception to this pattern occurs with cooking pots (table 2.5 and figure 2.7). Here, as expected, we see that local cooking pots are the most

61

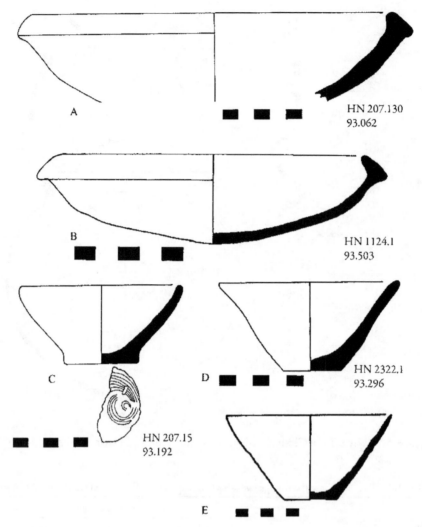

Figure 2.6. Local Late Chalcolithic (*A* and *B*) and Uruk (*C, D,* and *E*) serving vessels.

Table 2.4. Hacınebi Phase B2 Serving Vessels—Style Compared for Uruk and Local Contexts (*N*=1767)

Context	Ceramic Style		
	Local	*Uruk*	*Indeterminate*
Local	83.2%	16.8%	0%
Uruk	3.0 %	97.0%	0%

common forms (93.3 percent) in predominantly local contexts. However, the anomaly comes when we examine the predominantly Uruk contexts. It is highly significant that *local,* not Uruk, cooking pots are the most common forms, even

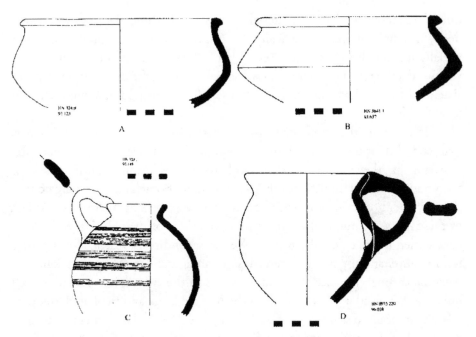

Figure 2.7. Local Late Chalcolithic (*A* and *B*) and Uruk (*C* and *D*) cooking vessels.

Table 2.5. Hacınebi Phase B2 Cooking Vessels—Style Compared for Uruk and Local Contexts (*N*=571)

Context	Ceramic Style		
	Local	*Uruk*	*Indeterminate*
Local	93.30%	2.20%	4.5%
Uruk	39.99%	23.40%	36.61%

in predominantly Uruk contexts. Cooking pots are the only functional class of ceramics for which local styles predominate in Uruk contexts.

In other words, local cooking pot forms predominated in kitchens all across Hacınebi—in both Uruk and local households. But in Uruk contexts, this predominance is *reversed* when one moves from the kitchen to the dining area, from cooking to serving, so that Uruk forms are most common in public social settings of feasting.

CONCLUSIONS

A holistic understanding of the archaeology of colonial encounters requires that we play close attention to gendered daily practice as a domain where social identities were expressed and transformed. However, we can understand this domain only if we recognize that the material expression of ethnic identities was dependent on social context—specifically the distinction between public and more socially restricted domestic spheres. When we examine the lithic, faunal, and ceramic data in terms of their gendered social contexts, the distributions are consistent with a model of intercultural households comprised of Uruk males and local females.

How would the Uruk colonists in these intercultural households have maintained their distinctive diasporic/foreign identity over time? One possible answer is that they maintained their Uruk identity by keeping continuous, long-term trading links with their south Mesopotamian homeland, involving not just the movement of goods, but periodic travel by the merchants themselves. As part of these links, we might also expect small numbers of new Uruk merchants to have settled in the colonial outposts. We can see indirect evidence for the long-term maintenance of ties between Mesopotamia and the colonies in southeast Anatolia through the fact that ceramic styles in the two regions remain closely linked and evolved in tandem in both the Middle Uruk and the Late Uruk periods, a span of up to seven centuries. If the two regions had *not* remained in close contact, then we would have seen a divergence in ceramic styles between the two regions rather than continuing close similarities.

A more complicated question relates to the social identity of children and the ways that intercultural households maintained their dual character over time. While it is tempting to suggest that the social reproduction of these households meant that the children of intercultural households took on explicitly Uruk Mesopotamian identities, the available evidence is simply not sufficient at this point to determine whether this was the case.

In the intercultural households that apparently characterized the Uruk enclave at Hacınebi, the social sphere of public food consumption—in the commensal politics of feasting and alliance—was male and Mesopotamian. By contrast, in the domestic sphere, we can see the expression of Mesopotamian identities for those aspects of food preparation that were male-gendered, while local Anatolian identities are visible in female-gendered food preparation activities such as cooking. If this interpretation is correct, then butchery, cooking, and serving in these households provide a crucial line of evidence to understand the alliance strategies that enabled a Mesopotamian trade diaspora to maintain peaceful long-term economic and social relations in the world's earliest colonial network.

Acknowledgments. This chapter is a revised version of the paper originally presented in the session "Archaeological Studies of Cooking and Food Preparation," organized for the annual meeting of the Society for American Archaeology on March 31, 2005. I want to thank Sarah Graff and Enrique Rodríguez-Alegría for inviting me to participate in this conference and for their useful editorial suggestions for revisions. I also thank two anonymous external reviewers for their comments.

I wish to express my appreciation to the Turkish Ministry of Culture, General Directorate of Monuments and Museums, for permission to conduct the excavations at Hacınebi from 1992 to 1997, with subsequent study seasons from 1998 to 2002. Thanks are also due to the staff of the Sanlıurfa Museum and its directors—the late Adnan Mısır and his successor, Eyüp Bucak—for their administrative assistance. The project was funded with support from the National Science Foundation (grant number SBR–9511329), the National Endowment for the Humanities (grant numbers RO–22448, RK–20133–94, and RZ–20120), the National Geographic Society (grant numbers 4853–92, 5057–93, 5295–94, and 5892–97), the Wenner-Gren Foundation for Anthropological Research (grant number 6309), the Kress Foundation, the American Research Institute in Turkey (ARIT), the de Groot Fund of the Metropolitan Museum of Art, Faculty Research Grants from Northwestern University, and the generosity of private donors, most notably Joseph and Laura Kiser, Bill and Sally Anderson, and Paul and Mary Webster. I thank Jeffrey Nicola and Lauren Bigelow for their assistance in the zooarchaeological analysis. The ceramic analyses were conducted initially by Susan Pollock and Cheryl Coursey, and then continued by Julie Pierce. Dr. Belinda Monahan played a crucial role in revising the ceramic typology, organizing the ceramic raw data, and creating the SPSS database used for the quantitative analysis presented here. Any errors of fact or interpretation are my own.

REFERENCES CITED

Algaze, Guillermo. 1993. *The Uruk World System*. Chicago: University of Chicago Press.

————. 2001 The Prehistory of Imperialism: The Case of Uruk Mesopotamia. In *Uruk Mesopotamia and Its Neighbors: Cross-Cultural Interactions in the Era of State Formation*, edited by M. Rothman, 27–83. Santa Fe, NM: School of American Research Press.

Behm-Blancke, Manfred. 1992. Hassek Höyük: Eine Uruk Station im Grenzland zu Anatolien. *Nürnberger Blätter zur Archäologie* 8:82–94.

Boese, Johannes. 1995. Ausgrabungen in Tell Sheikh Hassan I. *Vorläufige Berichte über die Ausgrabungskampagnen 1984–1990 und 1992–1994*. Saarbrücken, Germany: Saarbrücker Druckerei und Verlag.

Bottero, Jean. 2001. The Oldest Cuisine in the World. In *Everyday Life in Ancient Mesopotamia*, edited by J. Bottero, 43–64. Baltimore: Johns Hopkins University Press.

Coldstream, J. N. 1993. Mixed Marriages at the Frontiers of the Greek World. *Oxford Journal of Archaeology* 12:89–107.

Costin, Cathy. 1996. Exploring the Relationship between Gender and Craft in Complex Societies: Methodological and Theoretical Issues of Gender Attribution. In *Gender and Archaeology*, edited by Rita Wright, 111–142. Philadelphia: University of Pennsylvania Press.

Crabtree, Pam J. 1990. Zooarchaeology and Complex Societies: Some Uses of Faunal Analysis for the Study of Trade, Social Status, and Ethnicity. *Archaeological Method and Theory* 2:155–205.

Deagan, Kathleen. 1973. *Mestizaje* in Colonial St. Augustine. *Ethnohistory* 20:55–65.

———. 1983. *Spanish St. Augustine: The Archaeology of a Colonial Creole Community.* New York: Academic Press.

———. 1985. Spanish-Indian Interaction in Sixteenth-Century Florida and Hispaniola. In *Cultures in Contact*, edited by William W. Fitzhugh, 281–318. Washington, DC: Smithsonian Institution Press.

———. 1996. Colonial Transformation: Euro-American Cultural Genesis in the Early Spanish-American Colonies. *Journal of Anthropological Research* 52:135–160.

———. 2003. Colonial Origins and Colonial Transformations in Spanish America. *Historical Archaeology* 37:3–13.

Faragher, John Mack. 1988. The Custom of the Country: Cross-Cultural Marriage in the Far Western Fur Trade. In *Western Women: Their Land, Their Lives*, edited by Lillian Schlissel, Vicki Ruiz, and Janice Monk, 199–215. Albuquerque, NM: University of New Mexico Press.

Gumerman IV, George. 1997. Food and Complex Societies. *Journal of Archaeological Method and Theory* 4:105–139.

Helwing, B. 2002. *Hassek Höyük II. Die spätchalkolithische Keramik.* Tübingen: E. Wasmuth Verlag.

Ijzereef, Gerald. 1988. Animal Bones and Social Stratification: A Preliminary Analysis of the Faunal Remains from Cesspits in Amsterdam (1600–1850 AD). *Archaeozoologia* 2 (1, 2):283–292.

Jamieson, R. W. 2000. Doña Luisa and Her Two Houses. In *Lines that Divide: Historical Archaeologies of Race, Class, and Gender*, edited by J. A. Delle, S. A. Mrozowski, and R. Paynter, 142–167. Knoxville: University of Tennessee Press.

Kohlmeyer, Kay. 1996. Houses in Habuba Kabira-South: Spatial Organisation and Planning of Late Uruk Residential Architecture. In *Houses and Households in Ancient Mesopotamia*, edited by K. Veenhof, 89–103. Leiden: Nederlands Historisch-Archaeologisch Instituut te Istanbul.

Langenwalter, P. E. 1980. The Archaeology of 19th-Century Chinese Subsistence at the Lower China Store, Madera County, California. In *Archaeological Perspectives on Ethnicity in America*, edited by Robert L. Schuyler, 102–112. Farmingdale, NY: Baywood.

Lightfoot, Kent, Antoinette Martinez, and Ann Schiff. 1998. Daily Practice and Material Culture in Pluralistic Social Settings: An Archaeological Study of Culture Change and Persistence from Fort Ross, California. *American Antiquity* 63:199–222.

McEwan, Bonnie G. 1991. The Archaeology of Women in the Spanish New World. *Historical Archaeology* 25 (4):33–41.

Murdock, George P., and Caterina Provost. 1973. Factors in the Division of Labor by Sex: A Cross-Cultural Analysis. *Ethnology* 12:203–225.

Rodríguez-Alegría, Enrique. 2005a. Consumption and the Varied Ideologies of Domination in Colonial Mexico City. In *The Postclassic to Spanish-Era Transition in Meso-*

america: Archaeological Perspectives, edited by S. Kepecs and R. T. Alexander, 35–48. Albuquerque: University of New Mexico Press.

———. 2005b. Eating like an Indian: Negotiating Social Relations in the Spanish Colonies. *Current Anthropology* 46:551–73.

Rothman, Mitchell, ed. 2002. *Uruk Mesopotamia and Its Neighbors: Cross Cultural Interactions in the Era of State Formation*. Santa Fe, NM: School of American Research Press.

Stein, Gil. 1999a. Material Culture and Social Identity: The Evidence for a 4th Millennium BC Uruk Mesopotamian Colony at Hacınebi, Turkey. *Paléorient* 25:11–22.

———. 1999b. *Rethinking World Systems: Diasporas, Colonies, and Interaction in Uruk Mesopotamia*. Tucson: University of Arizona Press.

———. 2001. Indigenous Social Complexity at Hacınebi (Turkey) and the Organization of Colonial Contact in the Uruk Expansion. In *Uruk Mesopotamia and Its Neighbors: Cross-Cultural Interactions in the Era of State Formation,* edited by Mitchell Rothman, 265–305. Santa Fe, NM: School of American Research Press.

———. 2002. Colonies without Colonialism: A Trade Diaspora Model of Fourth Millennium BC Mesopotamian Enclaves in Anatolia. In *The Archaeology of Colonialism*, edited by Claire Lyons and John Papadopoulos, 27–64. Los Angeles: Getty Research Institute.

Strommenger, Eva. 1980. *Habuba Kabira, Eine Stadt vor 5000 Jahren*. Mainz am Rhein, Germany: Phillip von Zabern.

Sürenhagen, Dietrich. 1986. The Dry-Farming Belt: The Uruk Period and Subsequent Developments. In *The Origins of Cities in Dry Farming Syria and Mesopotamia in the Third Millennium BC*, edited by Harvey Weiss, 7–43. Guilford, CT: Four Quarters.

Van Buren, M. 1999. Tarapaya: An Elite Spanish Residence Near Colonial Potosí in Comparative Perspective. *Historical Archaeology* 33:101–15.

Voss, Barbara L. 2008. Gender, Race, and Labor in the Archaeology of the Spanish Colonial Americas. *Current Anthropology* 49 (5): 861–893.

Weiss, Harvey, and T. Cuyler Young. 1975. The Merchants of Susa: Godin V and Plateau-Lowland Relations in the Late Fourth Millennium BC. *Iran* 13:1–17.

Young, T. Cuyler. 1986. Godin Tepe VI/V and Central Western Iran at the End of the Fourth Millennium. In *Gamdat Nasr: Period or Regional Style?*, edited by U. Finkbeiner and W. Röllig, 212–228. Weisbaden, Germany: Dr. Ludwig Reichert Verlag.

Discussion Questions: Food Preparation, Social Context, and Ethnicity in a Prehistoric Mesopotamian Colony

1. How does knowing and understanding food, in any place, reveal one's culture and how it was developed?
2. What evidence of colonialism and interaction between different populations is present in the archaeological sites of Mesopotamia?
3. How are gender differences studied, discovered, and identified in archaeological sites? Provides examples from food processing behaviors.
4. How did the colonial invasion remain a calm and peaceful process? What behaviors or patterns of behavior were uncovered related to colonialism?

Theories of Food and the Social Meanings of Coffee

꒰꒱

Catherine M. Tucker

Food is always about more than simply what fills the stomach.

(Rouse and Hoskins 2004: 226)

Food has always been of interest to social scientists, but for many years, the study of food remained on the edges of scholarly theories and debates. Since the 1950s, however, food has become an increasingly pertinent topic for scholars studying globalization, cultural identity, and social change (Mintz and Du Bois 2002). Coffee, in particular, offers interesting opportunities for study because of its relationships to global markets as well as group and national identities, and it is a political commodity with great economic importance. Coffee is the second most valuable commodity traded on world markets (although in times of economic crisis, it occasionally falls to third place). The world's most valuable commodity is petroleum, our premier source of energy for transportation. Petroleum and its derivatives find their way into innumerable goods used in all facets of our lives—plastics, electronics, carpets, building materials, clothing, furniture, machinery, pesticides, and many chemical products. When compared with petroleum, coffee seems misplaced as a major generator of international trade dollars.

Coffee provides little nutritional benefit, and it is not a major component in any industrial product other than itself. While coffee can serve as a useful stimulant, a number of the world's coffee drinkers prefer decaffeinated coffees or prepare weak coffee to reduce caffeine content. Moreover, coffee is only one of many sources of caffeine, including tea, chocolate, sodas, diet aids, analgesics, and caffeine tablets. Therefore coffee's economic value, prevalence, and popularity must derive from more than its nutritional, medical, or stimulating qualities. In part, coffee is valuable because it is consumed by large numbers of people who live in places far from its points of origin. But more important, coffee's popularity and economic importance trace to its social utility and associated meanings and values. We drink coffee for many reasons beyond caffeine; like many things we eat, coffee evokes feelings and communicates values unrelated to nutritional content.

SOCIAL IMPLICATIONS OF FOOD

Food exists within complex webs of social relationships. Food provides nutrition for physical sustenance, but it also serves to support social and cultural survival. Food-sharing builds relationships within families and groups; food exchanges with people outside immediate social circles can help build social networks and develop political alliances (Bryant et al. 2003). From birth, the food we eat becomes associated with family, home, and shared experiences that go beyond meals. Our favorite "comfort food" is often a simple dish from childhood; its comfort derives not from novelty or elegance but from deep familiarity and often associations with love and security. A cup of coffee with milk and sugar signifies relaxation for me; it reminds me of the hours I spent talking with friends in graduate school while sipping coffee with free refills. We know we belong where we eat familiar foods in the company of people who share similar memories and experiences, and inviting people to share our meals can be a sign of friendship, or sometimes more. For example, inviting a boyfriend or girlfriend over for dinner with the family can imply that the relationship may be more than a transitory affection.

Food selection and preparation can communicate social skills, shared values, and cultural knowledge, which can be particularly important for women who are usually responsible for food preparation. Among African American women who convert to Islam, food selection and preparation can become empowering religious practices as they follow dietary principles while expressing their perspectives on the historical, symbolic, political, and cultural dimensions of African American "soul foods" (Rouse and Hoskins 2004). Across ethnic and religious backgrounds, bridal gift registries in the USA often include a coffee maker for soon-to-be married couples. Coffee-making may be seen as a necessary skill, depending on one's cultural background. One of my friends, Halima, is from Egypt but, due to her family circumstances, she grew up without learning how to make coffee. When Halima came to the USA as a young bride, she met an Egyptian woman who owned a coffee shop. Halima confided that she did not know how to make coffee, and the shop owner pulled her into the kitchen to teach her. An hour later, Halima knew how to make coffee, and had absorbed a cultural lesson as well: if she wanted to have a long and happy marriage, she needed to be able to make good Egyptian coffee.

Each coffee-consuming society tends have a dominant way to prepare coffee, even when there may be other options. In the USA, filtered coffee is the default form. In Mexico, Central America, and Scandinavia, boiled coffee dominated for many years. Instant coffee has become typical for many parts of South America. Thick boiled coffee, served in tiny cups, remains popular in the Middle East. Each brew carries its own consistency and range of flavors that seem "right" to the people who drink it; when offered a different brew, it may barely seem like coffee at all.

Acceptance or rejection of coffee, or any food, offered to guests may be seen as accepting or rejecting an offer of friendship. Guests who wish to develop friendly relationships with their hosts usually attempt to eat everything put before them, however unfamiliar or personally problematic. During my first fieldwork as a young anthropologist, I worked with a team of researchers in the highlands of Peru. While on an early visit to a family in the community, I was offered a plate of fried sheep's blood. They purchased the blood from the slaughterhouse because they could not afford meat. I had never eaten anything like it; reddish brown globules slid in grease around the plate and tasted like salty rust. I wanted very much to gain their trust and friendship, so I ate it with as much relish as I could muster. My introduction as a teenager to traditionally prepared Colombian coffee did not prove much easier; my hosts served me thick coffee, complete with the grounds, in a demitasse cup dosed liberally with sugar. I sipped it politely, but despite the small quantity, I felt a jolt of energy and did not get much sleep that night. I didn't care for fried blood or traditional Colombian coffee, but in accepting my hosts' gift of food without question, I symbolically accepted them and opened a door to friendship.

RAW, COOKED, OR ROTTEN? PERCEPTIONS OF FOOD, NATURE, AND CULTURE

The meanings and values ascribed to foods may relate to ways that the human mind interprets and categorizes the world. Lévi-Strauss, a renowned French anthropologist, proposed that foods fall into one of three broad categories: "raw," "cooked," or "rotted." By collecting information on myths and food beliefs around the world, he argued that while societies vary in how they interpret the meanings of food, they still deal with dualities such as raw/cooked, raw/rotted, and cooked/rotted, which symbolize and echo other oppositions: nature/culture, good/bad, edible/inedible, self/other, desirable/repulsive. Raw foods are "natural," "unprocessed," and "wild"; they often require some kind of preparation, such as washing, peeling, and cutting to be deemed edible. Cooked foods have been transformed through roasting, boiling, or smoking to become "civilized." Societies tend to regard roasting, boiling, or smoking as having different levels of prestige. Among western societies, roasting tends to have higher prestige than boiling. The relative status of these forms of cooking varies across history and people (Lévi-Strauss 1983, 2008). There is no universal way to ascertain a food's position in a cultural system of meaningful oppositions and dualities. Instead, it is necessary to understand a people's perspectives and experiences.

The way society categorizes a food reflects its prestige, usefulness, and potential risks, which reflect historical, political, and economic processes, and preferences whose roots may be long forgotten. Perceptions of food risks emerge because of the ways that society links potentially edible substances to social values and experiences. In the USA, edible food discarded by restaurants and groceries becomes "rotted" the moment it hits the dumpster. Insects are considered to be inedible in western society because they are associated with filth and decay (they are "raw" or "rotten"), but in most of the world, people recognize certain insects as delicious and nourishing foods (Bryant et al. 2003). A given food may take on multiple meanings as people negotiate its social values, political meanings, and symbolic representations. The television show "Fear Factor" played upon Western distastes by challenging contestants to do unpleasant things, such as eating insects while competing for monetary prizes. Contestants who chose to eat the insects symbolically and physically transformed the inedible ("raw" or "rotten") to the edible, defying one social norm in order to fulfill another social norm: willingness to sacrifice for monetary gain. In forcing contestants to choose between social norms, the show compelled the audience to question where their preferences and priorities lay. Can something repulsive be made tolerable by the possibility of enrichment (and fleeting fame)? Few westerners found the answers simple. Lévi-Strauss's perspective helps us to understand that the dilemma emerges from Western perceptions of underlying oppositions. For someone from an insect-eating society, there would be no opposition or repulsion, and no dilemma.

BREWING UP AN EDIBLE AND MEANINGFUL COMMODITY

Coffee does not present moral conundrums for most drinkers, but how does society interpret coffee? Clearly, coffee is "cooked." It has been roasted, ground, and mixed with water by some means—boiling, percolating, filtering, pressing, or steaming under pressure. In this sense, coffee is a complex culinary creation. Yet coffee is also represented as something "natural," "wild," and uncivilized in Western society, because of its associations with exotic origins and dangerous diseases that medical science does not understand well. The perceived risks of coffee led certain religions to ban it and some physicians to warn against it, while the perceived benefits of coffee resulted in the creation of coffee breaks.

Lévi-Strauss suggested that different social meanings map consistently to different types of food preparation: the high prestige activities involve greater patience, more complex technology and resources, or greater skill to carry out well (Lévi-Strauss 1983). Espresso drinks carry the highest social prestige for coffee preparation;

it requires special machinery and training to create a perfect shot of espresso, a fine latte, or a cappuccino. People who prefer these drinks may be perceived as more ambitious or wealthy than those who drink regular coffee; thus coffee can be a marker of socioeconomic class.

Yet because a shot of espresso or a cappuccino is within the economic grasp of nearly everyone, people may choose to consume these drinks not only out of enjoyment, but also to appear affluent, discriminating, or tasteful. Similarly, people of wealth may choose regular coffee in part to signal humility, lack of pretention, a connection to modest origins, or shared values with the middle and lower classes. The choice of coffee can thus signal membership in or identification with a social class, but it can also be used to transcend, contradict, or undermine social class divisions. The malleability of coffee to send many messages is part of what makes it so appealing to people of many social backgrounds.

Coffee is also subject to a multitude of opinions because people's experiences and reactions to it vary. The current multiplicity of meanings associated with coffee has emerged (or re-emerged) since the 1980s. Between 1960 and 1988, the percentage of coffee drinkers in the USA fell gradually from 74 percent to 50 percent (Roseberry 1996). Small coffee roasters and shop owners realized that they needed to expand their clientele, and attract young people who had grown up preferring soft drinks. Meanwhile, transnational food corporations that dominate coffee markets (Nestlé, General Foods, Sara Lee, Philip Morris, Proctor and Gamble) depended on their diversified business interests to protect them from declining coffee sales. The big companies' decisions to produce successively cheaper and therefore less flavorful coffee between the 1960s and 1980s most likely contributed to falling demand. Independent entrepreneurs took advantage of the lack of good coffee to draw clients who appreciated quality, flavor, and variety (Roseberry 1996).

COFFEE, IDENTITY, AND MEANING IN THE USA

In the USA, "regular" coffee typically means filtered or percolated coffee. But why coffee instead of tea? American preference for coffee emerged through specific historical events leading up to the Revolutionary War, but it endures because social values and national identity became linked to coffee drinking. In other places, tea, *mate*, or *qat* gained these meaningful linkages. Coffee, however, is unusual as a global commodity because food preferences usually arise when sources are nearby. Tea is native to Asia, where the majority of the world's tea drinkers reside. *Qat*, a popular beverage in the Middle East, grows natively in the region, as does cacao (chocolate) in Mexico, where hot chocolate emerged prehistorically as a favorite elite beverage. *Yerba mate* from local bushes remains a more popular drink in Uruguay and Argentina than coffee, which can be had from nearby Brazil. Instead, most of the world's coffee drinkers live half a world away from the people who produce coffee. Increasing recognition in the USA of coffee's origins now influences people's choices.

Coffee drinkers can choose fair trade, organic, and shade-grown coffees because they appreciate high quality coffee. Or they may see their choice, and their willingness to spend a bit more, as a way of showing solidarity with coffee growers, countering some of the inequities of the profit-driven global economy, and supporting environmental sustainability (Jaffee 2007). "Yuppies" who favor gourmet coffee may also be longing for a more genteel past before mass consumption, and endeavoring to reconstruct a more wholesome era by favoring whole-bean coffees, gourmet shops featuring antique coffee grinders, and diversity in coffee varietals and roasts (Roseberry 1996). Choosing fair trade or other specialty coffees can symbolize resistance to the dominant society. Within punk culture, the choice of fair trade and organic coffee symbolized opposition to capitalism, and rejection of a society characterized by profound social inequities (Clark 2004). In the past 20 years, fair trade and specialty coffees have become the fastest growing segment of the global coffee market. The success of these coffees in many "niche" markets reflects associations with social values and meanings held dear by people across a range of social groups and political perspectives.

The diversity of meanings associated with types of coffee is reinforced by the contrasts in public spaces in which coffee is consumed. Social meanings of place and space intersect with social class and individual identity. Upscale coffee shops contrast with working-class delicatessens; barbershops with coffee pots in waiting areas create an entirely different social space than elegant hair-styling salons with espresso makers in the foyer, even if both provide a similar service. Coffee is an equalizer as well as a marker of difference. Its omnipresence suggests cultural consensus, but it can also be an object of contention. Ironically, the cheapest, least flavorful coffee is associated with some of the world's wealthiest multinational conglomerates, while high quality coffee is associated with independent entrepreneurs, local cooperatives, small coffee shops, and not-for-profit environmental and social justice organizations.

COFFEE AND FETISHISM OF COMMODITIES

Through systems of production and distribution, our choices of food can transform the Earth, and may degrade or conserve the soil and water upon which we depend for sustenance. One of the results of the modern agroindustrial complex has been to separate people from food production. Many things that we consume, including coffee, come prepared and packaged in ways that utterly disguise or contain very little of its original content. A package of hamburger carries no element that implies a cow; a can of ground coffee represents nothing of the bush and cherry of its origins. Some prepared foodstuffs have more to do with laboratory processes and chemical additives than agricultural fields and pastures (Pollan 2008). Instant coffee derives from an industrial process of dehydrating or freeze-drying brewed coffee made from inferior beans, to form a powder that dissolves easily in water. While convenient, the resulting beverage offers a flavor barely reminiscent of fresh-brewed coffee, with less caffeine and a more bitter taste. Marx described this profound separation of the consumer from the producer, and the utter transformation of a final product from the original form, as "fetishism of commodities" (Marx 1978: 319–29). When coffee drinkers consume their brew without knowledge or concern for its origins, they deny their connections to any troubling truth of how it came to their table. Because coffee is produced far away from the majority of its consumers, it has been particularly vulnerable to these separations. But the growth in fair trade and specialty coffees is an attempt to reconnect consumers with producers. The Slow Food and local food movements that are spreading through Europe, the USA, Canada, and Japan in recent years reveal increasing awareness among consumers that they have lost ties to the producers of their food. This awareness has triggered a commitment to rebuild those linkages. The efforts present a humble challenge to the dominance of impersonal global markets, and have created opportunities to renegotiate the culturally specific and globally relevant significance of coffee and many other foods.

Coffee's popularity, however, can only be understood in relationship to global markets. While its origins precede the development of the modern world system, the use of coffee as a beverage apparently emerged not long before the time that European vessels began exploring the globe. Thereafter, the history of coffee becomes inseparable from the history of colonialism, imperialism and the rise of global capitalism. To comprehend the economic, social, and cultural significance of coffee, we must explore its history.

REFERENCES

Bryant, C.A., K.M. DeWalt, A. Courtney, and J. Schwartz. 2003. *The Cultural Feast: An Introduction to Food and Society*. Belmont, CA: Thomson Wadsworth.

Clark, D. 2004. "The Raw and the Rotten: Punk Cuisine." *Ethnology 43*: 19–31.

Jaffee, D. 2007. *Brewing Justice: Fair Trade Coffee, Sustainability, and Survival*. Berkeley: University of California Press.

Lévi-Strauss, C. 1983. *The Raw and the Cooked: Mythologiques Vol. I.* Chicago: University of Chicago Press.

———. 2008. "The Culinary Triangle." Pp. 36–43 in *Food and Culture: A Reader*, 2nd edition, eds. C. Counihan and P. Van Esterik. New York: Routledge.

Marx, K. 1978. Capital, Volume One. Pp. 294–439 in *The Marx-Engels Reader*, ed. R.C. Tucker. New York: W.W. Norton.

Mintz, S.W., and C.M. Du Bois. 2002. "The Anthropology of Food and Eating." *Annual Review of Anthropology 31*: 99–119.

Pollan, M. 2008. *In Defense of Food: An Eater's Manifesto.* New York: Penguin.

Roseberry, W. 1996. "The Rise of Yuppie Coffees and the Reimagination of Class in the United States." *American Anthropologist 98*: 762–75.

Rouse, C., and J. Hoskins. 2004. "Purity, Soul Food, and Sunni Islam: Explorations at the Intersection of Consumption and Resistance." *Cultural Anthropology 19*: 226–49.

Discussion Questions: Theories of Food and the Social Meanings of Coffee

1. Why is coffee consumed? Which coffee preparation is typically considered the most prestigious?
2. What is true of every coffee-consuming society or culture? How is coffee used?
3. When attempting to become a part of a host culture, what is important in terms of food and drink? What should one do?
4. Why aren't insects consumed in Western cultures and societies?

"I'll Have Whatever She's Having": Jews, Food, and Film*

NATHAN ABRAMS

A number of films in the last few decades have famously used food in their narratives to celebrate particular cultures. There is a deliciously long list of films in which foods—marked as Jewish and kosher, Jewish but not kosher, or non-Jewish, are not simply glimpsed as part of a film's setting but also employed as important plot devices that explore cultural, ethnic, and religious issues. Woody Allen, for example, makes much use of the nature and function of food and dining in his films. His movies abound with memorable moments and food allusions: the Chinese food scene in *Manhattan* (1979); the crazy seder in *Sleeper* (1973); the split-screen families and their foods in *Annie Hall* (1977); the serious discussion at the seder in *Crimes and Misdemeanors* (1989); the jokes about kosher food and fasting during Yom Kippur in *Radio Days* (1987); New York's Carnegie Deli and the plates of kosher meat in *Broadway Danny Rose* (1984), and so on. Certainly, Allen's use of food in his films intrinsically connects that food to Jewish culture.

Surprisingly, very little has been written about the topic of Jewish cultural representation through food in films. I will attempt here to begin filling this gap by exploring the ways in which "Jewish," kosher, and *treyf* (explicitly non-kosher) foods are represented in film. My discussion will include observations on the ways in which Jews have been represented and stereotyped in visual

*I would like to thank Alex Gordon, David Desser, Gail Samuelson, and all those who responded to my queries on the various H-NET discussion lists; without their help this essay would not have been possible. I am also extremely grateful to Douglas Brode and Terry Barr, who have written extensively about food in the films of Woody Allen and Jewish dining scenes, respectively.

popular culture through food. Specifically, I'll look at the connections among food and Jewish motherhood, cultural traditions, history, identity, sex, and nostalgia. Finally, I will also examine cinematic representations of the Jewish family meal as the primary site of philosophical debate about the Jewish condition and Jewish identity.

Motherhood

Much of Jewish humor is food related, and many traditional jokes are concerned with Jewish mothers. Likewise, film often plays with the traditional stereotype of the Jewish mother, usually presented as an overeating, overcaring, and overbearing matriarchal figure who stuffs her children with far more than they can possibly digest. As the poet Isaac Rosenfeld has put it, "the hysterical mother who stuffs her infant with forced feedings (thereby laying in, all unwittingly, the foundation for ulcers, diabetes, and intestinal cancer with each spoonful she crams down the hatch) is motivated by a desire to give security to her child."[1] At the same time that they denigrate the mother figure, however, such jokes are laced with a reverence for mother's cooking. She is known as the *baleboosteh*, a Yiddish term for a praiseworthy mother.

The stereotypical image of a Jewish mother is represented by the mother of Buddy Young Jr. (Billy Crystal) in *Mr. Saturday Night* (dir. Billy Crystal, 1992). This woman goes through a daily ritual of pushing food on all of her relatives particularly her sons, with the admonition, 'Eat, eat.' During Buddy's opening monologue, a close-up montage of the delicious and filling foods she has lovingly worked hard to prepare by hand for her family over the years is shown: matzo balls, onions, tomatoes, corned beef, stuffed turkey, stuffed cabbage, latkes, challah, matzo-ball soup, and all kinds of desserts. Buddy describes his mother forcing food on her family, quipping, "My mother was trying to kill us with fat." The same kind of stereotype occurs on American television. The sitcom *The Nanny* (1993–99) lampoons the loving Jewish mother character, in this case Fran's (the nanny's) mother, who is also stereotypically obsessed with food and is usually seen in the kitchen or around food. Interestingly, though, in an unusual inversion of the stereotypical self-abnegating Jewish mother who just pushes food on her kids, Fran's mother cooks (and eats) more for herself than for her child.

Identity and Culture

Foodstuffs are intimately related to Jewish identity and culture in film. Although many of these products have long been assimilated into mainstream American culture, on film a corned beef or pastrami sandwich on rye bread, bagels and lox, gefilte fish, chicken soup, or matzo typically code the Jewish world semiotically. Chicken soup might now be considered a universal panacea, popularized even further by the best-selling book series *Chicken Soup for the Soul*, but it has long been identified with Jewish culture. In the television program *Northern Exposure* (1990–95) chicken fat is described as "Jewish mayonnaise," and in *The Apartment* (dir. Billy Wilder, 1960) the Jewish neighbor character nurses Fran Kubelik (Shirley MacLaine) back to health with chicken soup. Authentic chicken soup often features dumplings or balls made from matzo meal (hence the apocryphal question Marilyn Monroe asked when visiting Arthur Miller's parents, "What kind of animal is a matzo?"), and because of matzo's connection to Passover it is also considered a trope for Jewishness. In *Torch Song Trilogy* (dir. Paul Bogart, 1988), Arnold Beckhoff's mother goes into the kitchen looking for matzo meal. When Arnold (Harvey Fierstein) tells her which shelf it is on, she says, "He has matzo meal! I brought him up right," suggesting that his ownership of a Jewish food product overrides his "deviant" (by Jewish religious law)—and thus disappointing—(homo)sexuality.

In Robert Redford's *Quiz Show* (1994), the Reuben sandwich is semiotically deployed to code Jewishness. The Reuben—a grilled combination of corned beef, Swiss cheese, and sauerkraut (or coleslaw) on sourdough pumpernickel bread—is a clear signifier of ethnicity; its origins are specific to Jewish delicatessens in New York. One theory even attributed its invention to the movies themselves when, in 1914, Annette Seelos, the leading lady in a Charlie Chaplin film, first ate the sandwich (albeit with Virginia baked ham rather than corned beef). The link between film and food was cemented when the New York delicatessen Reuben's began naming sandwiches after actors.[2] In *Quiz Show*, Dick Goodwin (Rob Morrow), a Jew, orders the sandwich as the special of the day at the Athenaeum, the elitist Manhattan club. Aware of his outsider status as a Jew and the unwillingness of white Anglo-Saxon Protestant (WASP) America to accept his ethnicity, Goodwin remarks that the sandwich was named after Reuben Kay of Nebraska, before wryly observing about the club, "Unfortunately, they have the sandwich here, but they don't seem to have any Reubens." Here the Reuben sandwich serves to code both his Jewishness and his interloper status, standing among the patrician elite. Later, the distance is emphasized when he is invited to the Van Doren estate in rural Connecticut, where he feasts on distinctly nonethnic and genteel fare such as fresh corn on the cob and tomato salad. Goodwin is slowly seduced by the gentile world of the Van Dorens, and this is emphasized in a key sequence featuring an exchange between him and the other main Jewish protagonist, Herb Stempel (John Tuturro). Goodwin goes to the Stempels' apartment to interview Stempel about his charges that the quiz shows are rigged. The gulf between them is signified when Stempel offers Goodwin some ruggelach, "a Jewish delicacy." Stempel has to explain this because to him, Goodwin carries all the signifiers of assimilation; indeed, he seems to be the epitome of the successful and accepted American who has escaped the bounds of his ethnic culture. Goodwin has an important government job; he has straight white teeth, wears well-made suits, and carries a briefcase. Stempel believes that Goodwin has forgotten, if indeed he ever knew, his traditional Jewish roots. When Goodwin disdainfully declines, Stempel rebukes him with the words:

"You don't know what you're missing." Goodwin contemptuously replies that he "knows ruggelach" and the point is made that Goodwin is perfectly aware of his ethnic roots but prefers the splendor of genteel and gentile rural Connecticut fare more than thoroughly ethnic pastries served from a tin in the middle of Queens.

Perhaps the most distinctively Jewish foodstuff is gefilte fish. *Gefilte* literally means "stuffed," and this specialty is basically a poached fishball made from whitefish, pike, and/or carp with filler (bread crumbs or matzo meal), served on the Sabbath and holy days among German and Eastern European Jews. Gefilte fish carries the mark of Jewish authenticity. Its preparation (when not bought ready-made in a jar) requires skill and patience. *The Jewish Home Beautiful*, the guide for aspiring Jewish mothers, states, "If there is any one particular food that might lay claim to being the Jewish national dish, gefilte fish is that food." One company, Mother's, once advertised its product by connecting it to history and tradition. It was "old-fashioned" and the "real" thing, made in the "finest tradition," and carried with it all of the symbols of *kashrut* (being kosher) and Jewish authenticity, including Hebrew writing. Gefilte fish was often upheld as a method of prevention against assimilation, as represented by the consumption of Chinese food by Ashkenazi urban Americans, and summed up in the words, "Down with chop suey! Long live gefilte fish!"[3] Since Gefilte fish is clearly and visibly Jewish, it is readily used in film and television. In the American television sitcom *The Nanny,* the characters worry over whether gefilte fish should be served at a favorite aunt's funeral. In one episode of *The Goldbergs* (1949–54), the immensely popular television sitcom that attracted some forty million viewers per week at its peak, the heroine of the show, Molly Goldberg, was invited by a leading food manufacturer to produce some of her own gefilte fish in his test kitchen.[4]

In contrast to such foods as Reuben sandwiches and gefilte fish, Wonder Bread, mayonnaise, pork and/or ham, and lobsters signify the non-Jewish world. Wonder Bread stands for whiteness because of its uniformly white nature and its origins in the Midwest. Comedian Lenny Bruce once quipped, "Pumpernickel is Jewish and, as you know, white bread is very goyish," and Nora Ephron has commented on the socioethnic construction of mayonnaise, in particular Hellman's, as gentile.[5] In *Hannah and Her Sisters* (dir. Woody Allen, 1986), Mickey (Allen), newly (and temporarily) converted to Catholicism, unloads a grocery bag, withdrawing a loaf of Wonder Bread and a jar of Hellman's mayonnaise, clear and humorous signifiers to any Jewish audience of Mickey's conversion. Along those lines, in Susan Mogul's taped performance *The Last Jew in America* (1984), the heroine Barbara is trying to attract a Jewish mate by pretending to be a Christian. As a consequence, she goes out and buys Wonder Bread and removes not only the matzo from her pantry, but also the Chinese food. And, although not about Jewishness (but similarly positing a distinct ethnicity—Greek in this case—as against "Americanness"), the film *My Big Fat Greek Wedding* (dir. Joel Zwick, 2002) perpetuates the link between Wonder Bread and whiteness. As its Greek protagonist moves into the American mainstream, she swaps moussaka for Wonder Bread sandwiches, and is hence accepted by her white peers whereas hitherto her consumption of ethnic foods symbolized her distance from the American mainstream.

Jewish versus Non-Jewish

In addition to serving as a cultural identifier of Jewishness, in many films food also stands as a trope for the clash between the Jewish and non-Jewish worlds. A scene used humorously by Allen (and others) features a non-Jew ordering a corned beef/pastrami sandwich and asking to have it with mayonnaise on white bread, thus violating Jewish tradition and *kashrut* laws, both of which "prescribe" that corned beef be eaten on rye bread with mustard. At dinner in a Jewish delicatessen in *Annie Hall*, Annie (Diane Keaton) clearly feels out of place and, with no idea of how to order "properly" in a deli, orders a WASPish meal—pastrami on white bread "with mayonnaise, tomatoes, and lettuce"—to Alvy's (Allen's) obvious disgust. A similar scene occurs in the (in)famous orgasm sequence in the famous (kosher) Katz's Deli on Manhattan's Lower East Side in *When Harry Met Sally* (dir. Rob Reiner, 1989), which begins with the eponymous gentile Sally (Meg Ryan) ordering a turkey sandwich on white bread with mayonnaise, while the overtly Jewish Harry (Billy Crystal) eats salt beef on rye. Harry visibly winces as she orders, as does Alvy in *Annie Hall;* in each case the girlfriend's sandwich becomes emblematic of the cultural clash between the male Jewish protagonist and his non-Jewish female partner, and suggests the problems that lie ahead for the relationship. In a later scene in *Annie Hall*, Alvy's discomfort with Annie's family is expressed through food and dining, when the use of a split screen, juxtaposing both families' mealtimes, reinforces their differences, like "oil and water."

The same kind of coding of simple foods showed up in the television series *Eight is Enough* (1977–81). In one episode, one of the eight daughters befriends a Jewish doctor, and a waitress at the hospital coaches her on how to eat a deli sandwich with mustard, rather than mayonnaise, and not with a glass of milk. This change of eating pattern caused her father to think she was converting to Judaism.

Pork, since Jewish *kashrut* laws proscribe it, also frequently occurs as a symbol of the cultural clash between Jews and gentiles. Comedian Lenny Bruce articulated the culinary side of this Jewish self-definition: "Spam is goyish and rye bread is Jewish." Pork and ham stand as tropes for all that is non-Jewish or *treyf.* "Pork," as Rosenfeld puts it, "means the uncircumcised."[6] *Big Boy* (dir. Alan Crosland, 1930), starring Al Jolson, ends with him singing about coming home to his little cabin, which he describes with vivid details, extolling the smell of the ham his mother is preparing in the kitchen. After a slight pause Jolson says: "Ham? . . . Wait a minute! That ain't my house!" Of course, simply because something is forbidden doesn't mean it isn't eaten. Indeed, probably because they are forbidden, some Jews will choose such foodstuffs.

Often the consumption of forbidden foods symbolizes rebellion and/or the rejection of traditional ethnic roots. In *Mr. Saturday Night*, Buddy Young Jr. invites a beautiful woman in the audience (who will later become his wife) to part with her traditional Jewish parents and treats her to a roast pork dinner. In Boaz Yakin's *A Price above Rubies* (1998), the main character uses food to demonstrate her rebellion againt the Hasidic tradition by buying a nonkosher hot dog on the street in Manhattan and loving it. Later, the effect is compounded when her husband and their rabbi/therapist are shocked when they learn that she's been keeping kosher only at home. In *The Jazz Singer* (dir. Alan Crosland, 1927), Al Jolson pointedly eats nonkosher food: in the first scene after he has left his Orthodox family to pursue his jazz singing career, he sits in a restaurant practically dancing in his chair with delight as he digs in to bacon, juicy pork sausages, and eggs. There is even a quasi-pornographic close-up of the plate. In Allen's *Radio Days*, eating pork chops as well as clams (which one character breaks the fast to eat with his Jewish communist neighbors) stands for conversion to atheistic communism.

Religious food restrictions limit gastronomic exploration, but more important, they can curtail social and geographic mobility, which has led many people in real life to break away from such religious sanctions. Therefore it is not surprising to find that, in order to achieve higher social identification, Jews in film have eaten forbidden foods, as the conspicuous consumption of such food is an important indicator of status. Consequently, the consumption of such products becomes emblematic of attempts to assimilate, to move away from Jewish origins. The pork-eating scene in *The Jazz Singer* also serves to underscore the protagonist's accelerating assimilation. In *Annie Hall*, Alvy is eating Easter dinner at his partner's very WASPish parents. He compliments her grandmother, Grammy Ann, on her "dynamite ham," even though he has no idea what he is talking about. He is simply trying to fit in, since everyone else is complimenting her, too. The failure of this gesture is underlined by her imagining him dressed in the long black coat and hat of an Orthodox Jew, complete with mustache and beard. In *Europa, Europa* (dir. Agnieska Holland, 1991), set in the Holocaust era, the Jewish hero, who is posing as a gentile, is served ham at his girlfriend's house, coding the dilemmas of that period between *kashrut* and survival. Here ham is used to disguise his Jewishness. And a similar situation takes place in *Chariots of Fire* (dir. Hugh Hudson, 1981) when the Jewish character inadvertently confronts pork that has been ordered for him.

Along with assimilationism, certain foods considered *treyf* by Jews are items that, in addition, signal sophistication and the desire to gentrify. In the leading and influential Jewish journal *Commentary*, a full-page color 1970s advertisement for Bolla Italian wine depicts lobster, clearly encoding it (along with other *treyf* foodstuffs, including various shellfish) as the epitome of worldliness and cosmopolitanism. But even as a food like lobster is coded to signal assimilation and sophistication, it can become emblematic of the cultural gap between Jews and non-Jews. In *Annie Hall*, Alvy and Annie spontaneously laugh at crawling crustaceans on the kitchen floor as they awkwardly prepare a lobster dinner at a beach house in the Hamptons: "Maybe we should just call the police. Dial 911. It's the lobster squad." Alvy is fearful of the creatures, and when he realizes that one big lobster has crawled behind the refrigerator, Alvy jokes: "It'll turn up in our bed at night. Talk to him. You speak shellfish...Annie, there's a big lobster behind the refrigerator. I can't get it out. . . . Maybe if I put a little dish of butter sauce here with a nutcracker, it will run out the other side? . . . We should have gotten steaks, 'cause they don't have legs. They don't run around." As with a similar scene in the British film *Leon the Pig Farmer* (dir. Vadim Jean and Gary Sinyor, 1992), lobsters symbolize the inherent distance between the male Jewish protagonist and the non-Jewish figure of his erotic infatuation.

Food and Sex

The link between dietary and sexual prohibition in Judaism is often repeated throughout Jewish culture, and interpretations linking sex and *kashrut* food regulations have long been made. Indeed, since Adam and Eve ate the apple in the Garden of Eden, food and sex have been inextricably linked. Rosenfeld adumbrates the link: "When the Lord forbade Adam and Eve to eat of the Tree, He started something which has persisted throughout our history: the attachment of all sorts of forbidden meanings to food, and the use of food in a system of taboos which, though meant to regulate diet, have also had as their function—perhaps the primary one—the regulation of sexual conduct."[7] Meat and milk in Jewish law cannot be mixed and/or eaten together, for example, deriving from the enigmatic Biblical injunction against "seething a kid in its mother's milk." In a 1979 article in the *New York Review of Books*, "The Dietary Prohibitions of the Hebrews," Jean Soler argued that this biblical ban on cooking a kid in its mother's milk was linked to an incest taboo, wittily observing, "You shall not put a mother and her son into the same pot, any more than into the same bed."[8] Many films have connected food and *kashrut* with sexuality. This sanction has provided further grist for the popular culture mill. It is no coincidence, for example, that Alisa Lebow and Cynthia Madansky named their 1998 documentary about Jewish lesbians *Treyf*. Similarly, growing sexual awareness is signaled in *A Walk on the Moon* (dir. Tony Goldwyn, 1999), when a young Orthodox girl eats bacon for the first time.

The classic incident connecting food and sex in a Jewish setting is the orgasm scene in *When Harry Met Sally*. Harry and Sally are discussing sex over a meal in a kosher deli; Sally has just ordered a "*treyfed*" version of a typically Jewish sandwich (as discussed earlier). Harry confidently believes that his sexual prowess satisfies his female partners and brings them to orgasm, until Sally explains how "most women, at one time or another, have faked it." Harry doesn't believe that he has been fooled because he "knows":

Sally: Oh right. That's right. I forgot. You're a man.

Harry: What is that supposed to mean?

Sally: Nothing. It's just that all men are sure it never happens to them, and most women at one time or another have done it, so you do the math.

Harry: You don't think that I can tell the difference?

Sally: No.

Harry: Get outta here.

Sally then looks at Harry seductively, and begins to illustrate, in the middle of the busy restaurant, how easily women can convincingly fake an orgasm. With a loud and long display of pants, groans, gasps, hair rufflings, caresses, table poundings, and ecstatic releases, she yells "Yes, Yes, YES! YES! YES!" as she brings herself to fake orgasm. The entire restaurant is quieted down and attentive to her realistic act. When she is finished with her demonstration, she calmly composes herself, picks up her fork and resumes eating. The sequence ends with an older woman customer (Estelle Reiner, director Rob Reiner's mother) requesting, "I'll have whatever she's having," thus implying the erotic effect of non-kosher food upon Jews; the *treyf* version of the traditional Jewish sandwich being inherently preferable to Jews than the kosher one. Likewise, a similar sequence in *Annie Hall* suddenly cuts from Annie and Alvy eating to the couple in bed, having just finished making love.

As seafood is only kosher if it has fins and scales, all shellfish are forbidden. The symbolic or allegorical interpretation of the *kashrut* laws has it that fins and scales on a fish are signs of endurance and self-control; the lack of them can be construed to mean wild, impetuous abandon. Shellfish—in particular the king of shellfish, lobster—stands as a code for wantonness and excess. In the musical *Funny Girl* (dir. William Wyler, 1968), which depicts the life of Jewish comedienne Fannie Brice (Barbra Streisand) from her early days in the Jewish slums of New York's Lower East Side to the height of her career with the Ziegfeld Follies, her future husband, Nick Arnstein (Omar Sharif), introduces Fanny to lobster. The scene opens on a close-up of a restaurant table covered with lobster debris (shells, crackers, butter, etc.). The camera pulls back to Nick and Fanny. She has a napkin round her neck. He watches her benignly as she licks her fingers and wipes her hands. Nick says, "You don't know how proud I am to think that I am the man who introduced you to your first lobster," to which Fanny giggles and replies, "Among other things." The restaurant owner/cook in the background says to her, "Lady, if you're game for this one, he's on the house. Nobody in history ever had three." Fanny responds, "Start boiling the water!" Fanny directly equates the loss of her gastronomic virginity with the loss of her sexual virginity, and her appetite for both is seemingly insatiable. In *Portnoy's Complaint* (dir. Ernest Lehman, 1972), the protagonist's mother connects lobster with sexual temptation and urges restraint. But when the fifteen-year-old Alex Portnoy sucks on a lobster claw one night, within the hour "his cock is out and aimed at a shiksa on a Public Service bus." Along the same line, for Woody Allen, lobsters are the symbol of insatiable sexual attraction; they symbolize love affairs, as opposed to the more humdrum foods of marriage. In *A Midsummer's Night Sex Comedy* (1982), when his wife interrogates him about a previous relationship, Allen's character nervously replies, "I went out with her *once* . . . and had a couple of *lobsters* . . . that's *it!*"

Lobster's role as signifier of temptation also occurs in an episode of the television series *Seinfeld* (1990–98). Jerry Seinfeld, who plays himself in the series, is dating a Jewish girl who maintains a strictly kosher diet and refuses to eat the lobster that they catch out on Long Island when they—Jerry, George (Jason Alexander), Elaine (Julia Louis-Dreyfus), and Kramer (Michael Richards)—are spending the weekend at a friend's place. All evening the friends talk of how delicious and succulent the lobster is and the temptation proves too difficult to resist. In the middle of the night, Jerry's girlfriend creeps down to the kitchen to sneak some of the lobster without anyone else seeing. Kramer, guessing that this would happen, is guarding the refrigerator and refuses to let her eat it, essentially becoming the self-appointed guardian of her morals. The next day, however, in an act of revenge for an earlier transgression, George puts the leftover lobster in the scrambled eggs without her knowledge. On hearing of this, she feels defiled. Lobster here clearly signifies temptation and abandon. The girlfriend's attempts to avoid eating it symbolize her efforts to remain ritually pure. *Treyf* foods like lobster thus signify, in the words of Rosenfeld, "the whole world of forbidden sexuality, the sexuality of the *goyim*, and there all the delights are imagined to lie, with the *shiksas* and *shkotzim* who are unrestrained and not made kosher."[9]

Whether involving *treyf* foods or acceptable ones, one sees that connections between food and sex abound in films about Jews. In *Once upon a Time In America* (1984), Sergio Leone's epic about Jewish gangsters, a young gang member buys an ornate and nonkosher pastry in order to obtain sexual favors from the neighborhood sweetheart. As he waits outside her door, his desire for the pastry proves stronger than his lust for the girl: he begins licking the cream from his fingertips and ends up wolfing down the whole thing.

Allen's entire oeuvre is shot through with references to food and sex; indeed, the two become synonymous in his work. In *Annie Hall* he says, "We'll kiss now . . . then go eat." When he arrives at Diane Keaton's character's apartment in *Manhattan*, hoping to have sex, he asks, "Have you got anything to eat here?" Lunch, in particular, has sexual connotations: in *Manhattan* he tells his young date, "You'll have lunch—and attachments form," while in *The Purple Rose of Cairo* (1985) he suggests buying lunch as a prelude to sex.

The link between food and sex in film has further been explored through the use of certain settings as part of a film's mise-en-scène. Although not a Jewish invention, the delicatessen often symbolizes Jewish space; it is no coincidence that Katz's Deli is the site of the orgasm sequence in *When Harry Met Sally.* The prominence of Jewish summer resorts in the Catskills has continued the connection between kosher food and kosher dating since such places consciously linked Jewish traditions of matchmaking with kosher cuisine. The advertising for the most famous of them, Grossinger's, suggested that under this hotel's guidance, food was an opportunity for sociability and the means to endogamous marriage and reproduction. Indeed, Grossinger's enjoyed a high reputation as an ideal place to look for a mate. *Sweet Lorraine* (dir. Steve Gomer, 1987), *The Apprenticeship of Duddy Kravitz* (dir. Ted Kotcheff, 1974), *Dirty Dancing* (dir. Emile Ardolino, 1987), and *A Walk on the Moon* are all films situated at kosher resort hotels in which a protagonist is often either seeking love or is eligible marriage material. In such settings, food is frequently used to woo affections, as in *Dirty Dancing*, when the nerdy hotel owner's son takes the heroine, Baby (Jennifer Grey), into the hotel kitchen for a snack as part of his maladapted amatory efforts.

Key love scenes often take place in sites of food preparation or retailing. There is food in almost every Yiddish feature film: *Mamele* (dir. Joseph Green, 1938), for example, has such a scene at the end, when Khavtshi Samet (Molly Picon) is running off to get married; first she stops to check the chicken in the oven. In Joan Micklin Silver's *Crossing Delancey* (1988) the too-Jewish suitor is a kosher pickle salesman and wooing scenes take place in his store.

On a different note, it may even be argued that the movie and theater industries could not have functioned without Jewish delis. *Broadway Danny Rose* features the quintessential Jewish "kosher style" delicatessen, the Carnegie Deli on Fifty-Fifth Street and Seventh Avenue in New York. Its proximity to Broadway means that it has over the years been filled with regulars like actors Warren Beatty, Dustin Hoffman, and Burt Lancaster. Barbra Streisand, Kathleen Turner, Bruce Willis, and Dan Akyroyd are just a few of the stars that have lunched at Katz's. And when Johnny Depp met with his FBI contact in *Donnie Brasco* (dir. Mike Newell, 1997), it was at Katz's, as it was when Judge Reinhold went out to eat in *Off Beat* (dir. Michael Dinner, 1986). "We get a good deal of Jewish delicatessen in Hollywood," wrote Orson Welles. "Without pastrami sandwiches there could be no picture-making."[10]

Food and Nostalgia

Yet another function of Jewish foods in movies and television shows involves the expression of nostalgia for a somehow happier past. Here, "the Jewish *bagel* stands out like a golden vision of the bygone days when life was better, when things had substance, staying power, and an honest flavor of their own."[11] The bagel symbolizes the past not just because of its sixteenth-century origins but also because its preparation is difficult work that takes a good deal of time to learn. Until the invention of machine techniques, bagel making couldn't have been accomplished by just anyone—it required skill and patience. The skilled craft of making bagels by hand, which had defied the age of machine techniques, contrasted with the mass production of American bread—what Irving Pfefferblit has called "that tasteless, flavorless, bodiless miracle of modern science."[12] The bagels and lox, in *Down and Out in Beverly*

Hills (dir. Paul Mazursky, 1986), as well as the knishes and the jar of real kosher-from-Brooklyn and U-Bet chocolate syrup in *A Walk on the Moon*, all address concerns about holding onto traditions. Food in movies sometimes focuses on the issue of continuing or losing or changing Jewish cultural traditions and thus express a desire to preserve the past, as if in a sterilized jar.

The Dinner Table

Traditional Jewish culture focuses on the importance of family. After decades of ignoring such issues, in the 1960s Jewish American filmmakers began making movies that explored Jewish self-definition. A key part of this exploration was the depiction of eating as not only an important ritual for Jewish families but also a key signifier of their difference from the gentile world. Some Jewish American filmmakers looked back to remember the past nostalgically as a golden age, depicting family life with dashes of sentimentality, bitterness, longing, and, at times, ridicule. Thus, the Jewish family's partaking of food together, particularly on ritual occasions, has become a cherished filmic ritual. The Jewish Sabbath and Passover meals show up, in particular, as obvious cultural expressions. In *A Stranger among Us* (dir. Sidney Lumet, 1992) many explanations about food and other customs are given, including a detailed sequence about food preparation for the Sabbath. The various versions of *The Jazz Singer* films (1927, 1953, 1980) each have Passover seder scenes. In *Tevye* (dir. Maurice Schwartz, 1939) there is a scene during a Passover seder in which the daughter who intermarried is looking in on her family through a window and crying hysterically. There are several scenes in the *Revolt of Job* (dir. Imre Gyöngyössy, 1983), where food, around Jewish religious holidays, is eaten and discussed by the elderly Jewish couple and the Christian child they raise before the Holocaust. In the 1998 British film *The Governess* (dir. Sandra Goldbacher), a young woman, Rosina da Silva (Minnie Driver), passes herself off as the gentile Mary Blackchurch. As her Jewish identity is unknown to her employer, she celebrates Passover alone and the salt water included in her meal proves to be a fixative for photographic images. This ritual element, therefore, is an important part of the plot, which revolves around the invention of photography. In such films, what is stressed concerns the specific cultural aspects of the ritual meals.

Key filmic scenes are situated at the Jewish dinner table, a suitable location for the delivery of scenes worthy of the Socratic dialogue. Filmmakers clearly intend to show that important matters are discussed with the entire family present, and the entire family must be present for the evening and/or ritual meal. An extended family discusses morality, among other issues, over a meal in *A Price above Rubies*. In Allen's *Crimes and Misdemeanors* a Passover meal is the setting for debates about the nature of murder, ethics, and divine punishment; the character Judah Rosenthal flashes back to a Passover seder of his youth, during which he remembers his extended family arguing over complex moral issues like religion, Marxism, the Holocaust, and the "eyes of

God." While his father Sol insists that God's justice will ultimately rule, Judah's Aunt May believes that human beings can and will commit any crime they can get away with, and that they can even live peacefully with their crimes if they choose to. The seder scene is particularly important because the family is together, united around the observation of the traditional rituals. Even though the family members argue over complex moral issues and cannot reconcile their views, this is regarded as normal, for arguing is often presented as being a staple of the Jewish diet. In *My Favorite Year* (1982) directed and written by Richard Benjamin, the Jewish family meal offers a debate on the meaning of love and the importance of family. And, in *Avalon* (dir. Barry Levinson, 1990), the Jewish family meal includes commentary on Jewish culture and eating that reveals the legacy of immigration and the history of family assimilation into an American mainstream and the divesting of ethnic traits. Dining scene after dining scene in *Goodbye Columbus* (dir. Larry Peerce, 1969), the film based upon the story by Philip Roth, satirically portrays Jews and food (in particular, in the quasi-orgiastic wedding feast scene, as all the relatives stuff themselves at the big buffet), caricaturing Jewish food obsessions as a ridiculous abundance of food paired with greed. The movie *Wedding in Galilee* (dir. Michel Khleifi, 1987) illustrates a very different sort of clash of cultural identities between Israeli Jews and Palestinians. A Palestinian seeks Israeli permission to waive curfew in order to give his son a fine wedding, but the military governor's condition is that he and his officers attend, leading to a banquet full of tension. In *The Last Supper* (1995), a dark comedy directed by Stacy Title, a group of graduate students—one of whom is Jewish—use the dinner table to articulate their belief system and to convert nonbelievers. They invite a variety of politically inappropriate—sexist, racist, fundamentalist, politically conservative, and so on—individuals to supper to try to persuade them to change their ideas, but poison them and bury them in the back yard if they don't.

The dinner table also becomes the arena for articulating competing versions of Jewishness. For the Jewish characters, the conflicts with their ethnic and sexual selves are staged most pointedly at meals. In *The Last Supper* the Jewish character kills the first guest, a vicious anti-Semite, thereby reversing the stereotype of Jewish physical weakness. In *Kissing Jessica Stein* (dir. Charles Herman-Wurmfeld, 2001), the Jewish family dining scenes become an arena in which the Jewish daughter strives to assert her lesbian sexuality against the obvious wishes of her parents, who use these same mealtimes to try to match her with more suitable partners. Similar issues are dealt with in *What's Cooking?* (dir. Gurinder Chadha, 2000), where Herb and Ruth Seelig (Maury Chaykin and Lainie Kazan) are unwilling to discuss openly their grown lesbian daughter's relationship with her lover around the Thanksgiving dinner table. In both scenes, we witness an intergenerational clash, with daughters bringing home doubly "unsuitable" partners, both ethnically and sexually. In such dining scenes, it is usual for the gentile to be subject to parental interrogation, assessing whether she is fit/kosher enough to marry into the family. *Kosher* is also slang for "A-OK"; literally, it means "fitting and proper" in Hebrew (during the 1970s, advertisements for the Israeli national air carrier El Al would promise, "We don't take off until everything is Kosher").

The checking-out-the-gentile-at-the-Jewish-family-table formula is reversed to great effect in *Meet the Parents* (dir. Jay Roach, 2000), a comedy about a Jew, Greg Focker (Ben Stiller), who wants to marry a rich, WASPy blonde and accompanies her to visit her parents on the north shore of Long Island. In scenes reminiscent of *Quiz Show*, everything there conspires to remind him that he's a Jew of low status. The girlfriend's ex-CIA father Jack Byrnes (Robert De Niro) puts Greg under constant scrutiny and surveillance (he even has a series of hidden cameras rigged up to spy on the unwitting Stiller) and thus the seemingly simplest situations, like using the toilet, conceal hidden traps. The sequence around the dinner table is particularly important for establishing the cultural distance between the Jewish Focker and the WASP Byrnes family. Greg is asked by Jack to say grace at dinner. "Greg is Jewish," Jack is told. "I'm sure Jews bless their food," Jack smiles, and Greg launches into a tortured prayer that segues, to his own horror, into lyrics from *Godspell*. Mealtimes continue to be fraught with social danger. At breakfast, he is the last to arrive; still wearing his pajamas, he is the only person shown eating a bagel—a clear signifier of Jewishness—further widening the social gap between him and the Byrnes family.

Interestingly, Jewish families on film are often depicted celebrating the all-American and secular holidays of Thanksgiving and Independence Day rather than their own Jewish ritual holidays, suggesting their assimilation into the mainstream culture. In *Avalon*, the Thanksgiving meal serves as the pivotal point at which the extended Russian-Jewish Krichinsky family, now living in Baltimore, disintegrates into the separate, nuclear-family structure of the dominant culture. This also hints at the demise of the traditional Jewish, family-centered culture.

Conclusion

Food has become a means to explore Jewish identity visually, whether the food itself is "Jewish," kosher, or *treyf*. In this essay, I have tried to bring together a variety of films and topics as a step toward beefing up the study of visual victuals, giving some illustrative (and hopefully tasty) examples of the rich selection of films to be productively researched further from a variety of perspectives—social, cultural, religious, class, gender, and even sexual. Clearly, there is plenty of material for further exploration, and I hope that, in the future, the links among film, food, and Jewish social dynamics will be confronted. Even as we "consume" films, we can also "read" them, discovering much about both culture and filmmaking.

Notes

1. Isaac Rosenfeld, "Adam and Eve on Delancey Street," *Commentary*, no. 8 (1949): 386.
2. Alan Davidson, *The Penguin Companion to Food* (London: Penguin, 2002), 829.
3. Jenna Weissman Joselit, *The Wonders of America: Reinventing Jewish Culture 1880–1950* (New York: Hill and Wang, 1995), 215.
4. See Donald Weber, "Memory and Repression in Early Ethnic Television: The Example of Gertrude Berg and *The Goldbergs*," in *The Other Fifties: Interrogating Midcentury American Icons*, ed. Joel Foreman (Urbana: University of Illinois Press, 1997), 159–61.
5. Lenny Bruce, quoted in William Novak and Moshe Waldoks, eds., *The Big Book of Jewish Humor* (New York: Harper and Row, 1981), 60; for Ephron, see Deborah Tannen, *Talking Voices: Repetition, Dialogue, and Imagery in Conversational Discourse* (Cambridge: Cambridge University Press, 1989), 156.
6. Rosenfeld, "Adam and Eve," 387.
7. Ibid., 385–86.
8. Jean Soler, "The Dietary Prohibitions of the Hebrews," *New York Review of Books*, 14 June 1979, online at http://www.columbia.edu/itc/religion/segal/v3201/soler.html; accessed 2 December 2003.
9. Rosenfeld, "Adam and Eve," 387.
10. Welles, Orson. "From Mars," *Commentary*, no. 2 (1946): 70.
11. Irving Pfefferblit, "The Bagel: On This Rock . . . ," *Commentary*, no. 11 (1951): 475.
12. Ibid.

Further Reading

Barr, Terry. "Eating Kosher, Staying Closer," *Journal of Popular Film and Television* 24, no. 3 (1996): 134–144.

Brode, Douglas. *Woody Allen: His Films and Career*. London: Columbus Books, 1985.

Cohen, Sarah Blacher, ed. *From Hester Street to Hollywood: The Jewish-American Stage and Screen*. Bloomington: Indiana University Press, 1983.

Davidson, Alan. *The Penguin Companion to Food*. London: Penguin, 2002.

Desser, David, and Lester Friedman. *American-Jewish Filmmakers*. Urbana: University of Illinois Press, 1993.

Friedman, Lester D. *The Jewish Image in American Film*. Secaucus, N.J.: Citadel Press, 1987.

Gabler, Neal. *An Empire of Their Own: How the Jews Invented Hollywood*. New York: Anchor Books, 1988.

Girgus, Sam. *The Films of Woody Allen*. New York: Cambridge University Press, 1993.

Greenberg, Betty D., and Althea O. Silverman. *The Jewish Home Beautiful*, 9th ed. New York: National Women's League of the United Synagogue of America, 1958.

Joselit, Jenna Weissman. *The Wonders of America: Reinventing Jewish Culture 1880–1950*. New York: Hill & Wang, 1995.

Nathan, Joan. *Jewish Cooking in America*. New York: Alfred A. Knopf, 1995.

Novak, William, and Moshe Waldoks, eds. *The Big Book of Jewish Humor*. New York: Harper and Row, 1981.

Paskin, Sylvia, ed. *When Joseph Met Molly: A Reader on Yiddish Film*. Nittingham: Five Leaves, 1999.

Pfefferblit, Irving "The Bagel: On This Rock..." *Commentary* 11 (April 1951).

Rogin, Michael. *Blackface, White Noise: Jewish Immigrants in the Hollywood Melting Pot*. Berkeley and Los Angeles: University of California Press, 1996.

Rosenfeld, Isaac. "Adam and Eve on Delancey Street," *Commentary* 8 (October 1949).

Soler, Jean. "The Dietary Prohibitions of the Hebrews," *The New York Review of Books* (June 14, 1979).

Tannen, Deborah. *Talking Voices: Repetition, dialogue, and imagery in conversational discourse* (Cambridge: Cambridge University Press, 1989).

Weber, Donald. "Memory and Repression in Early Ethnic Television: The Example of Gertrude Berg and *The Goldbergs*," in *The Other Fifties: Interrogating Midcentury American Icons*, ed. Joel Foreman (Urbana and Chicago: University of Illinois Press, 1997).

Welles, Orson. "From Mars," *Commentary* 2 (July 1946).

Whitfield, Stephen J. *In Search of American Jewish Culture*. Hanover, N.H.: University Press of New England, 1999.

Discussion Questions: "I'll Have Whatever She's Having": Jews, Food, and Film

1. List the foods in this article that are associated with Jewish identity.
2. Designate which ones you have eaten and where you consumed these items.
3. List the foods that are mentioned in this article and said to represent the non-Jewish world and list why they would not be a part of Jewish food and identity.
4. How does religion guide or direct or constrain food consumption or basic habits around food?

Topic IV: Food and Nutrition in Africa

In *Out of Africa: A Brief Guide to African Food History*, we learn about the great diversity present on the African continent, and how little has been done to uncover what must be an extraordinary history of agriculture among the 54 countries that comprise Africa. Much of this could be due to the long history of the slave trade, however, because all African countries (with the exception of Ethiopia) were colonized by European nations, there may be little that is evident or discoverable about traditional food ways. The continent, as a whole, was the last of the continents colonized, late in the 19th century, and independence would have done little to resurrect traditional food systems.

Termites Tell the Tale: Globalization of an Indigenous Food System among Abaluyia of Western Kenya provides an example of a food context whereby eating locally available insects, in a particular way, is a long-held tradition for a particular ethnic group of Kenya. The reader learns about the staple and typical foods of contemporary Kenya, and the traditions of the Abaluyia. Most of Kenya's now common foods are actually from other world regions. The selection includes descriptions of some of the methods employed to study food culture. The reader also has the opportunity to examine the many ways in which food is produced, processed, and consumed. In the meantime, there is a detailed description of the actual context in Western Kenya where the Abaluyia live and work. In other words, food culture is situated within the whole of the lifestyle for this single Kenya population, providing an example of intra-specific variation for food and culture within Kenya.

Indigenous crops are a central element to food and culture in a particular country or place. In *Neglected Indigenous Food Crops that Could be a Savior*, the author reviews perspectives held by the Food and Agriculture Organization (FAO) on improving 'food security' globally. The focus on sub-Saharan Africa is for illustrative purposes only. It is suggested that one way to ensure that the world's people are fed in the coming years is to return to the indigenous crops that were once found exclusively in each landmass, region, and country, and on every continent. Indigenous crops were adapted to their place of origin, are often resistant to drought-prone areas, and able to grow best in the conditions that they evolved in. Moreover, a diversity of food crops improves the nutritional intake of the population and intercropping, rather than monocropping, reduces the need for pesticides.

Out of Africa

A Brief Guide to African Food History

JESSICA B. HARRIS

Balkanized by Victorian politicians at the 1884 Berlin Conference, disparaged by ethnographers of the same period, and laid open to colonial acquisition and subsequent imperial incursions, the African continent remains under-acknowledged and unsung. The continent, though, provides some of humanity's earliest food history and also offers indications of some of the world's pressing contemporary food issues and innovative food solutions.

The African continent is one of astonishing diversity. It is made up of hundreds of ethnic groups speaking a Babel of languages and is of such a geographical vastness that no one can truly claim to understand the whole. Over the centuries, a combination of misconceptions, fanciful inventions, and trite inaccuracies has muddled the world's vision and come to represent the continent. The first step, therefore, is to return to a tabula rasa and begin anew.

A few basic facts:

1. Africa is a continent, NOT a country.

2. The African landmass is more than three times the size of Europe and four times that of the United States.

3. Madagascar, an island off the east coast of Africa that is culturally and historically considered part of the continent, is the fourth largest island in the world.

4. More than one thousand languages are spoken on the continent.

5. North Africa and sub-Saharan Africa share history and have long been in communication with each other.

Given the variety of climates and cultures, whatever sure knowledge exists about one part of the continent can be contradicted somewhere else on the continent. Africa has many entry points. Nowhere is its diversity better expressed than in the history of its food.

The African continent has a lengthy culinary history that stretches from earliest prehistory to current culinary developments. In *Africans: The History of a Continent,* John Iliffe notes that "there is evidence as early as 20,000 to 19,000 years ago of intense exploitation of tubers and fish at waterside settlements in southern Egypt near the First Cataract, soon followed by the collection of wild grain."[1] However, the early sources for agricultural history are few.

James C. McCann, in *Stirring The Pot: A History of African Cuisine,* underscores our relative ignorance: "While Africa is now universally understood to be the place of humankind's origin, our knowledge of its agricultural history of food is more limited than that of other world areas." He goes on to discuss Africa's "limited genetic endowments of the flora and fauna of food sources," but cautions that "Africa has always been part of a global system of biological and human exchange."[2] It is from these exchanges that the multiple cuisines of the continent grew.

Primatologist Richard Wrangham informs us, in his groundbreaking *Catching Fire: How Cooking Made Us Human,* that from earliest record, humans were using fire on the continent to cook food. Burnt shells and fish bones have been found near family-sized hearths at a coastal archeological site in Klasies River, South Africa, dating from sixty thousand to ninety thousand years ago and "charred logs, together with charcoal, reddened areas, and carbonized grass stems and plants [dating to] 180,000 years ago [have been found] at Kalambo Falls in Zambia."[3] These sites indicate that fires may have been used for weeks or months at a time to cook. Wrangham postulates that the softer, more nutritious food that cooking provided gave *Homo sapiens* advantages that resulted in the social development of humans as a species. Cooking allowed humans to devote less time and energy to digestion, allowing more scope for the development of the brain.[4]

The history of food on the African continent has also been studied by archaeologists. Certainly one of the most complete records of early foodways on the African continent is that of ancient Egypt. Several noted

Egyptologists have studied the food culture of Pharaonic Egypt using the abundant available remains. In Egyptian archaeological sites, food is featured prominently in wall paintings and reliefs of all periods. From funerary art we deduce that the ancient Egyptians were gourmets and indulged in a wide range of foods. It is believed that they were the first to make leavened bread as we know it, flavoring loaves with spices and honey. They also used bread to brew beer and sometimes drank to excess.

Archaeologists and art historians have also explored ancient Roman cuisine in North Africa by investigating a number of sources including excavations of floor mosaics that were features in the Hellenistic villas of the rich in Tunisia. The mosaics in the Bardo Museum in Tunis, for example, depict the detritus that would have remained on the floor after a feast ended: fish heads, eggshells, cherry pits, and other discarded food scraps. Other mosaics depict actual banquets with bibulous guests, providing food historians with a sense of how art can inform their research.[5]

Travelers' accounts of Africa are another useful source for understanding the continent's culinary history. Travelers think of food, both foods they have tasted and foods they have observed, and their writings have provided some of the best descriptions of the food and foodways of the premodern African continent. Leo Africanus and Ibn Battutta, two early Arab travelers who ventured into sub-Saharan Africa, offer their views of the food and foodways they observed in their travel books. Polish scholar Thadeusz Lewicki's *West African Food in the Middle Ages: According to Arab Sources* mines Arab travel literature in an attempt to reconstruct the food of the western part of the continent before European contact.[6] The work, however, is seen as flawed by contemporary scholars for its inaccurate identification of plant species based on flawed translations. It also demonstrates the difficulty of reconstructing the foodways of the past based on travelers' observations.

The voyages of exploration brought Europeans to sub-Saharan Africa. Accounts of meals abound in their travelogues. One such travel journal, the 1687 *Descrição Histórica dos Três Reinos do Congo, Matamba e Angola*, written by a papal envoy, describes in great detail the pomp and ceremony of the dining habits of the Mbundu queen Nzinga.[7] Other journals depict daily life through the lens of European travelers such as Abbé Boilat, who described life in eighteenth-century Senegambia. Most European travelers in the eighteenth century stayed on the coast and didn't venture inland. Only in the nineteenth century with the scramble for colonial empires did this change. Explorers and missionaries, travelers and traders all wrote about the foods they saw, the meals they ate, and the crops they encountered, both familiar and strange.

Along with the explorers and the missionaries came the slave traders. The history of enslaved Africans has long infl u enced the developed world's opinion and images of the continent. The transatlantic slave trade spread Africa's culinary legacy wider than that of almost any other continent and has made possible a geographically extensive study of African culinary history. Over the modern centuries, Africans in diaspora and their descendants have formed major segments of the population in virtually all the countries in the western hemisphere, Brazil leading with almost ninety-seven million people of full or mixed African descent and the United States second with forty-two million.[8]

This African diaspora transformed the food of the western hemisphere. The conditions of enslavement meant that for more than three centuries, enslaved Africans and their descendants were in charge of kitchens throughout the hemisphere. They were also involved in the agricultural pursuits and animal husbandry of the lands to which they journeyed. However there are virtually no culinary histories and few cookbooks that document the African contribution to what have become the national cuisines of many New World nations. This is most likely because in most cases the dishes prepared by Africans have become inseparable from the national cuisine. Some dishes, though, maintain a manifestly African character and in more than a few instances can be traced to specifi c points of origin on the African continent. Here historians have looked for information on the origins of slave ships and the destinations of captives to trace culinary connections between Africa and the New World.

Many in the West think of the African continent monolithically when it comes to culinary culture. While certain generalities can be drawn, the foods of the African continent that traveled to the Americas are as regionally distinctive as are those brought by European settlers. Details are offered by slavers' records like *A Slaver's Log* by Theophilus Conneau, as well as by ships' provisioning manifests and other crucial sources. Studies like *The Atlas of the Transatlantic Slave Trade* by David Eltis and David Richardson give a sense of the scattering of slaves and the surprising culinary connectedness of their cultures.[9] To be sure, not all of the enslaved who shipped from a given port were from the region of that port. Conversely not all who survived the voyage remained at or near their port of entry, or even in the country in which they fi rst arrived. It is probable, however, that there were enough in one place from a particular ethnic group to ensure a cultural critical mass. To take one example, Senegambia, the Bight of Benin, Angola, and Cameroon further to the south are famed for their leafy green soupy stews commonly referred to as *sauce feuilles* (leaf sauce), *sauce gombos* (okra sauce), and *soupikandia* (*kandia* means okra in Senegal's Wolof language). Those regions sent many captives to Saint Domingue, Salvador da Bahia in Brazil, Martinique, Guadeloupe, and the Gulf Coast and Charleston in the United States.[10] It is not surprising then that green soups and stew-like dishes abound in these areas: the *efo* of Brazil, the *callaloo* of the southern English-speaking Caribbean, the *calalou* of the French-speaking Caribbean, and the gumbos of Charleston and New Orleans to name but a few. Some dishes like *efo, dukonoo* (from Jamaica), and *callaloo* even retain names that correspond to African points of origin.[11]

Along with green soupy stews came rice dishes. Low Country rice planters appear to have preferred slaves from rice-growing regions in western Africa, especially Liberia, Sierra Leone, Guinea, and southern Senegambia. These rice-growing regions have long had a considerable repertoire of rice recipes that are at the origin of some of South Carolina's favorite dishes. Along with the leafy greens and composed rice dishes, several other western and central African culinary paradigms apply in general throughout the western hemisphere and demonstrate how African culinary style influenced food culture in the Americas: the use of okra as a thickener, a taste for small pieces, a love of fritters, and a lively tradition of street vending.[12]

Along with key dishes and cooking techniques, the Americas also received plants and livestock from the African continent. Geographer Judith Carney's works investigate the botanical connections between the Old and New Worlds. Looking at plants in the Americas, she points out the African origins of several plants that have become emblematic of the African experience not only in the United States, but also throughout the Americas, and postulates several methods of plant transference.[13] Okra is perhaps a primary example, as the pod originates on the African continent and is a key ingredient in many African-inspired New World dishes. Rice however may be the most important contribution. West African rice *oryza glabberima* and a discussion of African-inspired methods of rice growing throughout the western hemisphere form the subject of Carney's first work, *Black Rice*.[14]

At the same time the continent was being depopulated by the trans-atlantic slave trade, exploration continued, along with trade and settlement. Again, travelers' tales, journals, and letters home from the likes of

Sir Richard Burton and René Caillié provide information about the interior of Africa. At the Berlin Conference of 1884, the map of the continent was redrawn, dominated by French Imperial turquoise and British Imperial pink. The Congo constituted an immense private possession of King Leopold of Belgium. The Congress preserved old, smaller holdings of the Portuguese and Spanish and confirmed new claims by Germany. Later the Italians would claim Somalia and Libya but fail to take over Ethiopia. Colonial divisions would leave marks on the food cultures of the continent that remain evident to this day and that have enriched the foodways of individual countries everywhere.

Colonization signaled the arrival of significant numbers of European women to Africa. They set up households and tried to recreate European life as they knew it in African urban centers as well as in more remote outposts of the continent. Cities were established on European models with special food markets catering to European colonists. Some, like Dakar's Marché Kermel, were designated for Europeans and differed from local markets in size and in the goods they carried. Trading posts grew into colonial stores bringing European products to Africa, and some cities saw the establishment of European-style restaurants. Cookbooks for departing colonial wives offered advice on purifying water by boiling it, de-contaminating fruit with potassium permanganate, and making substitutions with local products, such as using yams to replace mashed potatoes and plantains to make game chips to serve with the antelope that replaced venison on settlers' tables. These cookbooks also demonstrate that the resourceful colonial wives learned from their African cooks and houseboys and discovered that they could, for example, use papaya leaves as tenderizers and roselle pods instead of lemon juice. Some even feature adaptations of local dishes.

Colonial cookbooks offer a view into not only the larders and kitchens of colonial cooks, but also a vision of how households were run. More than a few of them deal with how to negotiate with recalcitrant houseboys and cooks. When they include traditional recipes from the colonial territories they also give a glimpse of what these traditional dishes were like at a given time (albeit through the eyes of the foreign other). Some examples of these books are: *The Kenya's Settlers' Book and Household Guide* published in 1928 by the Church of Scotland's Women's Guild; *A Household Book for Tropical Colonies* by E. G. Bradley, published by Oxford University Press in 1948; and Hildagonda Duckitt's *Hilda's Where Is It?*[15] This last is one of the oldest African colonial cookbooks. Born in 1840 in the Cape region of South Africa,

Duckitt collected recipes from her area of the country. The book, first published in 1891, is arranged in alphabetical order and offers a selection of European, Indian, Cape Malay, and other recipes from South Africa. There are also hints about food for invalids, and advice about how to make furniture polish and home remedies.

As colonial inhabitants migrated to other colonies and civil servants were transferred from post to post, culinary cross-fertilization took place as well. Workers too were transferred and South Africa's Durban, for example, took on an air of the Indian subcontinent. Soon Indians were middlemen shopkeepers in Uganda and Kenya, and Syrians and Lebanese became storeowners in the Ivory Coast and Senegal. Dishes like South Africa's bunny chow (bread hollowed out and filled with a kind of curry)—which may be named for the Indian Bania caste who originally prepared and consumed it—hark back to this era and tell their own culinary tale of diaspora.[16]

In English colonies, African home economists published books in traditional and colonial languages and crossed countries speaking to women's groups in an effort to improve sanitary conditions. They too influenced the cooking of the continent in that they relied heavily on European models and championed standardization, although they made a point of including traditional dishes in their collections. In the early twentieth century, the Players cigarette tin become a standard household measure in British colonies.

Independence for much of the continent began in 1957 when the Union Jack was lowered over the Gold Coast and the red, yellow, and green flag with its central black star proclaimed the birth of Ghana, a new nation and a new era for the continent. With independence came national pride and with national pride came a need to celebrate and codify traditional dishes like Ghana's jollof rice, a vegetable-filled rice dish made red with the addition of tomatoes, and the chicken and peanut-butter stew known as groundnut stew. In many of English-speaking countries, home economists continued their quest for food safety and hygienic conditions. In the English-speaking nations, books like Nigeria's *Miss Williams' Cookery Book* and the *Ghana Nutrition Cookery Book* (initially published in 1953) became staples among the emerging middle and upper classes.[17] In the French-speaking nations, Paris had been the focal point and Gallic culinary conventions became accepted for middle and upper class entertaining, albeit with traditional dishes filling the plates and bowls. Regardless of colonial language and country, throughout the continent and across classes, less formal meals were often eaten with the right hand from a communal bowl in the traditional style. Regional specialties developed into nationally beloved dishes across ethnic lines. The *soupikandia* of the Diola of southern Senegal became a dish served around the country along with the *thieboudienne* of the Wolof and the *mafe* that Senegal shares with neighboring Mali. *Soupikandia* is an okra-based soupy stew often served with rice. It is an ancestor to New World gumbo. *Thieboudienne,* the national dish of Senegal, is a red rice and fi sh dish, and *mafe* is a stew based on peanut butter, usually made with lamb.

The African American Civil Rights movement shared a kinship with the African independence movements. In fact, several of the leaders of the new emerging English-speaking nations had spent time in the United States. The fi rst Black Arts Festival, convened in Dakar in 1966, brought a returning wave of Africans in diaspora from the United States, Brazil, and the Caribbean in what would signal the birth of cultural tourism.

Unlike previous tourists who had come in search of game preserves and safaris, these tourists came mainly to the western areas of Africa and were looking for cultural connections in all realms, including food. This period, which witnessed the fi rst Peace Corps volunteers and groups such as Crossroads Africa, also saw the publication of some of the fi rst national cookbooks designed for visitors. Monique Biarnès' *La Cuisine senegalaise* and other works like it codifi ed national classics.[18] This epoch would expand even further with the airing of the television show *Roots* in 1977.

The 1970s and 1980s also saw the growth of African tourism agencies devoted to promoting tourism to the continent. Culinary endeavors formed a large part of their initiatives, and the resulting pamphlets on food and restaurants offer material for study. Hotel and tourism schools were also created. Untapped sources for study of this period include travel journals, cookbooks created by Peace Corps personnel for use by newly arriving volunteers, as well as restaurant information in contemporary African media. Publications like *Africa World News* and woman's magazines like *Amina* in the French-speaking countries offered recipes, and *Jeune Afrique* published a cookbook including recipes from all over the continent. Time Life included an African volume in its Foods of the World series (1970), written by Laurens Van der Post, a white South African who gave scant attention to the cuisines of West Africa.

The closing decades of the twentieth century saw an increasing number of African cookbooks in both French and English written by Africans, African Americans, and West Indians with connections to the continent. Books by authors ranging from Senegalese singer Youssou

N'dour and British television presenter Rosamund Grant, and African Americans such as Bea Sandler, Vertamae Grosvenor, and Jessica Harris explored the food of the continent, and its connections to the foods of the African diaspora. Former expatriates and those, like Fran Osseo-Asare, married to Africans, explored the cultures and cuisines of the part of the continent with which they were most familiar; still others, like Judith Carney, explored plant origins and diffusion to the New World from Africa.[19] Other writers present the food of specific regions.

In addition to its food history, the African continent has a great variety of beverages dating back to the ancient Egyptians. Wines are produced in the continent's temperate areas, notably in Tunisia, Morocco, and South Africa, and beer is common, both traditional styles prepared from millet and other grains and more European-derived styles. Ethiopia's *tej* is a variety of mead, and the country is also the birthplace of coffee. Roselle, called *bissap rouge* in Senegal and *karkade* in Egypt, is popular, as are a number of herbal teas and drinks both alcoholic and nonalcoholic, ranging from Benin's *sodabi* (fermented palm wine) to Morocco's *thé naanaa* (mint tea). Topics for possible study range from the importance of rum in the slave trade to the medicinal properties of Senegal's *kinkeliba* tea.

As the continent that evidences some of humankind's earliest foodways, Africa also records some of the world's earliest documented famines, beginning with ancient Egypt. However, beyond mentions in early Egypt, there is little information about early famines. Accounts do exist of later food crises in medieval Egypt as well as in precolonial Zimbabwe, Nigeria, and Mali, and the continent remains one of those most at risk for famine in the twentieth century. Famine—its causes ranging from drought and crop failure to colonialism and genocide to the spread of the Sahara—has changed the face of the continent into modern times. Contemporary, haunting images of the starving define Africa and food for many.[20]

At the beginning of the second decade of the twenty-first century, a singular food history of the African continent remains to be written. The scope of the subject is vast, encompassing as it does not only sub-Saharan Africa but also North Africa, which is the southern rim of the Mediterranean basin. While the countries of North Africa have had more thorough individual documentation through the work of contemporary chroniclers, ethnographers, and food scholars, such as Moroccan writer Fatema Hal, and Americans such as Copeland Marks and Paula Wolfert, the ebb and flow of the food of the entire continent has yet to be covered in a single volume. But then again, few comprehensive volumes present the food of Europe, South America, or Asia. James C. McCann's previously cited work, *Stirring the Pot: A History of African Cuisine,* runs a scant 184 pages, of which about twenty deal with the African diaspora and forty with Ethiopia. McCann offers an overview as well as insights into the difficulty of attempting to write a comprehensive history of African cuisine. Some of the problems preventing such a volume include the difficulties of synthesizing multiple languages, cultures, and religions, and of writing history based on sources that are largely secondary accounts, as records of African food history often come from colonizers or visitors. Perhaps, it is best to hope for a multilingual series of volumes that might present the history of the food and foodways of individual countries or groups of people. What is clear is that there is ample material for study, a rich culinary matrix, and a need to understand better the food and foodways of a continent that has not only nourished itself for millennia, but has also had a major influence on the food of the western hemisphere.

NOTES

1. John Iliffe, *Africans: The History of a Continent* (Cambridge: Cambridge University Press, 1995), 12.

2. James McCann, *Stirring The Pot: A History of African Cuisine* (London: Hurst, 2010), 22–23.

3. Richard Wrangham, *Catching Fire: How Cooking Made Us Human* (New York: Basic Books, 2009), 84–85.

4. Wrangham, *Catching Fire,* 84–85.

5. Phyllis Pray Bober, *Art, Culture and Cuisine: Gastronomy Ancient and Medieval* (Chicago: University of Chicago Press, 1999), 134.

6. Tadeusz Lewicki, *West African Food in the Middle Ages: According to Arab Sources* (London: Cambridge University Press, 1974).

7. João Antonio Cavassi de Montecuccolo, *Descrição Histórica dos Três Reinos do Congo, Matamba e Angola,* vol. 1 (1687; Lisbon: Junto de Investigacoes do Ultramar, 1965), 139–40.

8. CIA, *World Factbook,* 11 March 2014.

9. David Eltis and David Richardson, *Atlas of the Transatlantic Slave Trade* (New Haven: Yale University Press, 2010), 87–137.

10. Gwendolyn Midlo Hall, *Slavery and African Ethnicities in the Americas: Restoring the Links* (Chapel Hill: University of North Carolina Press, 2007), 91, 93.

11. Jessica B. Harris, "Food of the Scattered People," in *Food and Drink: The Cultural Context,* ed. Donald Sloan (Abingdon: Goodfellows, 2013), 98–114.

12. Jessica B. Harris, *Beyond Gumbo: Creole Fusion Food from the Atlantic Rim* (New York: Simon and Schuster, 2003).

13. Judith Carney and Richard Nicholas Rosomoff, *In the Shadow of Slavery: Africa's Botanical Legacy in the Atlantic World* (Berkley: University of California Press, 2011), 123–34.

14. Judith Carney, *Black Rice: The African Origins of Rice Cultivation in the Americas* (Cambridge, MA: Harvard University Press, 2002).

15. *The Kenya Cookery Book and Household Guide* (Nairobi: Kenway Publications, 1970; first printed as *The Kenya Settler's Cookery Book* in 1928); E.G. Bradley, *A Household Book for Tropical Colonies* (Oxford: Oxford University Press, 1948); Hildagonda Duckitt, *Hilda's Where Is It of Recipes* (London: Chapman and Hill, 1891).

16. Brij V. Lal, ed., *The Encyclopedia of the Indian Diaspora* (Honolulu: University of Hawai'i Press, 2006).

17. Omosunlola R. Williams, *Miss Williams' Cookery Book* (1953; repr. London: Longmans, Green and Co., 1957).

18. Monique Biarnès, *La cuisine sénégalaise* (Dakar: Société africaine d'édition, 1972).

19. Carney and Rosomoff, *In the Shadow of Slavery;* Fran Osseo-Asare, *A Good Soup Attracts Chairs: A First African Cookbook for American Kids* (Gretna: Pelican Press, 1993).

20. Cormac Ó'Gráda, *Famine: A Short History* (Princeton: Princeton University Press, 2009).

BIBLIOGRAPHY

Africa News Service. *The Africa News Cookbook: African Cooking for Western Audiences.* Edited by Tami Hultman. New York: Viking, 1986.

Amina. www.amina-mag.com.

Biarnès, Monique. *La cuisine sénégalaise.* Dakar: Société africaine d'édition, 1972.

Boilat, Abbé David. *Esquisses sénégalaises.* 1853. Reprint, Paris: Karthala, 1984.

Bradley, E.G. *A Household Book for Tropical Colonies.* London: Oxford University Press, 1948.

Caillié, René. *Travels through Central Africa to Timbuctoo, and across the Great Desert, to Morocco, Performed in the Years 1824–1828.* 2 vols. 1830. Facsimile of the first edition. New York: Cambridge University Press, 2013.

Carney, Judith. *Black Rice: The African Origins of Rice Cultivation in The Americas.* Cambridge, MA: Harvard University Press, 2002.

Carney, Judith, and Richard Nicholas Rosomoff. *In the Shadow of Slavery: Africa's Botanical Legacy in the Atlantic World.* Berkeley: University of California Press, 2011.

Cavassi de Montecuccolo, João Antonio. *Descrição Histórica dos Três Reinos do Congo, Matamba e Angola.* 1687. 2 vols. Reprint, Lisbon: Junto de Investigações do Ultramar, 1965.

CIA. *The World Factbook,* 2014. www.cia.gov/library/publications/the-world-factbook/index.html.

The Church of Scotland's Women's Guild. *The Kenya Cookery Book and Household Guide.* Nairobi: Kenway Publications, 1970. First published as *The Kenya Settlers' Cookery Book,* 1928.

Conneau, Theophilus. *A Slaver's Log Book or 20 Years Residence in Africa: The Original Manuscript.* Englewood Cliffs: Prentice Hall, 1976.

Duckitt, Hildagonda. *Hilda's "Where Is It?" of Recipes.* 1891. Reprint, London: Chapman and Hill, 1914.

Eltis, David, and David Richardson. *The Atlas of the Transatlantic Slave Trade.* New Haven: Yale University Press, 2010.

Grime, William Ed. *The EthnoBotany of the Black Americans.* Algonac: Reference Publications, 1979.

Hal, Fatéma. *Les Saveurs et les gestes: Cuisines et traditions du Maroc.* Paris: Stock, 1995.

Harris, Jessica B. *Iron Pots and Wooden Spoons: Africa's Gifts to New World Cooking.* New York: Atheneum, 1989.

———. *Beyond Gumbo: Creole Fusion Food from the Atlantic Rim.* New York: Simon and Schuster, 2003.

———. *The Africa Cookbook: Tastes of a Continent.* New York: Simon and Schuster, 2010.

———. "Food of the Scattered People." In *Food and Drink: The Cultural Context*, edited by Donald Sloan, 98–114. Abingdon: Goodfellows, 2013.

Ibn Battuta. *The Travels of Ibn Battuta.* Translated by H.A.R. Gibb. 3 vols. Cambridge: Hakluyt Society; Cambridge University Press, 1958–2000.

Iliffe, John. *Africans: The History of a Continent.* Cambridge: Cambridge University Press, 1995.

Leo Africanus. *The History and Description of Africa.* Edited by Robert Brown. 3 vols. 1896. Reprint, New York: B. Franklin, 1963.

Lewicki, Tadeusz. *West African Food in the Middle Ages: According to Arabic Sources.* London: Cambridge University Press, 1974.

McCann, James C. *Stirring the Pot: A History of African Cuisine.* London: Hurst and Co, 2010.

Midlo Hall, Gwendolyn. *Slavery and African Ethnicities in the Americas: Restoring the Links.* Chapel Hill: University of North Carolina Press, 2005.

National Research Council. *Lost Crops of Africa.* Vol. 1. *Grains.* Washington, DC: National Academy Press, 1996.

N'Dour, Youssou. *Sénégal: La cuisine de ma mère.* Paris, Minerva, 2004.

Ó'Gráda, Cormac. *Famine: A Short History.* Princeton: Princeton University Press, 2009.

Osseo-Asare, Fran. *A Good Soup Attracts Chairs: A First African Cookbook for American Kids.* Gretna: Pelican, 1993.

Saffery, David, ed. *The Ghana Cookery Book.* 1953. Reprint, London: Jeppestown Press, 2007. First published as *The Gold Coast Cookery Book,* British Red Cross Society: Government Printing Office, Accra, 1933.

Williams, R. Omosunlola. *Miss Williams' Cookery Book.* London: Longmans, Green and Co., 1957.

Wilson, Hilary. *Egyptian Food and Drink.* Aylesbury, Bucks: Shire, 1988.

Wrangham, Richard. *Catching Fire: How Cooking Made Us Human.* New York: Basic Books, 2009.

Discussion Questions: Out of Africa: A Brief Guide to African Food History

1. When is there the first evidence for food preparation in Africa? What kind of evidence was uncovered?
2. Why is it difficult to write a food history for the continent?
3. What is *soupikandia*? What is it made with and how is it served? If you were served this dish, where might you be?
4. What are some of the fermented drinks of Africa? What are major sauces found on the African continent?

Termites Tell the Tale

Globalization of an Indigenous Food System
among Abaluyia of Western Kenya

Maria G. Cattell

Biographical sketch. Maria Cattell has done research among Zulus in South Africa and older white ethnics in Philadelphia, but Kenya remains her first love. She lived among Abaluyia in rural western Kenya for two years and has made a number of four- to six-week return visits to renew friendships and carry out short-term research projects on issues of current interest, such as place and identity (Cattell 2005). When she returned for the first time in 1987, Maria was amazed when people hugged her. Kenyans are publicly undemonstrative, and these were big hugs—in public! Finally someone told her, "Now we know you really love us because you have come back." And so Maria has gone back, many times, and has shared many more meals (and hugs) with her Kenyan friends.

ADVENTURES WITH TERMITES

One day my co-researcher, John Barasa "JB" Owiti, and I were walking through the Nangina Hospital's grounds in rural western Kenya. As we approached the outpatient clinic, JB rushed to the side to a large hole in the ground. He squatted, then reached toward the hole, and put his hands to his mouth again and again. I squatted beside him. JB was catching little white-bodied insects as they flew from the hole—and he was indeed eating them! "Termites?" I asked. "Yes," said he, throwing a few more into his mouth. I watched for some time, longing to try them because I was born with an adventurous palate and love trying new foods—but termites? Do they bite? Taste awful? An image popped into my head: the man in the seat ahead of me on the country bus who bought a bag of live termites from one of the women who appear at every bus stop to sell snacks like bananas, popcorn, and roasted groundnuts (peanuts). As the man popped handfuls of the termites into his mouth, some escaped and crawled over his head and the back of his neck. He paid no attention to them. But I wondered, how can he eat those things? And how can he let them crawl all over him?

But in spite of that memory, suddenly my hand reached out, almost on its own, grabbed one termite, flung it into my mouth—and I ate it. Just that one, but I ate it. When we stood up, I heard a voice behind me: "Maria, did you eat?" I turned around. "Yes, I ate!" I told the inquirer, my friend Fosca, a nurse's aide. She was with a small crowd that had gathered on the veranda of the outpatient clinic to watch the *musungu* (European or American) at the termite hole. I am sure word quickly spread far and wide by "bush telegraph" about my exploit: "The *musungu* eats termites!"

For the most part I had no problem with Kenyan foods. The staple *ugali* (in Swahili; *obusuma* in Luyia), a stiff porridge made by boiling white maize-meal and water, was easy. Ugali is similar in flavor to grits, which my family ate often although we lived among meat-and-potatoes Pennsylvania Dutch farmers (my father was a Southerner). When people served "black ugali" made with millet or sorghum or stickier ugali made with cassava, it was no problem. Goat meat—again, no problem; we had eaten goats on our Pennsylvania farm. The ubiquitous *sukuma wiki* (collards or kale), chopped, boiled, and seasoned with onion and tomato—no problem; my father grew these greens in his garden. New foods, like *emjombola* (a fruit) and "slippery vegetable" (*omutere*), also offered no challenges because of my eagerness to try new foods. So after eating that one live termite, I was sure I could eat anything my Kenyan friends offered me, including termites. So I ate termites, lightly fried and salted, as often as I could. I ate them with pleasure, enjoying their flavor and preserving my self-image as someone who can eat anything.

But then I met my comeuppance. Occasionally I visited Gladys, the eighteen-year-old "matron" who supervised the boarding students after the day scholars went home from Nangina Girls' Primary School. One day, as we drank the super-sweet tea she always served, Gladys opened a paper bag and took out a largish insect, about an inch long, which she popped into her mouth and crunched like a potato chip. "Dried termites," she said, offering me one. I took one and held it in my hand for a long time, staring at it. The longer I looked at that termite, the more it looked like a cockroach. My stomach was telling me, "If you put that thing down here, it's coming right back up." Whoops! What about the person who can eat anything? But finally, reluctantly—but also with relief—I held the termite out to Gladys as I said: "Sorry, Gladys, I just can't eat that. I'd like to, but my stomach is refusing." Luckily, Gladys was not offended—although since this was a private occasion and Gladys was a very junior person, and in fact was from another Luyia area, it would not have mattered if she had been. But we remained friends, and I drank many more cups of overly sweet tea with her. To this day I doubt I could eat one of those termites! Well, maybe . . . I'd like to think I could. But I doubt it.

TERMITES ARE GOOD TO THINK

Even if the occasional termite is not good for me to eat, termites are "good to think" about food in the social life and cultural imagination of Luyia people. Food sustains life. But food is never just food. It is rich with meaning and power. It is woven into history, into the fabric of daily work and social relations, hospitality and special occasions. It is used for gifts and as a medium of exchange. It figures in stories grandmothers tell grandchildren about *amanani*, the antisocial ogres who overeat, consuming even the plates and also humans. It is embedded in ordinary speech as metaphors, as when someone remarks that so-and-so is "only cooking" for her husband (meaning that she is refusing sex) or a widow says, "I refuse the brothers-in-law because they would just eat me" (meaning that she refuses to marry her deceased husband's brother, as is the custom, because he would consume her resources and give nothing in return). Plenty of food makes a person's body fat, and a fat body signifies good health, wealth, power, and authority. So if you lose weight, people worry and ask if you are ill. Thus, "you are fat" is a compliment. I wish I could discuss this, and more, in this chapter, but doing so would probably take half the book, so I will stick to the theme of the transformation of the Luyia food system from localized to globalized and how that process has resonated in social relations.

Initially my research was inspired partly by modernization theories, which grapple with issues such as the impact of modernization on family structures and social roles. Although these theories have inspired a great deal of research, modernization remains hard to define because of the complexity and ever-changing nature of the processes involved. But surely *something* is going on as indigenous societies move from relatively closed subsistence economies following local customs and lifeways into societies connected to the wider world and the global economic system. We can name that something "modernization" or "social change" or "globalization" (the preferred term now).

There have been many factors influencing the enormous changes Abaluyia have experienced since about the 1880s, when the first Europeans arrived in their land. The environment—droughts, floods, locusts, epidemics, epizootics, soil degradation—plays a part. Demography figures in the story, especially in regard to the people/land ratio (land abundance or scarcity). The impacts of colonialism and postcolonialism have reached into every aspect of life, including governance, education, healing practices, religion, and incorporation into the global capitalist political economy. Incorporation into the global economy involves such things as the introduction of money and commodification of goods, labor, and land, which have led to extensive labor migration and the development of cash crops and agricultural exports to other nations. Among other things, the modernization (or globalization) of the food system has changed people's relationships to food and their relations with each other as expressed through food. Because food is fundamental to life and an ongoing daily concern for everyone, it is an excellent lens for examining these changes.

RESEARCH SITE AND METHODS

My adventures with termites occurred in the mid-1980s when I was doing my dissertation research on aging, gender, family life, and the lives of older persons under circumstances of far-reaching socioeconomic, political, and cultural change (Cattell 1989). For two years I lived among Samia (Abasamia, Basamia) people in rural western Kenya, in Busia District (county), in the land they call Samia or Busamia. I also made brief visits to Banyala, culturally similar neighbors to the south, in the land called Bunyala. Since then, return visits have enabled me to keep my knowledge up-to-date, develop longitudinal data on contemporary life and individuals and families I have known for over a quarter century, and investigate special issues and events as they have arisen.

Samia and Banyala are two of seventeen subgroups of Abaluyia (or Luyia, also spelled Luhya), who together numbered about 4 million persons in the 1999 Kenya census. Abaluyia means "Luyia people," which is indicated by the "Aba" prefix. (Luyia can refer to the people or be used as an adjective; the "Bu" prefix indicates place.) Luyia homelands are in Kenya's Western Province, bordered on the west by Uganda. Bunyala and Samia (or Busamia) lie along the northeastern shores of Lake Victoria. Most Luyia women and men are peasant farmers and use hand-tools (such as hoes and machetes) on small acreages to grow food and cash crops. Poverty is widespread and persistent. To increase incomes many people make and sell artisanal items (such as baskets and clay pots), engage in petty trading (especially of food), and are active in a variety of self-help groups. Some are employed in the modern sector as teachers, medical workers, or government administrators. Some practice a trade such as tailoring or carpentry. Others are shopkeepers or traders in local markets. Near Lake Victoria men and women work in the fishing industry. Theft (another form of self-help) is also common. Many become migrant laborers, going to Kenyan cities like Mombasa and Nairobi or cities in nearby Uganda and elsewhere in Africa and beyond to look for hard-to-find employment.

In my research I have used field-designed formal instruments (including, in 1985, an Old People of Samia survey of 200 women and 216 men aged fifty years and older), but my knowledge has come mostly from participant observation: being with people in various settings, watching what they do and how they interact with each other, trying some of their activities myself, talking with them (often with JB or someone else as interpreter, since my ability to speak the Samia language was not as good as I would have liked), and, of course, eating with them.

Kinship is a primary determinant of position among Luyia (and other Kenyans and Africans generally), and—like many anthropologists—I was "adopted" by two Samia families, JB's and the family of Tadeyo and Regina Makokha, whose daughter Teresa worked for me in 1984. The Mahagas of Bunyala also made me one of theirs. These relationships are not mere formality; I am expected to behave appropriately with other family members and participate in family reciprocity. For example, I have contributed to educational fees for family members and have been asked for money for a really important event such as a funeral, which I hear about quickly now via cell phone and e-mail. I have learned much through these relationships. I have also observed and interacted with numerous other people in homes, on roads and footpaths, and in public places such as markets, churches, and schools. I have shared many meals and daily activities, joys, and problems including serious illness, marriages, births and deaths, theft, house fires, and the struggle to educate children. My contacts have included females and males of all ages with a range of social and economic characteristics.

Relative age is another important determinant of an individual's social status. Being older brings respect and, often, authority. In many encounters, like the one with Gladys and her crunchy termites, I was the elder (I was then in my mid-forties). Other characteristics frequently put me on the top of the social ladder, even with persons older than myself, because I was an educated person with a college degree and an American and, therefore, wealthy according to local standards (I always had money for food, bus fare, and so on). Another source of respect was being a white person, a *musungu* (*mzungu* in Swahili, the lingua franca of East Africa). Probably this was in part a colonial hangover but most of the thirty-five or forty other whites in the county (Busia District) were nuns or priests, and I was commonly thought to be a nun. People called me "sistah" (sister) even when I said, "No, I am not a sistah, and I even have a husband and four adult children, including three sons" (another source of respect). As JB said to me in a recent visit, "You know, with you people [whites], we always have to respect you." Respect keeps distance between people.

Years ago JB asked if he could call me mama. I replied, "Yes, but I'll be your American mama, which means we can talk about many things, even sex, which you cannot discuss with your really mama." (I had my research needs in mind.) So JB called me mama or mom, but we developed a relaxed, comfortable joking relationship, like that between grandparent and grandchild (Cattell 1994). With some people it has been difficult or impossible to get beyond the respect relationship, although older people often are willing to talk about many things regardless of status difference. Elders have fewer behavioral constraints, and as people age they become more self-confident and ready to speak out (this is especially true of women, who as girls are taught to be meek and submissive).

Sometimes I have used my high status (or perhaps, as I am not easily put into a category, it is more of an anomalous status) to escape from rules of behavior. For example, the custom is to leave visitors alone in a house to eat, not to isolate them but as a sign of respect. Families usually do not eat together. Men and older sons eat in the house while women, older girls, and young children eat in the kitchen. But Samia say that if you have "eaten from the same pot" (even if not in the same space), you have strengthened your relationship with everyone who ate from that pot. So being left alone is a courtesy, and you have eaten with the family symbolically. But when I finish my meal, I often go out and walk around the homestead. That way I catch people living their daily lives—bathing a child, peeling cassava, eating the chicken I had left in the serving bowl, washing dishes—and daily lives are what I want to learn about.

GLOBALIZATION OF AN INDIGENOUS FOOD SYSTEM

As a culinary item, termites are a vestige of the nearly self-sufficient indigenous food system of Abaluyia and other peoples of the East African interior. In the indigenous system, termites were one among many wild foods, including other insects (such as locusts, beetles, moths, and bees), birds, fish, mammals, and plants. Domesticated livestock and cultivated crops provided other foods. The main cereal crops, finger millet and sorghum, are native to East Africa. Cowpeas and probably sesame are also of African origin. But other foods had non-African origins and reached East Africa in the distant past. Goats, sheep, and zebu cattle were domesticated in India and Southwest Asia about 10,000 years ago. Bananas (including plantains) came from Southeast Asia. New World foods—beans, groundnuts (peanuts), maize (corn), peppers, squash, and sweet potatoes—first reached Africa (often via Portuguese traders) in the sixteenth century as part of the "Columbian exchange" (Plotnicov and Scaglion 2002 [1999]; Viola and Margolis 1991). The globalization of East African diets began long before the British arrived.

In the nineteenth century, people had a local orientation and met nearly all their needs from local resources and their own labor. In addition to producing food, they built houses, tools, and other utilitarian items from local materials. Education, carried out by parents and grandparents, taught the technical and social skills needed for daily living with no schools or books, no reading, writing or arithmetic. There was no money. Chickens, livestock, grains, and iron hoes (*embako*) and other items made by Samia blacksmiths served as media of exchange. Regional exchange systems with regular markets and long-distance traders moved food, livestock, and locally made goods throughout the Lake Victoria region (Alpers 1974; Ndege 1990). Famous rainmakers also traveled far beyond their homes to provide their services. But for the most part, the orientation was local.

Historians portray nineteenth-century Samia as turbulent and dangerous, with cattle raiders, ivory hunters, slavers, and people of different ethnicities moving over the land in numerous local migrations (Seitz 1979; Were 1967).[1] Consequently, people lived in fortified villages (*olukoba*, pl. *engoba*) surrounded by mud walls, a yard wide and about fifteen feet high (1 by 4.5 meters), and dry ditches (fosses) of a similar depth. These villages were symbolic of the relatively closed world in which people lived. An olukoba village contained ten to twenty households and 200 or more inhabitants (Soper 1986). Inside the walls, people lived in extended family groups: a husband, two or more wives, their children, and elderly parents (and probably other kin too). These families were the basic social and production units of Luyia societies. During the day people went outside the walls to graze their cattle, sheep, and goats; cultivate their crops; and hunt and gather wild foods. By sundown people and livestock returned to the village and the gates were shut (Wandibba 1985). Men and older boys gathered in the male space of cowsheds around a fire called *esiosio* to eat their evening meal and chat, while women, older girls, and young children ate in the preeminent female space, the kitchen (*amaika*)—gendered eating spaces that reflected the gendered nature of work and other activities.

Daily, people ate *obusuma*, the stiff porridge made from flour cooked with water or milk that is still the daily staple. (Luyia today say, "If you haven't eaten obusuma, you haven't eaten.") Obusuma was eaten with side dishes such as meat, chicken, peanut sauce, and leafy greens. People cultivated bananas, beans and other legumes, grains (millet, sorghum, maize), and sweet potatoes.

From livestock they got blood, milk, butter, and meat. They ate fish, insects, honey, wild-collected fruits and vegetables, and wild birds and animals. Drinks included water, milk (often soured), and *amalwa*, beer prepared from finger millet in a large pot and drunk through long reeds by men (a privilege of gender) and older women (a privilege of age).

The first European explorers appeared in the 1880s. Twenty-five years later, British control over western Kenya was firmly established (Maxon 2002). The British colonial government brought radical changes to the indigenous economy, including the introduction of money, wage labor, and cash crops, which the colonial government pushed aggressively. Among these cash crops was white maize, which displaced what were regarded as local varieties of colored maize (maize that had originated in Mesoamerica). White maize eventually became the staple food throughout Kenya and much of eastern and southern Africa. Other new foods (such as kale, onions, white potatoes, tomatoes) and ways of preparing foods came with the influx of administrators, missionaries, traders, and laborers from England, the United States, and India. Indians brought chapattis and samosas, which became nearly ubiquitous in Kenya. Imported salt from mineral sources saved women the work of producing salt from the water-filtered ashes of various plants, but it had to be purchased—like so many things in the new cash economy. Tea was established as a commercial crop in Kenya by about 1925. By the mid-1930s, *chai* (tea) was the main drink served to visitors in Christian and "progressive pagan" households among Bukusu and Maragoli (Luyia subgroups). It was served in proper British style, in imported china cups (not in the homegrown gourds that served as local "cups") with plenty of milk and sugar, the sugar also being new (Wagner 1956:74). Serving a proper cup of chai required money.

European and U.S. missionaries brought Christianity. Their daily lives modeled a very different lifestyle. They also promoted "the gospel of domesticity" as part of the process of "civilizing" Africans. For example, in the 1920s, Quaker missionaries at the Girls' Boarding School in Maragoli (in Luyialand) taught African girls domestic skills including U.S.-style cooking, cleaning, and sewing (Thomas 2000). They promoted the notion of woman as housewife, ignoring Luyia women's productive roles, which were as, or more, important as men's, since women contributed the bulk of agricultural labor in addition to doing domestic work and childcare (Cattell 2002).

As Abaluyia became increasingly integrated into the global political economy, they added new foods to their diet and ate fewer wild foods, a process of dietary change still going on—and not always for the better. For example, today people eat more cassava and maize than the more productive and nutritious local grains, millet and sorghum. Cohen and Odhiambo (1989), writing about Luo people in Siaya District (in western Kenya, not far from Samia), show how "maize means hunger" because Kenyan governments (colonial and independent) have pushed maize as both local staple and export crop. This has led to maize largely replacing local grains in people's diets.

As food became a commodity (something bought and sold) and new foods became available, more and more food was purchased rather than grown at home. And eating wild foods has come to be regarded with scorn as something poor people must do. People have taken to many nonlocal foods such as bakery products like bread and cookies, fat for cooking, and margarine for bread, sodas, and fruit drinks. Some innovations I have noticed since the mid-1980s include Knorr's dry soup mixes, peanut butter, rice pilau seasoned with Mchuzi mix (packaged spices), and spaghetti. But when times are hard, food becomes expensive, even unaffordable. In a 2004 tour of the small market town of Funyula, I noticed many small packets of things—like a sliver of soap, a bit of salt, a little sugar—so a person could buy just enough for a day instead of larger, more economical sizes (Cattell 2008). Thieves steal ripening crops from fields as well as anything they can get by breaking into houses—and so more and more homes are surrounded by fences and high walls. There is less sharing of food within extended families. That old enemy *enjala* (hunger) used to show up seasonally or in drought years. Today enjala has become a more constant companion for many people. While much of the world is experiencing the "nutrition transition," the shift from under-nutrition to over-nutrition and obesity (Popkin 2007), in western Kenya over-nutrition is not a problem. Rather, endemic under-nutrition and child malnutrition are ongoing problems. Most people are struggling just to survive.

FROM ABUNDANCE TO SCARCITY

Overwhelmingly, the images of pre-colonial and early colonial western Kenya are images of abundance, whether they come from the writings of Europeans who first went there or the memories of older Kenyans. Although people everywhere have a tendency to romanticize the past, to remember the best and forget difficulties, there is much evidence supporting the view of past abundance. For example, Joseph Thomson (1885), a British geographer who in 1883 walked on a mapping expedition through Luyialand (including Samia and Bunyala), was impressed with "the surprising number of villages, and the generally contented and well-to-do air of the inhabitants" (481). "Food at Kwa-Sundu [a trading center about twenty-five or thirty miles from Samia, now called Mumias] was surprisingly cheap and apparently inexhaustible . . . we were in a veritable land of Goshen" (487–488). Thomson remarked on the number of cattle, the vast expanses of cultivated fields, and the abundance of food, which local people were happy to exchange for beads.

In the 1980s many Luyia elders remembered food being abundant in the past. "Food was plenty," they said, or "food was cheap" or "food was free." In 1985, in response to the survey question, "Was life better in the old days?," 77 percent of 122 elders in my Old People of Samia survey said yes, life was better in the old days. They gave two main reasons: greater material prosperity (more food, more land, less need for money) and better relationships. A woman born around 1934 said: "Long ago food was easy. We harvested much and food was cheap. Or you could be given sorghum or maize free; nowadays that is not easy, not even with relatives" (Agneta interview, September 1984). At a group interview in a private home, an old Samia man (age not recorded) recalled: "Long ago life was good. There was organization in the home and people stayed together, worked together, ate together. Brothers and cousins [half-brothers] might stay in the same home. All the wives cooked for a meal, and all the men ate together, and all the women, and all the children [in separate groups]. There used to be much milk, and after a meal we drank milk. And there was much meat, especially *emitanda* [dried meat]" (Then and Now interview, June 4, 1984). Others spoke longingly of emitanda and of having so much milk that obusuma was cooked with it. Today, obusuma is always cooked with water.

Over beer and food in a Nairobi hotel, Paul Okumu Oyiikamo described the feasts of his grandfather Omonyo, who was a very old man when he died in 1954 (Okumu interview, January 1985). Omonyo, a blacksmith with twelve wives, lived a life of abundance and generous hospitality. "Three times a year he had his wives brew much beer and killed a bull or even two. Then he invited his relatives and neighbors to his home, and they would pass two days eating and drinking and doing no work." On ordinary working days, Omonyo had six wives cook food just for the men working at his forge: "Food was ever there. First one wife would bring obusuma and beef, then another brought sweet potatoes, another brought *amayengere* [maize and beans]. So people were enjoying to eat."

Weddings and funerals were also occasions for feasts. Traditional Luyia wedding ceremonies included several feasts and a procession from the bride's home to her new husband's home. The bride's body was oiled and covered with sesame seeds, symbolizing health, wealth, and fertility. In the 1980s many old people described their own weddings as having been like that, in the early to mid-twentieth century. But by the 1980s, marriages often began with no ceremony: the woman simply moved into the man's house one night, and if she was still there in the morning, that was it.[2] In 1985 I attended a church wedding followed by a feast (for which I made the wedding cake), but the old-style ceremonies and multiple feasts were a thing of the past. I never saw or heard tell of a modern bride covered by the sesame seeds of abundance.

When I first went to Kenya, funerals were major social occasions. They took place over three or four days (three for a woman, four for a man), with all the mourners being fed by the family of the deceased—a heavy burden for the family. But now, thanks in part to the efforts of saved (born-again) Christians (Cattell 1992) and stimulated by the increased numbers of deaths because of AIDS, funerals take only one afternoon, and people may not be fed even one meal. That reduces the burden on the family but also diminishes the sociability that used to be an important aspect of funerals.

Other food customs have also changed in the direction of reduced sharing. Older men described the elaborate protocol for sharing meat when a man slaughtered one of his cows. But today few people have cows, and meat sharing is virtually unknown. Older people also said that beer groups were common when they were younger. At the end of the day, men sat on their four-legged stools (symbols of male authority, even today) with their senior wives sitting at their feet. They sipped beer through long reeds and discussed everything. Now such beer drinking is almost gone—in part because of the cost of brewing beer, but also because the Kenyan government requires a person to get a permit for such a party. Beer drinking in Africa as a significant social activity has been much written about by anthropologists, but in Samia, at least, it seems to be a fading custom. In all my years in Kenya I have seen only two such parties. (And yes, I sipped the beer—which is thick, milky-colored, and a bit sour—through a reed.)

In 1984 and 1985 I often walked by the fields of Leo Balongo, then about eighty years old. Sometimes Balongo would be there, sitting on the ground to weed his cassava (he sat because he was nearly blind and needed to get close to see what to pull). One day Balongo told me: "Modern life is terrible in that relationship is slow. People used to visit each other and converse, especially in the cowsheds at the time of eating. Now people have a gap, they don't visit each other" (Balongo interview, October 1984). All but a few of the 216 old men in my survey said that when they were young, they took their evening meals at the men's *esiosio* fire (at the cowsheds, as Balongo said) and learned from the discussions and advice of the older men present. Nearby neighbors and relatives would gather at one fire or another, so the practice helped build community. That custom was gone probably by the 1950s, and today a man eats in his own house with his older sons while his wife, daughters, and young sons eat in the kitchen (a separate building because of the hazard of cooking with open fires under a grass-thatched roof). Or families even eat all together behind the closed door of their house, because they have so little they cannot feed visitors who might drop in, or even share food with others (especially elderly parents) in the extended family homestead (Cattell 2008).

Günter Wagner (1956), in his research among Bukusu and Maragoli (other Luyia groups) in the 1930s, observed much informal hospitality with neighbors and relatives moving about and freely dropping in on other households to share food and conversation. He took this to be "an indication of a quantitatively fairly high level of food supply, which allows people to display a certain generosity" (73). In the 1980s I observed such behaviors in Samia. But in western Kenya today, poverty and scarcity have become the norm.[3] Food sharing is much diminished, not just within a family but at public events such as funerals and community gatherings. And as food sharing has diminished, what Balongo said—"relationship is slow"—seems ever more true.

GLOBALIZATION AND ENJALA (HUNGER)

"In the old days food was free," the old people told me, meaning if you cultivated your crops, you would eat. "But today it is a world of money." The old people were right. Globalization changed people's relationships to the land, to food, and to each other, in the sense that today they are mediated by money. Today is indeed a world of money. And without money there is hunger.

With a declining national economy and high unemployment, many Kenyans are unable to earn enough money to meet even minimal needs. Although the majority of Kenyans live in rural areas, many experience hunger even when there is no drought (or, in Bunyala, floods) because of the competition for limited cropland between cash and food crops. Also, people may sell their food crops to get money for daily necessities—and later buy the same foods back at high prices or go hungry. Inflation has played a part in making things more expensive, but also people now buy many things they once made themselves or simply did not have, such as salt, sugar, cooking fat, kerosene, matches, soap, TVs, cell phones, clothing, and furniture. Today most people buy even meat and milk, when they can afford them, since many do not have cows. And they pay for services that used to be done by family labor, such as grinding maize into flour. In the 1980s most homes had grinding stones (and I learned the womanly skill of grinding from Marita, an old woman who earned money by selling *obusara*, a thin porridge similar to cream of wheat, served in dried gourds). Today, women pay a small fee to have their grain ground mechanically—and very fast. By the end of the twentieth century, grinding stones—like so much else of indigenous origin—were things of the past.

As farmers, Abaluyia are accustomed to seasons of lean and plenty. A pre-harvest *enjala* (hunger) is normal. In 1992 I was in Kenya in August, the month of maize harvest. There was plenty of maize obusuma in homes but also much "strong tea" (*echai strongi*), tea with neither milk nor sugar. Most people prefer "milk tea," tea that is half milk and sweet with sugar. The strong tea made me suspect that people were really struggling. The abundant maize harvest compensated for that temporarily, but many people no doubt experienced hunger once the maize was eaten (or sold). The next year was a drought year. When I visited in July, it was obvious people were struggling. They were eating obusuma of cassava, sometimes with sorghum, sometimes just cassava. Cassava (introduced around 1915) is a famine food, because its roots keep in the ground for up to five years. Magoba Anyango (then in her late sixties) told me: "We have enjala nowadays because there is very little cassava. If you don't want enjala to invade your house, then you plant cassava. So you can be adding there just a little sorghum and that will chase away enjala" (Magoba interview, May 1985). Cassava keeps hunger at bay but is not very nutritious.

In July 1993, Nangina Hospital administrator Nicholas Habala told me, "We're already seeing malnutrition"—well ahead of the maize harvest, which might be "zero yield" because of drought. Everywhere, people were talking of money, rising prices, and how they could not afford this and that. One man went without lunch every day so his wife, who was breastfeeding, and children could eat. I also noticed the absence of sodas. In earlier years when I visited homes, I would usually be offered sodas, two at a time. I would arrive and a kid would be sent off, on foot or bike, to buy sodas (you do not buy the sodas or catch the chicken till the visitor reaches the homestead, as you cannot be sure when or if the visitor will show up). I recalled that in 1992 only one person served me a soda. The same thing happened in 1993. Sodas remained nearly absent from the hospitality scene until 2004. In that year I was served sodas (and once, Dasani mineral water, something new on the scene) on a number of occasions but only by people who were better off than average. Perhaps my "soda-meter" indicator of prosperity (or diminished adversity) was pointing the right way in 2004, as the Kenyan economy has experienced growth since then. I hope that means less enjala for my Luyia friends.

GLOBALIZATION AND SOCIAL CHANGE

The processes of modernization/globalization have had many social impacts. For example, in pre-colonial Luyialand elders (male and female) were the advisers and decision makers. But intergenerational and gender relationships were transformed as young men gained access to money through education, employment, and political power in the colonial government and then in Kenya's independent government. Wealth and power shifted from older to younger generations and particularly to males (it is likely that British gender ideology and practices strengthened indigenous patriarchal leanings). At the same time, with most men engaged in labor migration, women found themselves as household heads and having to make decisions and do the work that would have been the husbands' responsibility.[4] These days some women are also labor migrants or join their husbands away from home. And in recent decades women (especially older women) have been taking more leadership roles in their families and communities (Cattell 1992, 2002).

In family and community life, the giving of food has been fundamental to relationships. When food is plentiful it can help expand or strengthen relationships. When food is scarce, it has a diminished role in relationships. In prosperous times, food is given as gifts in many situations. A visitor may take a gift of food to the host and receive a gift of food when departing. During my two years in Kenya I was given various foods, including several kilograms of beans—enough to last me for months!—and a number of chickens (which rode home on my hip and then I doubled the gift by giving them to someone else). Grandmothers like to give visiting grandchildren eggs, and adults remember fondly the food they received from grandmothers as being "very sweet." Family members carry food from home when they visit family members working away from home. But nowadays migrant workers may not go home even for Christmas because they have no money for gifts, not even a kilo of sugar, and home folks may not visit the migrants because they have no food to give.

Food giving is an intensely emotional means of creating, maintaining, and strengthening relationships. It is preeminently a female activity. Indeed, a woman becomes a mother not just by giving birth but by feeding her children, day after day, year after year. And a mother's curse is much feared. She will shake her breasts at you and say: "With these breasts I fed you! How can you deny me now?" Many people, when asked about caring for their frail old parents, say simply: "They fed me when I was young. Now they should be able to just sit and eat." This is the obligation of the gift and the emotional basis of female power (Counihan 1999). But in these difficult modern times, people lament their inability to care properly for their old parents—although they do what they can. In some cases the old parents themselves are caring for grandchildren orphaned by AIDS, which strikes hardest among middle-generation adults who provide most of a family's labor and income. Parental deaths from AIDS have created many orphans among Abaluyia (and neighboring Luo too)—and have left many grandparents struggling to feed their grandchildren (Nyambedha, Wandibba, and Aagaard-Hansen 2003). Such grandparents cannot just sit and eat.

Women grow food, decide what foods to eat every day, and prepare and apportion the food. The kitchen is female space, the domain of women and usually not entered by men, not even by a woman's husband. One evening JB and I made a "pop-in" (unannounced) visit to his cousin Michael. I was invited to visit Michael's wife, Beatrice, in her kitchen. It was a big kitchen, dark but for the light from the cooking fire. Kitchen things and seven of Beatrice's nine kids were scattered about the room. Beatrice sat in one corner, stirring a big pot of obusuma. She mounded the obusuma on two plates, one big mound (about two quarts) and one huge (more than three quarts). The big obusuma went into the house for Michael, JB, and me, along with a huge *embuta* (Nile perch)—enough food for five or six people. The huge obusuma and a small embuta remained behind for Beatrice and her children to eat. I am sure they also got to eat what JB, Michael, and I did not eat, which was most of what was served to us. But the nutritional hierarchy was clear: the man of the home and visitors came first.

In cooking and distributing food as Beatrice did, women are daily structuring or reaffirming (or denying) relationships, each individual's status, and the nutritional hierarchy within their families. But when money and food are in short supply, their decisions about who gets what are made more difficult. It may be that only the nuclear family eats together, and there is no food to share with the extended family (such as old parents) in the homestead. So the widespread, persistent poverty that has developed with globalization has made food giving difficult and has impoverished relationships—within the family and beyond, at public occasions such as weddings and funerals, and in the diminution of gifts of food.

EPILOGUE: BECOMING MUSAMIA, OR WE ARE WHAT WE EAT

In 1985, toward the end of my two-year stay among Samia people, I was visiting JB's family as I had done many times before. When it came time to eat, everyone except JB left the house. JB, as the "owner" of the visitor, was to eat with me. On this day we got chicken, which is often served to visitors, especially in-laws (for whom it is mandatory). The chicken was prepared the usual way, cut into chunks, boiled, and served with the broth. It was accompanied by rice. We were being served by JB's younger sister Pauleen, who added a bowl of fat-bodied termites to the table—live termites, crawling around their dish and onto the tablecloth! By then I had eaten termites several times but always sautéed and sprinkled with salt (they taste rather like mushrooms). The only live termite I had eaten was that one caught on the wing as it flew from its underground nest two years earlier. I had no problem looking at the termites crawling around the bowl, nor did my stomach issue any warnings, but they did not look all that appetizing. I certainly did not want to pop some in my mouth and have escapees crawling around my neck and down my shirt, like the man on the bus! But even more, I did not want to insult JB's sister (by kinship, my daughter), who had gone to some trouble to please me because she had heard I liked termites. What to do?

My solution was to mix things up. I poured chicken broth over my rice, added a couple spoons of termites, and stirred everything up. The hot broth and rice slowed the termites down—and it tasted delicious. After a few bites, I did not really mind the crawling critters. Then JB, who had been quietly watching me, said: "That looks like an interesting recipe. May I try it too?" I felt I had truly learned to eat local food if I could create a new recipe for termites! And that, because we are what we eat in more ways than one, I had become—as JB put it—"almost Musamia" (a Samia person).

Acknowledgments. I am most grateful for the invaluable help over the past quarter century of my Luyia co-researchers, especially my son John Barasa "JB" Owiti of Siwongo village in Samia and my daughter Frankline Teresa Mahaga of Port Victoria (in Bunyala) and Nairobi. Special thanks to Frankie and JB and their extended families for their love and hospitality over the years, and also to the family of Tadeyo and Regina Makokha of Samia. I especially recognize here JB's real mama, Nabwire, who died in October 2007. She hosted me for many a meal. Sadly, I salute JB himself, who died unexpectedly at the age of forty-eight in August 2008. For a quarter century, JB fed my anthropological inquiries and his wife, Mary, fed my body. *Pole sana*, Mary, and JB—*mareba*! Thanks also to Medical Mission Sisters at Nangina Holy Family Hospital (especially Sr. Marianna Hulshof, now retired); the many pupils and staff at Nangina Girls' Primary School (now St. Catherine's) who have welcomed me over the years; and Samia officials, particularly my old friend, Fred Wandera Oseno, once a teacher at Nangina and now retired as Chief of Funyula Division. Above all, mutio muno to the many people in the Luyia areas known as Samia, Bunyala, and Bungoma (and the Kisumu and Nairobi families of some) who have allowed me to share their lives in various ways. The research was partially funded by the National Science Foundation (grant BNS-8306802), the Wenner-Gren Foundation for Anthropological Research (grant 4506), a Frederica de Laguna Fund grant from Bryn Mawr College, and the generosity of my late husband, Bob Moss, who loved to teach at Nangina Girls' Primary School. I was a research associate at the University of Nairobi's Institute of African Studies in 1984 and 1985.

NOTES

1. Although there were no written languages in East Africa (except for Swahili at the coast) and hence no written records before the British came, research has unearthed much information on life in western Kenya during pre-colonial times. Reconstructions of African history depend on a variety of sources including colonial documents, missionaries' and travelers' accounts and other written materials (e.g., Jackson 1930; Thomson 1885), archeological and linguistic evidence, oral traditions (proverbs, stories, songs, etc.), and field research conducted by anthropologists, historians, and others and usually involving interviews with older persons in a community. To reconstruct

political and economic history, Gideon Were, a Luyia historian, interviewed Luyia clan elders, probably all men (Were 1967); and U.S. historian Jacob Seitz interviewed Samia individuals (mostly men) of various ages and social statuses (Seitz 1979). A research team from the University of Nairobi's Institute of African Studies interviewed women and men during field research in Busia District in the mid-1980s. Their report (Soper 1986) provides much information about daily life among pre-colonial Abaluyia. In the mid-1980s I too asked Samia women and men about life "in the old days" in what I called "then and now" interviews (Cattell 1989).

2. The woman's family will still expect bridewealth (cattle and/or money), which is likely to be paid over many years (if at all). Some have civil or church weddings—although sometimes after years of living together as spouses.

3. For a history of the growth of widespread poverty in colonial and postcolonial sub-Saharan Africa, see Iliffe (1987).

4. In my Old People of Samia survey, 187 of the 216 male interviewees had been labor migrants (only 7 of the 200 women had done this).

REFERENCES

Alpers, Edward A.
1974   The Nineteenth Century: Prelude to Colonialism. In *Zamani: A Survey of East African History*, ed. B. A. Ogot, 229–248. EAPH/Longman Kenya, Nairobi.

Cattell, Maria G.
1989   Old Age in Rural Kenya: Gender, the Life Course and Social Change. Ph.D. dissertation. Department of Anthropology, Bryn Mawr College, Bryn Mawr, PA.
1992   Praise the Lord and Say No to Men: Older Samia Women Empowering Themselves. *Journal of Cross-Cultural Gerontology* 7(4):307–330.
1994   "Nowadays It Isn't Easy to Advise the Young": Grandmothers and Granddaughters among Abaluyia of Kenya. *Journal of Cross-Cultural Gerontology* 9(2):157–178.
2002   Holding Up the Sky: Gender, Age and Work among Abaluyia of Kenya. In *Ageing in Africa: Sociolinguistic and Anthropological Approaches*, ed. Sinfree Makoni and Koen Stroeken, 157–177. Ashgate, Aldershot, England.
2005   African Reinventions: Home, Place and Kinship among Abaluyia of Kenya. In *Home and Identity in Late Life: International Perspectives*, ed. Graham D. Rowles and Habib Chaudhury, 219–235. Springer, New York.
2008   Aging and Social Change among Abaluyia in Western Kenya: Anthropological and Historical Perspectives. *Journal of Cross-Cultural Gerontology* 23(2):181–197 (DOI 10.1007/s10823–008–9062-x).

Cohen, David William, and E. S. Atieno Odhiambo
1989   *Siaya: The Historical Anthropology of an African Landscape*. James Currey, London.

Counihan, Carole M.
    1999   Food, Power, and Female Identity in Contemporary Florence. In *The Anthropology of Food and Body: Gender, Meaning, and Power*, ed. Carole M. Counihan, 43–60. New York, Routledge.

Iliffe, John
    1987   *The African Poor: A History*. Cambridge University Press, New York.

Jackson, Frederick
    1930   *Early Days in East Africa*. Edward Arnold, London.

Maxon, Robert M.
    2002   Colonial Conquest and Administration. In *Historical Studies and Social Change in Western Kenya: Essays in Memory of Professor Gideon S. Were*, ed. William R. Ochieng', 93–109. East African Educational Publishers, Nairobi.

Ndege, P. O.
    1990   Trade since the Early Times. In *Themes in Kenyan History*, ed. William R. Ochieng', 117–132. Heinemann Kenya, Nairobi.

Nyambedha, Erick O., Simiyu Wandibba, and Jens Aagaard-Hansen
    2003   "Retirement Lost": The New Role of the Elderly as Caretakers for Orphans in Western Kenya. *Journal of Cross-Cultural Gerontology* 18(1):33–52.

Plotnicov, Leonard, and Richard Scaglion
    2002   *The Globalization of Food*. Waveland Press, Prospect Heights, IL.
    [1999]

Popkin, Barry M.
    2007   The World Is Fat. *Scientific American* 297(3):88–95.

Seitz, Jacob
    1979   A History of the Samia Location in Western Kenya: 1890–1930. Ph.D. dissertation. Department of History, West Virginia University, Morgantown.

Soper, Robert W. (editor)
    1986   *Kenya Socio-Cultural Profiles: Busia District*. Republic of Kenya, Ministry of Planning and National Development, Nairobi.

Thomas, Samuel S.
    2000   Transforming the Gospel of Domesticity: Luhya Girls and the Friends Africa Mission, 1917–1926. *African Studies Review* 42(3):1–27.

Thomson, Joseph
    1885   *Through Masai Land*. Edward Arnold, London.

Viola, Herman J., and Carolyn Margolis (editors)
    1991   *Seeds of Change: A Quincentennial Commemoration*. Smithsonian Institution, Washington, DC.

Wagner, Günter

1956   *The Bantu of North Kavirondo*, Vol. 2: *Economic Life*. Oxford University Press, Oxford.

Wandibba, Simiyu

1985   Some Aspects of Pre-colonial Architecture. In *History and Culture in Western Kenya: The People of Bungoma District through Time*, ed. Simiyu Wandibba, 34–41. Gideon S. Were Press, Nairobi.

Were, Gideon S.

1967   *A History of the Abaluyia of Western Kenya: c. 1500–1930*. East African Publishing House, Nairobi.

Discussion Questions: Termites Tell the Tale: Globalization of an Indigenous Food System among Abaluyia of Western Kenya

1. What is now the staple food in Kenya and what is it called in Swahili? What are other common foods and their Swahili names in contemporary Kenya?
2. According to the author, how can food be described and defined, and what does it represent, based on the entire chapter?
3. What are foods that are indigenous to Africa and part of the diet for the Abaluyia? When did the diets change for East Africans?
4. How did food systems in Kenya change and who introduced the changes through time?

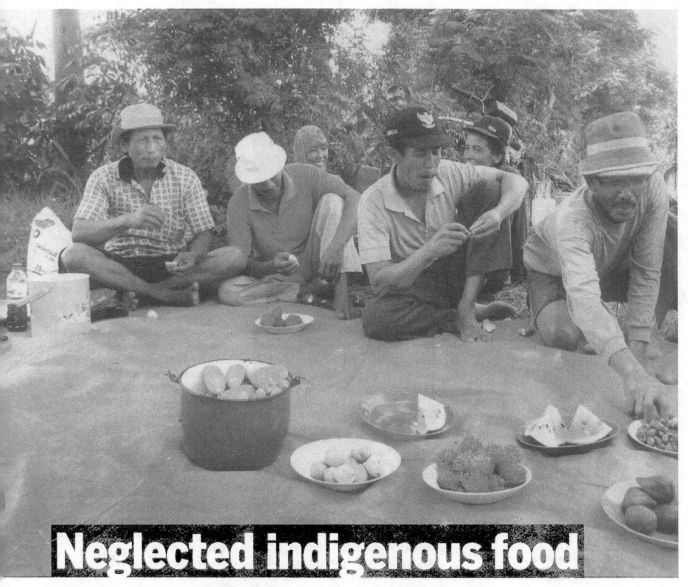

Neglected indigenous food crops could be a saviour

Underutilised food crops (also called neglected or indigenous crops) can save the world, especially Sub-Saharan Africa, from hunger. So why have African scientists rarely looked to their neglected indigenous crops to provide solutions to their food needs and for export? **Curtis Abraham** went to find out.

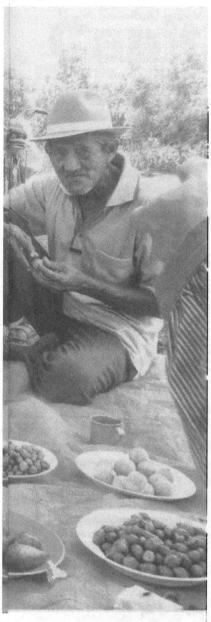

THE UN FOOD AND AGRICULTURE Organisation of the United Nations (FAO), which is headed by the Senegalese-born Jacques Diouf, estimates that over 800 million people do not meet their daily required energy needs from their diets. But that is not the worst of it. Millions of people around the world and particularly in sub-Saharan Africa suffer more acute malnutrition during transitory or seasonal food insecurity.

Around the world, the vast majority of people rely heavily on the trio of wheat, rice and maize. In fact, over 50% of the global requirement for proteins and calories is met by these three foods, according to the FAO.

But what if humanity was able to add another three or four more important food crops to its list? It could happen. And if it does, chances are that these new crops will come from arid or semi-arid parts of Africa, South Asia, and Southeast Asia, where they would first be commercialised.

Underutilised food crops (also called neglected or indigenous crops) are plant species that are little used, or which were grown traditionally but have fallen into disuse. These species have been proved to have food or energy value, and were widely cultivated in the past or are currently being cultivated in a limited geographical area.

Furthermore, such crop species have enormous potential for contributing to improved financial situations, food security and nutrition and for combating "hidden hunger" caused by micronutrient (vitamin and mineral) deficiencies.

These crops also consist of local and traditional varieties or wild species whose distribution, biology, cultivation and uses are poorly documented. Underutilised crops are strongly linked to the cultural heritage of their place of origin; and tend to be adapted to specific agro-ecological niches and marginal land.

It is estimated that globally, over 7,000 wild plant species have been grown or collected, but amazingly, only less than 150 have been commercialised. And out of these the world's food needs are provided for by just 30 species of plants.

But throughout sub-Saharan Africa, for example, there are more than 2,000 native grains, legumes, roots, vegetables, cereals, fruits and other food crops that have been feeding people for thousands of years.

Placing too much reliance on just a few crops is risky even at the best of times, especially in developing regions, which are presently almost twice as dependent on wheat, rice and corn as richer nations. Much else can go wrong including crop failure, civil wars, commodity price fluctuation, climate change leading to destabilised food crop production, etc.

Furthermore, the "Green Revolution" is said to be reaching its limits in generating the ever-increasing amounts of food needed to feed a growing global population. It's a warning that Professor M. S. Swaminathan, one of the Green Revolution's leaders, and now chairman of the non-profit NGO trust, M. S. Swaminathan Research Foundation in India, gave farmers in the developing world 40 years ago. "I cautioned our farmers that single varieties, genetic homogeneity – these are the words I used – would increase vulnerability to pest and disease. Therefore you must have varietal diversity, you must conserve agro-biodiversity," he says.

However, crucial problems exist. Some of the shortcomings in harnessing these neglected food crop species to feed the world's poor are based on sheer ignorance. Surprisingly, mainstream international science as well as people living outside the rural regions of the world, have had little knowledge about these forgotten species. Furthermore, there has been a loss of traditional knowledge in growing such plants.

"If we see the farmer who is more than 50 or 60 years old, he still recalls the traditional farming systems in his memory," says Dr Oliver King, senior scientist at the M. S. Swaminathan Research Foundation, referring to millet farmers of the Kolli Hills in the Tamil Nadu region of India. "But when we interact with the younger girls or boys or younger youths, they really don't know about the farming system for millet. It's a kind of cultural erosion."

Food insecurity is a routine fact of life for many of the world's poorest people in the best of times, and the global food crisis, which has been brought about by a combination of food scarcity and rising food prices, has only made matters worse.

As the food crisis is not about to disappear any time soon, scientists are searching for new ways to utilise these neglected food crops. Among other things these forgotten species could be essential components in helping to diversify farming systems in the developing world and thus contribute to global food security. In recent years, however, neglected food crops have come out of the shadows and are moving fast into the limelight of rural development in some Least Developed Countries (LDCs) in East Africa and elsewhere.

Several national research systems are supporting research on these forgotten species, though by no means to the same extent as research on industrial and staple crops such as palm oil, rubber, cocoa, tea, wheat, and rice. Nevertheless, global ef-

for Underutilised Species (GFU) and the International Centre for Underutilised Crops (ICUC).

Indigenous food crop research has concentrated so far on a small number of key activities. But there have been numerous success stories in the reintroduction and commercialisation of underutilised indigenous food crops in places such as Ghana and India. In Ghana, for example, people are beginning to utilise the Bambara Groundnut, a legume related to cowpea and found locally throughout sub-

recent study identified 57 indigenous fruit species in Mwingi District and showed that wild fruits form a key safety net for rural Kenyans during times of food shortage. Kenya is also reintroducing African Leafy Vegetables (ALV) to urban areas.

Indigenous food crops might also have strong export value to Western countries. Proponents of the "Slow Food" movement, an international association that aims to counteract the "Fast Food" culture, also seek to protect cultural identities linked to food and gastronomic traditions worldwide. The movement was founded by Carlo Petrini in Italy in 1986. It has more than 800 local groups in 50 countries.

Some neglected non-food crops have also proved beneficial to Africa's agricultural sector. There are several examples of oil-producing crops that can be used for cosmetics. Some of them double as food crops as well. The Shea butter tree in West Africa is a good example. There are also many plants with medicinal properties that have potential for further production, especially by small-scale producers.

So why have African scientists rarely looked to their neglected indigenous crops to provide solutions to their food needs and for export?

"One of the issues is that government funding is usually provided for the main staple crops and only small amounts of funding are available to research the potential of new crops," says Dr Hannah Jaenicke, Global Coordinator at Crops for the Future. "Whilst there are a number of researchers looking into indigenous crops, the hurdles to overcome are plenty: selections need to be made, production and propagation systems to be studied, seeds or seedlings to be produced in significant quantities and good quality."

Dr Jaenicke also mentioned that often large distances need to be covered to the research sites, which are usually located in less accessible parts of the country. Furthermore, it is also a matter of perception by the African crop scientists themselves: they see indigenous crops as old-fashioned and less attractive to the "sophisticated" urban population.

"It is important to address all of these issues through raising awareness using information that is based on solid data. This is one of the priority mandate areas of Crops for the Future," says Dr Jaenicke. ■MA

"Neglected food crops could be essential in helping to diversify farming systems and thus contribute to global food security."

●●●●●●●●●●●●●●●●●●●●

Jacques Diouf's Food and Agricultural Organisation (FAO) estimates that over 800 million people do not meet their daily required energy needs from their diets

forts are underway to get these forgotten species onto the research and development track so that they can be improved, cultivated, sold and consumed once again.

Some of the organisations that have supported the research and development of indigenous crops include ACIAR (Australia), CTA, DFID (UK), the International Fund for Agricultural Development (IFAD), the Mac Knight Foundation, the Syngenta Foundation and USAID.

Research into the utilisation of Africa's neglected crops was boosted in late 2008 with the launch of a new organisation called Crops for the Future, which is set to further explore the potential of underutilised food species in the developing world. The establishment of Crops for the Future came about through a merger of the Rome-based Global Facilitation Unit

Saharan Africa. Scientists at the University of Nottingham believe that it may well be the future of vegetable protein in countries with particularly dry climates. It is a crop that grows where other legumes cannot.

"What is significant, and what is unusual about it, of course, is that it is drought-tolerant and is grown in areas which are too dry for other legumes," says Dr Azam-Ali of the University of Nottingham, "and that's very important because most people's food, certainly in developing countries, comes from vegetable protein, so you need a source of this in a dry climate. Bambara Groundnut provides that."

Funded by the European Union, researchers at the University of Nottingham have carried out highly targeted research on Bambara Groundnut using special climate-controlled greenhouses.

Computer modelling based on their research and field experiments predicts that the crop could be suitable for a number of locations outside Africa.

But it is not only Bambara Groundnut that is making a comeback. In Kenya, a

Discussion Questions: Neglected Indigenous Food Crops that Could be a Savior

1. What are the three major food crops that most of the world's people consume?
2. What are indigenous crops and why might they be important?
3. How many plants provide the world's food needs versus how many have been commercialized?
4. What are some examples of indigenous crops that are being reintroduced to improve nutrition?

Topic V: Food and Nutrition in the Americas

The world is obsessed with quinoa, but the trendy crop is an important food in the Andes, where it is indigenous. There are many factors to consider when a crop of any kind is cultivated miles from its place of origin. This includes maximizing the nutritional content, maintaining the genetic diversity, and ensuring access for those who have always grown and consumed the crop. In *From Lost Crop to Lucrative Commodity: Conservation Implications of the Quinoa Renaissance*, the world's discovery of quinoa is discussed in terms of the cost to those who know it best. We have the opportunity to learn the history of this now famous crop, starting with its origin in the Andes. We study quinoa's nutrition, as well as its botanical history. Then we examine the efforts to discourage the production of quinoa and the promotion of other crops by outside forces. Finally, we see how a renaissance is born, outside of the long cultural process that creates a human-plant interaction in the first place, and the resulting dependence developed by both humans and plants to sustain life.

We learn, in *Ode to a Chuno: Learning to Love Freeze-Dried Potatoes in Highland Bolivia*, that potatoes, now part of the cuisine on every continent, are grown, processed, and consumed in very different ways in their region of origin. We also discover, through reading *Ode to the Chuno*, that a single food can look, feel, and taste differently from one place to the next, based on its growing conditions and preparation. But we also learn that it carries very different social meanings. Differences in the types of proteins, fats, and carbohydrates that are prized in Bolivia, based on a particular culture and context, are described in depth. Consequently, one learns about the history and association that a single food item can have on all aspects of life, and how that meaning and appreciation for a beloved food is not easily translated to a visitor.

The diversity of plant life that exists in the Caribbean is sustained through a variety of climate variations throughout the tropical islands. In *Caribbean Food Plants*, we learn of the food histories that existed before and after colonization, differences between indigenous versus introduced foods, and the many cultural traditions that came together to form Caribbean cuisine. There are longs lists of all of the food types that locals consume, their nutritional value, and the ways in which they are used and prepared. This reading reinforces the idea that food security is critical for the independence of any nation. But colonization and world food policies driven by the largest populations can create macro and micronutrient deficiencies among those forced in any way to produce food for others.

Within *Tomatoes: Immigration and the Global Food Supply*, the author describes one of the most common fruits (or vegetables) in the world, the tomato. The article is comprehensive in that it includes a botanical description, a nutritional breakdown, a discussion of the plant's origin and subsequent distribution, the patterns of consumption, and a review of production and pricing of the crop around the world. Terms such as 'locavore', GMO, and 'globavore' are discussed, as is the import of immigrant labor to the production of this ubiquitous fruit. The pros and cons of different types of production are outlined.

Nutrition & the Indigenous Body: A Genetic Concept of Food reminds the reader that Native peoples of North America, and particularly those of the US, are still alive and well. This is in spite of the high rate of diabetes among most indigenous people of the Americas. The myth of the 'indigenous body' is described, and one learns about the theoretical perspective, the 'thrifty genotype' that has driven most research into the topic. Dietary shifts among the indigenous peoples of the US are detailed from the 17th century, when access to traditional foodways became impossible to sustain. The Tohono O'odham are used to illustrate the connection between food, health, and culture and the time necessary to create balance.

On Eating Animals takes the reader on a journey to consider the way in which livestock rearing has changed through time. The author highlights the changes that have occurred with the American consumer in terms of what is important, from the quality of the product to the cost. We are forced to consider a process for creating meat that did not exist a few decades ago. Our recent change in lifestyle, and the limited contribution made in agriculture by the American public, has allowed the act of animal consumption to be done outside of and away from our hearts and minds.

From Lost Crop to Lucrative Commodity: Conservation Implications of the Quinoa Renaissance

Kristine Skarbø

This paper examines the conservation implications of initiatives to invigorate the cultivation of quinoa in the Andes. Two decades back, quinoa was considered a "lost crop of the Incas"—ceding ground to Old World grains within the Andes and remaining undiscovered beyond the region. Yet, the following years were to witness a grand quinoa renaissance. A series of campaigns were initiated to conserve the crop and reinforce its role in Andean fields. Quinoa caught the attention of chefs and consumers across the world, and production and exports rose rapidly. While research on other crops often has associated increased commercialization with the loss of crop diversity from farmers' fields, few have considered the impact of the above development on quinoa diversity. This article addresses this issue through a case study in Northern Ecuador, employing ethnographic and survey data. Assessments of quinoa varietal diversity before and after the implementation of several quinoa projects reveal that a new formally bred variety has substantially increased its role, while the number of landrace seed lots has been reduced. This indicates that the efforts emanating from a concern regarding the crop's genetic erosion actually might, in the longer term, contribute to accelerate this process.

Key words: agrobiodiversity, Andes, crop diversity, genetic erosion, quinoa

Introduction

Quinoa (*Chenopodium quinoa*) was a central crop in Andean highlands through several pre-conquest millennia (Morris 1999; Tapia 1979) but ceded ground to Old World grains after Spanish colonization (NRC 1989). In 1989, the crop was identified by the US National Research Council (1989) as a "lost crop of the Incas." Since then, it has been rescued from oblivion and attained the status of a global gourmet grain. Nutritious and tasty, it is now found in many nations' markets and touted in a plethora of cookbooks and websites as a miracle heritage food. This development has been accompanied by a keen interest in the crop among research and development agencies and also led to a renaissance for quinoa in its native Andes. Numerous projects have been put in place to recuperate its cultivation in the Andean countryside, and new harvests feed an increasingly quinoa-hungry international market. Quinoa's renaissance reached a highpoint with the United Nation's declaration of 2013 as the International Year of Quinoa (United Nations General Assembly 2011).

The recent surge in quinoa's popularity, production, and price levels has not gone unnoted among social scientists working in the realm of food and agriculture; it has been critically examined in terms of its effects on local economic relations and nutrition (Brett 2010; Friedman-Rudovsky 2012; Ofstehage 2012). Yet, while research on other crops in other settings often has linked commercialization of cultivated crops with reduced on-farm varietal diversity (Abbott 2005; Brush and Meng 1998; Brush, Taylor, and Bellon 1992; Nazarea 1998; Rana et al. 2007), few have so far paid attention to potential consequences for the conservation of quinoa biodiversity.

The maintenance of a genetically broad quinoa diversity in its Andean center of origin and diversity holds central importance for the crop's future sustainability. Along the Andean mountain range, the crop is grown on altitudes from sea level and up to 4,000 m, and different landraces[2] are adapted to the varying environmental and

Kristine Skarbø is currently a Postdoctoral Fellow with the Department of International Environment and Development Studies at the Norwegian University of Life Sciences. This research was supported by the US National Science Foundation under Grant No. 0921859 and an Andrew E. and G. Norman Wigeland Fellowship from the American-Scandinavian Foundation. I extend my gratitude to the many people in Cotacachi contributing to the project. In particular, I thank Rosa Ramos for research assistance and the Unión de Organizaciones Campesinas e Indigenas de Cotacachi for facilitating the work. I appreciate feedback on earlier versions of the paper from Virginia Nazarea, Susannah Chapman, Jon Holtzman, Trygve Berg, and two anonymous reviewers for Human Organization. Any errors of fact or interpretation remain those of the author.

climatic parameters along these gradients (Rojas, Pinto, and Soto 2010). As with other crops, the continued cultivation of diverse landraces is crucial in order for the crop to be able to adapt to changing environmental conditions and societal needs; a wide varietal diversity provides farmers and breeders with options and raw materials for crop development and food production now and in the future (FAO 2010).

Accordingly, the main objective of the present paper is to investigate whether and how quinoa's renaissance influences the crop diversity under cultivation. The objective is pursued through a case study in Cotacachi, a site in the Ecuadorian Andes where several quinoa projects have been implemented during the recent past.

Below, I begin with an overview of quinoa's past and present situation in an Andean and global perspective. I then present the case study area and methods, report on quinoa's traditional role in the study area, and show how the quinoa renaissance has played out locally through the description of two recent quinoa projects. Next, I present data on changes in farmers' quinoa agrobiodiversity following the projects. Finally, I discuss the observed processes and conclude with some implications for further conservation and development work.

Quinoa's Past: Glory and Neglect

Quinoa is not a grass like most of our major staple grains but belongs to the goosefoot-family. Because of this heritage, it is classified a "pseudo-cereal," together with other related American domesticates (Harlan 1995). Quinoa exhibits nutritive qualities superior to most cereals. Its protein contains a remarkably balanced set of essential amino acids, similar to milk's caseine (Repo-Carrasco, Espinoza, and Jacobsen 2003). It is also rich in polyunsaturated oil, vitamins, minerals, and antioxidants (Abugoch James 2009; Repo-Carrasco, Espinoza, and Jacobsen 2003). The catch is that each seed is enveloped in a bitter, saponine-containing coating. The saponine protects the plant against pests and must be removed before cooking.

Quinoa was domesticated about 5,000 BP, probably on the high plateaus of Southern Peru and Bolivia (Bruno 2006; Pearsall 2008). At the time of the Inca Empire in the 14th-15th centuries, it was grown along the whole Andean mountain range, from Colombia to southern Chile (NRC 1989). So central was its importance in the reign that the emperor ceremonially broke soil with a golden spade and planted each season's first quinoa seed (NRC 1989). But its public celebration was to fade. Together with a number of other native crops, quinoa became one of those disdained by Spanish conquerors' successors. Instead, Old World imports, notably wheat and barley, grew in importance as highland grains (Hernández Bermejo and León 1994). In the second half of the 20th century, quinoa's competitive pressure was increased as wheat gained even further stronghold as a food in the Andes, linked to the initiation of large-scale import programs (Tapia 1979). Protected under the United States Law PL480, massive amounts of wheat were cheaply or freely provided to Andean governments by the United States, and white bread and pasta rose in importance in urban as well as rural diets (Brett 2010). Quinoa continued to be considered an inferior *food of the Indians* along with certain other foods (Weismantel 1988), and while still grown by part of the rural population for subsistence purposes, some farm households opted for more prestigious purchased food alternatives, like rice and pasta, as they became available and accessible through market expansions and cash incomes from off-farm employment (Skarbø 2012).

The Quinoa Renaissance

During the 1980s, quinoa entered a new era of celebration. Andean researchers realized that quinoa, along with other native crops largely neglected by urban and scientific communities, carried potential for future agriculture (Mujica 1994; Peralta 1985; Tapia et al. 1979). Its retreat from Andean fields was characterized as worrisome; instead of further stimulating its take-over by wheat and barley, these scientists saw a need to promote its conservation and cultivation. Foreign observers also sparked interest in the crop. In the US National Research Council's (1989:3) book *Lost Crops of the Incas*, quinoa was listed among 30 other Andean domesticates that had largely been "lost to the outside world." But, the authors urged, "It is not too late to rescue these crops from oblivion" (NRC 1989:3). Quinoa was posed "a grain of the future" (NRC 1989:150); in addition to a potentially increased importance in the Andes, it was considered a promising crop for other marginal highland areas, as well as an interesting and novel product for consumers in developed countries.

Since the 1980s, Andean research institutions have, with the support of foreign donors and collaborating institutions, invested considerably in the development and conservation of native crops, and among them, quinoa has played a prominent role. In Ecuador, breeding efforts began already in the 1960s (McElhinny et al. 2007), but it was not until the 1980s that a concerted research program was formed (Nieto 1993). Backed by foreign funds, in particular from the Canadian International Development Research Centre (IDRC), the Ecuadorian National Institute for Agricultural and Livestock Investigation (INIAP) began a series of activities to recuperate quinoa diversity and cultivation. These included the systematic collection of germplasm, breeding of improved varieties, development of harvest and postharvest technology and new food products, and promotion of the crop among producers and consumers (Nieto 1990). By 1993, Carlos Nieto, (1993:185-188) one of INIAP's researchers, had already declared that in this "recovery of native mountain species from their imminent genetic erosion... quinoa has been transformed from an almost forgotten crop to a commercially valuable crop in the Ecuadorian mountain

Figure 1. Global Quinoa Exports, 1980-2010. Source: FAOSTAT 2013

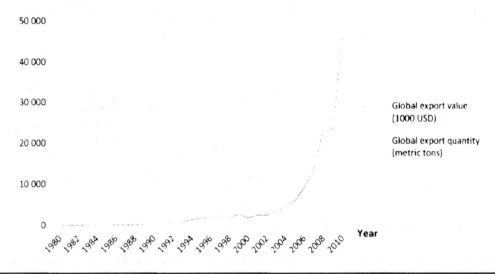

range." Major achievements included the release of two near saponine-free formally bred varieties, *Tunkahuan* and *Ingapirca* (Nieto et al. 1992). Research, development, and extension programs involving quinoa continue today and involve numerous foreign and local NGOs and institutions (McElhinny et al. 2007; Peralta et al. 2009; Villacrés et al. 2011). A number of businesses for processing and export have also appeared (BCE 2013). Quinoa's remarkable attractiveness to research and development agencies seems to stem from its dual potential to improve diets and raise incomes (Jacobsen and Sherwood 2002; McKnight Foundation n.d.).

In tandem with the above development, an international market for quinoa has taken form and grown. Quinoa can be said to have it all for the modern, conscious consumer; a mouthful of the grain is a piece of healthy and tasty gourmet gastronomy and simultaneously a heritage food that might even be organically produced and fairly traded. According to data from the Food and Agriculture Organization of the United Nations Statistics Division (FAOSTAT), 15,363 metric tons of quinoa was traded internationally in 2010, up from 177 in 1980 (Figure 1). Most of this global market has been fed by rising production in Bolivia and Peru (Figure 2). However, exports have risen in Ecuador as well (Figure

Figure 2. Quinoa Production in Bolivia, Peru, and Ecuador, 1980-2012. Source: FAOSTAT 2014

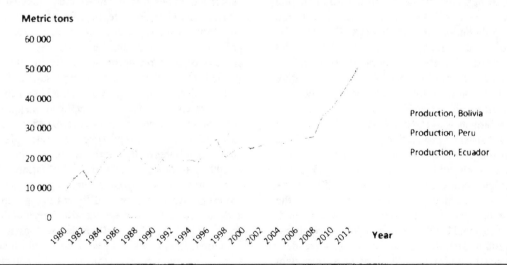

Figure 3. Ecuador's Quinoa Exports, 1980-2009. Source: FAOSTAT 2013

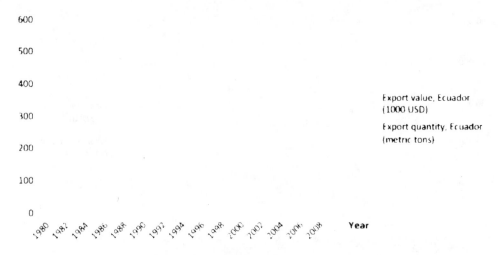

3). Data from Ecuador's Central Bank show that the most important importers of Ecuadorian quinoa are the United States, the United Kingdom, France, Spain, and Colombia (BCE 2013).

Study Area and Methods

Study Area

This research was carried out in Cotacachi, a *cantón*[1] in Northern Ecuador's Imbabura province, about 80 km from the capital Quito. While the cantón also includes a subtropical zone, the study is focused on the cantón's Andean part, an area of about 219 km², spanning altitudes from 2,080 m and up to the peak of the landmark volcano Cotacachi at 4,939 m (Zapata Ríos et al. 2006). The population is mainly divided between three urban centers, Cotacachi, Quiroga, and Imantag, with an estimated total of 9,000 inhabitants, and 43 rural communities, with a combined population of some 15,884 (INEC 2011; UN-ORCAC 2007). The majority of urban dwellers consider themselves mestizo, while most community members identify as indigenous Kichwa (INEC 2011). Agriculture remains an important livelihood strategy among rural households, although some 70 percent have members that work off-farm as well (UNORCAC 2007). The main focus is on subsistence production, but those who have more land also cultivate for the market. Fields and communities span an altitudinal belt from about 2,300m in the Inter-Andean valley bottom and up to 3,300 m. As temperature regimes change up the slope, so does the complex of crops grown. Agrobiodiversity is high, both on a farm and regional level, reflecting a long agricultural heritage. In 2009-2010, 103 cultivated species were identified in Cotacachi, and within 20 of the most important crop species, a total of 367 varieties were documented (Skarbø 2012). Most of these (87%) were landraces; formally bred varieties were only found in commercially important crops. Intercropping is common, in particular in subsistence oriented farms and fields. Agriculture and agrobiodiversity play central roles in local cultural and culinary traditions. Farmers further recognize several agronomic and dietary advantages of growing a diverse crop portfolio. Nevertheless, other current factors, including market demand and time constraints, compel many to limit the number of crops and varieties grown (Skarbø 2014).

Methods

This study builds on data collected by the author during a total of 16 months of ethnographic fieldwork in Cotacachi in 2003-2004 and 2009-2010. Participant observation in the cantón's communities and urban areas allowed for insight into quinoa's changing roles in different settings. Interviews with farmers and representatives of institutions and NGOs provided information about quinoa-related projects. Finally, surveys of on-farm agrobiodiversity in 2003 and 2009 yielded data on changes in the composition of local quinoa diversity during this period. Of Cotacachi's 43 communities, five representing different geographical and agroecological zones were selected for the surveys. Of 45 farms originally surveyed in 2003, it was possible to relocate and survey 37 in 2009. For a fuller picture of the recent situation, the sample in 2009 was expanded to a total of 89 farms. Within each community, purposive quota sampling was used to ensure representative inclusion of different age groups (Teddlie and Yu 2007). The surveys identified agrobiodiversity on crop and intracrop (varietal) levels and consisted of semi-structured interviews with farm household heads. In the surveys, interviewees were asked to identify all crops grown for food during the previous 1-year period. A crop list compiled during initial stages of the fieldwork was subsequently used to prompt for any forgotten crops. For a subset of the crops, including quinoa, interviewed farmers were further asked to identify the crop varieties they had planted during the same one-year period. Whenever possible, the information was triangulated with field and seed store inventories. For each variety grown, farmers were also asked about the number of consecutive years they had grown and saved seed from this particular variety and the original sources of the seed. Here, presentation of survey data is focused on that covering quinoa production and varieties. All interviews were conducted by the author, either in Spanish or a combination of Spanish and Kichwa, and in most cases accompanied by a bilingual research assistant.

Quinoa Traditions in Cotacachi

Despite competition, quinoa was never quite lost from Cotacachi. In kitchens, it continues to be an appreciated ingredient in savory and sweetened soups, considered especially hearty and tasty. In the field, the plant is prized for its frost resistance. Traditionally, quinoa has most often been intercropped with maize, beans, squashes, faba beans, and other crops. Alternatively, it is planted with lupines or fabas only or as a monocrop. When intercropped, farmers consider the plant to protect the whole field from night frosts. The crop's exceptional frost resistance has also been recognized by scientists, and some varieties have been measured to avoid freezing at temperatures as low as -8°C, linked to the plant's ability to supercool (Jacobsen et al. 2007). Recent research further shows that in quinoa monocultures, tall plants provide shade and radiative protection for lower plants, such that night temperatures often are 2-3°C higher in their shade than on the top of the tallest plants' canopy (Winkel et al. 2009). This ability to provide radiative shade corresponds well to Cotacachi farmers' consideration of quinoa as a frost protector of other crop species as well. Quinoa is adapted to all of Cotacachi's agroecological zones and does not require highly fertile soil to produce well. The crop requires much labor, especially during its harvest and food preparation. Panicles are hand cut, dried, and threshed. Prior to cooking, the bitter seed coat is removed by packing the amount of seed needed for a pot of soup into a piece of cloth and scrubbing and washing arduously for about one hour. According to local legends, quinoa's bitter coat is a curse from *Achi tayta* (Father God), from a time when the quinoa plant disclosed his path to his persecutors, the malevolent *aukas*, by shivering and thereby shedding its seeds to the ground as Achi tayta passed. As a result of the curse, quinoa has to suffer lengthy scrubbing before it serves as food. The crop's legendary inscription attests to its deeply held position in local culture and agriculture. In 2003, 26 of 45 surveyed farms (58%) in Cotacachi grew quinoa (Skarbø 2006). The crop ranked 5th in popularity among 17 field crops; in terms of proportion of farms cultivating a crop, it was only surpassed by maize,

beans, potatoes, and peas. Still, people reported its role to have declined during the past generation, a trend especially attributed to its heavy labor requirements. In 2003, quinoa's renaissance had yet to reach the region; however, that was soon to come.

Quinoa's Renaissance in Cotacachi

After 2003, several quinoa-focused projects have played out in local fields. Cotacachi is a worksite for a variety of organizations, and a number of them have taken part in promoting the crop. For some illustration of this process, we shall here look into two projects, one led by an Italian NGO and one by an Ecuadorian entrepreneur. They are chosen as examples because of their large sizes and because they display the variation in recent years' quinoa initiatives.

Project 1: The NGO Example

The Italian NGO Unity and Cooperation for the Development of Peoples (UCODEP)[3] has worked in Ecuador since 1993, with the objective of "strengthening the capacities of indigenous and peasant organizations, recuperating and valuing local resources and knowledge" (UCODEP 2010:2). Cotacachi has been one of their main sites to undertake this task in the country. In collaboration with the local farmer union *Unión de Organizaciones Campesinas e Indígenas de Cotacachi* (UNORCAC) and other organizations, UCODEP has been involved in varied rural development projects in the cantón's communities. Several of these have been specifically focused on the conservation and use of agrobiodiversity, in their Program of Neglected and/or Underutilized Crops. Among the program goals is "rescuing forgotten and underutilized traditional crops such as amaranth, quinoa, lupines among others" (UCODEP 2010:4). Their quinoa initiative, begun in 2007, has been carried out under two project umbrellas, one supported by the International Fund for Agricultural Development (IFAD) and Bioversity International, and the other by *Cooperazione Italiana*—the Italian government's aid and development agency. UCODEP has acted as a bridge between the Quito-based company *Cereales Andinos* (CA) and local farmers. The company provides seed (INIAP's low-saponine variety Tunkahuan) and technical advice to farmers, who in turn commit to sell 80 percent of their harvest to CA and in addition return an amount equivalent to the seed they received. UCODEP has invested in two threshers, which they move around to the different communities during harvest time. In 2010, farmers were paid $70/quintal,[4] of which $5 went towards covering threshing and transport costs. CA processes the grain into a suit of quinoa-based products for the national market, including granola, quinoa flakes, and energy bars (Cereales Andinos 2011). UCODEP reports of a rapidly growing interest among farmers to participate in the project—by May 2010,

Table 1. Characteristics of Quinoa Varieties in Cotacachi

Name (Kichwa)	Chawcha	Puka chawcha	Hatun	Mishki
Name (Spanish)	Chaucha	Chaucha rojo	Grande	Dulce
Name (English)	Fertile	Red fertile	Large	Sweet
Name (formal)	-	-	-	Tunkahuan
Origin	Native	Native	Native	INiAP
Plant description	Short plant	Short plant	Tall plant	Tall plant
	Slender stem	Slender stem	Thick stem	Thick stem
	Dark green leaves with red powder	Pale green leaves with white powder	Dark green leaves with white powder	Green leaves with pink powder
Grain color	White	Reddish	Yellow	White
Medicinal properties	No	No	Yes	No
Rinsing requirements	Relatively quick	Long time	Long time	Very brief
Cooking quality	Soft	Hard; longer time needed	Soft	Soft
Market acceptance	Low	Low	Low	High
Dominant production	Intercrop	Intercrop	Intercrop	Monocrop

134 farmers had joined, of these 74 as individuals and the rest organized in five community associations. In total, they were cultivating 60 ha of quinoa.

The NGO's staff explains that whereas projects typically have been oriented exclusively toward export markets, they intend to change this, focusing instead first on food for the families themselves, then on local markets, and third, on export. Thus, they have campaigned to foment local rural and urban consumption of quinoa and other native crops. They have worked with chefs to develop new and modern recipes, printed posters and recipe cards, arranged meetings, tasting events, and culinary contests with the participation of local restaurants. Their engaged efforts have not been in vain—local cafés are starting to offer modern quinoa inventions on their menus, and customers are curious to try things such as quinoa-filled empanadas and cakes. Finally, it should be noted that this rising interest in products from an indigenous crop is also related to broader societal reconfigurations in Cotacachi and beyond, entailing a new appreciation for indigeneity in general and indigenous foods in particular (Skarbø 2012).

Project 2: The Entrepreneur Example

A second quinoa production project in Cotacachi consists of community based women farmer associations producing on rented hacienda land. Behind this initiative stands an entrepreneur from the regional capital Ibarra, also seat of the region's branch of the Ministry of Agriculture, Livestock, and Fisheries (MAGAP). In 2008, he contacted women in two of Cotacachi's communities, encouraging them to form associations of about 20 members and co-cultivate quinoa with him on land rented from adjacent haciendas. Seed (again the variety Tunkahuan) and agronomic advice was provided by a MAGAP employee. The entrepreneur arranged the land rent and hired someone to plow the fields with a tractor, and the

women were responsible for all remaining work, including preparing furrows, planting, weeding, pesticide application if deemed necessary by the agronomist, harvesting, drying, threshing, and packing the quinoa in sacks. Of the harvest, 25-40 percent went to cover land rent and the remaining 60-75 percent was divided in two equally sized shares, one for the entrepreneur and one for the women's association. The women further divided their share between them according to labor input logs. The entrepreneur then purchased any quinoa they did not want to keep, for $100/quintal. This may appear as an appealingly high price, but if one considers that the women collectively only gained rights to about one third of the total harvest and each woman only to about 1.5-2 percent, the deal appears less just. I learned of at least one community where during the course of my field work the same entrepreneur was turned away by women not willing to accept his conditions. While initially enticed to participate in a quinoa project, these women refused upon learning the details, pointing out the reminiscence of hacienda owners' exploitation of indigenous communities' labor force two generations ago. His successful negotiations in other communities nevertheless demonstrate people's high interest in the "new" quinoa and the income generating opportunity presented, even despite these terms.

Quinoa Varieties in Cotacachi

Table 1 presents a comparison of the characteristics of different quinoa varieties grown in Cotacachi, based on farmers' classifications during workshop exercises in 2009-2010. Farmers distinguish between three main landraces, varying in size and coloration of plant and grain, cooking quality, and other characteristics. For example, one of them, *hatun kinuwa* (large quinoa), has local value not only as food but also as medicine—for curing human fever and pigs' trichinosis. In addition to these landraces, the formally bred Tunkahuan variety has

Figure 4. Venn Diagram of the Partly Overlapping Farm Samples from 2003 and 2009

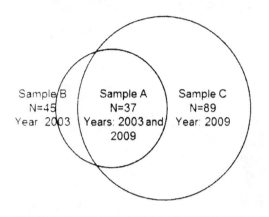

recently entered the local ethnobotanical classification system. Tunkahuan is called *mishki kinuwa* and *quinoa dulce* (both meaning "sweet quinoa") in the local Kichwa and Spanish vocabularies, respectively, for its exceptionally low content of bitter saponine. While seed from the landrace varieties has limited market acceptance, the slightly larger, whiter, and near saponine-free Tunkahuan seed is rather easily sold for a decent price. Farmers do not report differences in terms of agroecological fitness between varieties; rather, all can be grown across Cotacachi's different agroecological zones. On the other hand, they explain that while quinoa landraces are best intercropped with maize, beans, and other crops, Tunkahuan is preferably grown in monoculture.

Change Over Time in the Composition of Quinoa Agrobiodiversity

In what follows, I will report data on the composition of local quinoa agrobiodiversity before and after the project's implementation. As explained above under *Methods*, the data come from two rounds of surveys in Cotacachi, one in 2003 and one in 2009, documenting the crops and varieties planted by each farm household during the previous agricultural year. The total sample sizes were 45 in 2003 (Sample B) and 89 in 2009 (Sample C). The two samples partly overlap—37 farms were surveyed in both years (Sample A) (Figure 4). I report data on changes for both the core sample where the farms are the same in both years and the extended samples. The data cover changes in agrobiodiversity on the crop and variety levels. To complement and triangulate, I also report data on seed sources and the number of years each variety has been saved on-farm.

Changes at the Crop Level

Table 2 and Figure 5 show that there was a decline in the portion of farmers growing quinoa from 2003 to 2009, both when considering the smaller and the larger samples in each year. In 2003, close to 60 percent of surveyed farmers grew quinoa, while the figure was reduced to near 40 percent in 2009. Farmers themselves explained that their abandonment of the crop was related to its high labor requirements. The decline in the number of quinoa producers resonates with a decline in the number of farmers growing several other field crops during the same period, a complex process that is linked to reduction in available labor, increasing importance of off-farm work and

Table 2. Proportions of Farmers Growing Quinoa in 2003 and 2009

Grows quinoa?	Yes		No		Total	
Sample	N	%	N	%	N	%
Sample A - 2003	21	57	16	43	37	100
Sample B - 2003	26	58	19	42	45	100
Sample A - 2009	15	41	22	59	37	100
Sample C - 2009	33	37	56	63	89	100

Table 3. Relative Distribution of Quinoa Varieties in Recorded Seed Lots, 2003 and 2009

Sample/Variety	No. of Seed Lots	Tunkahuan (%)	Chawcha (%)	Puka chawcha (%)	Hatun (%)	Unspecified Landrace (%)
Sample A – 2003	23	4.3	35	8.7	35	17
Sample B – 2003	30	3.3	40	6.7	33	17
Sample A – 2009	19	42	26	5.3	26	0
Sample C – 2009	42	43	26	4.8	26	0

Figure 5. Proportion of Farmers Growing Quinoa in 2003 and 2009. See Table 3 for frequencies.

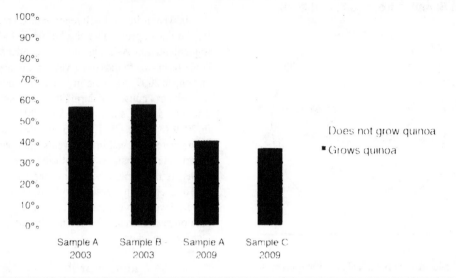

purchased foods, climatic calamities, and the lack of regeneration of local planting material (Skarbø 2012).

Changes at the Varietal Level

Changes in the distribution of varieties are reported in Table 3 and Figure 6. Most quinoa-growing farmers planted only one variety, but some planted two or even three different varieties. Thus, the total number of *seed lots*, defined as "seed of one variety, selected and planted on a specific farm during a season" (Louette 1999:112), slightly exceeds the number of surveyed farms. In 2003, the seed lots planted were almost exclusively landraces; only one sampled farm household had planted the Tunkahuan variety, acquired on a trip to another region of the country. The situation was turned on its head in 2009, when over 40 percent of the seed lots were made up by this new variety. Both among the subset of farmers sampled in both years (Sample A), as well as in the larger sample (Sample C), Tunkahuan had become the most popular variety.

Data on the age of each seed lot from the extended 2009 sample confirm the recent introduction of Tunkahuan in the local farming system. Table 4 shows summary data on farmers' reports of how many consecutive years they had planted and saved seed of their currently grown quinoa varieties. While the mean number of years for landraces ranged from 8.5 to 17.6, with a maximum of 60, the average number of years Tunkahuan had been planted and saved was two, with a maximum of seven.

Seed Sources

Data on seed sources underline the central importance of projects and NGOs in facilitating the entry of Tunkahuan

seed to Cotacachi's farms. Table 5 and Figure 7 present an overview of where farmers originally obtained the quinoa seed they planted in 2009. While family (including parents, grandparents, and fictive kin) was the chief source of landrace seed (71%), NGOs or other projects were the most important sources of Tunkahuan seed (50%). In addition to the two projects described above, farmers had received seed directly from the farmer union UNORCAC, from a project in a community school, and

---

Figure 6. The Proportion of Different Varieties Making Up Sampled Farmers' Seed Lots in 2003 and 2009. See Table 3 for exact percentages.

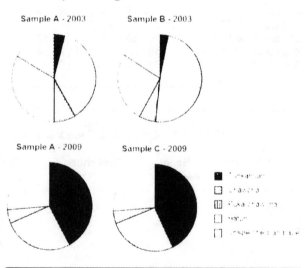

Table 4. Number of Consecutive Years Seed of Different Varieties Have Been Planted on Farm—Summary Data Based on 42 Seed Lots from 33 Farms, 2009

Variety	Tunkahuan	Chawcha	Puka chawcha	Hatun	Total
Mean	2	17.6	8.5	14.7	9.6
Median	1	5	8.5	10	2
Min.	1	1	2	1	1
Max.	7	60	15	40	60

from organized visits to project sites in other areas. Others had obtained Tunkahuan seed through exchanges or gifts from neighbors or family members, most of whom had received seed from organizations. Thus, seed introduced through projects rather rapidly move on to non-participating farmers interested in testing the variety. At the time of research, local markets had played no role in the spread of Tunkahuan, while they played a minor role as a source of landrace material.

Discussion

The two project examples illustrate the ample set of actors riding the quinoa wave in Cotacachi and beyond: farmers, governmental and non-governmental organizations from local to global levels, processing companies, restaurants, and entrepreneurs. A range of intentions is involved—from earnest attempts to improve others' livelihoods and maintain the cultivation of an eroding crop to pure profit making. The two initiatives are

Figure 7. Reported Sources of Quinoa Seed, 2009, Graphic Presentation

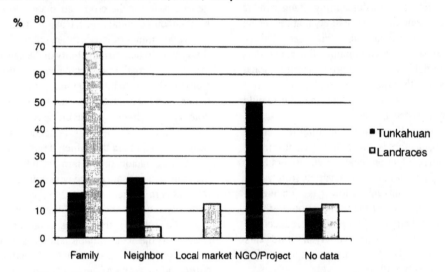

Table 5. Reported Sources of Quinoa Seed, 2009

Varieties	Tunkahuan		All Landraces		Total	
Seed source	N	%	N	%	N	%
Family	3	17	17	71	20	48
Neighbor	4	22	1	4	5	12
Local market	0	0	3	13	3	7
NGO/Project	9	50	0	0	9	21
No data	2	11	3	13	5	12
Total	18	100	24	100	42	100

quite different in the aims and motivation of their architects, as well as the distribution of benefits—but not so unlike in practice when it comes down to agricultural production. In both cases, the formally bred Tunkahuan variety is grown in monoculture; none of the projects involve landraces. The main focus is on market production, and only a small part of the harvest is kept for home consumption. Some level of mechanization is involved, including tractors for field preparation and mechanical threshers. In addition, the cultivation is supervised by external institutions' technical staff. This stands in rather sharp contrast to the traditional way of growing quinoa in Cotacachi described above—where landrace varieties of quinoa are intercropped with other plants, primarily for subsistence purposes, employing low levels of mechanization, guided by traditional knowledge.

What, then, are the conservation implications of quinoa's renaissance in Cotacachi? Do the initiatives emanating from a growing concern about the loss of this crop contribute to conserving it? The answer depends on how we direct our gaze—whether on the crop, varietal, or genetic level.

On an overall crop level, it is likely that the initiatives have had a positive effect—both in terms of number of cultivators and in the crop's extension. The observed decline in number of quinoa cultivators between 2003 and 2009 might have been steeper if the campaigns and projects were not in place. Although I do not have data concerning changes in the area under quinoa cultivation, it is very likely that the recent developments have led to an expansion in this regard. This is, first, because Tunkahuan is grown in monoculture, and thus with more plants per field than quinoa grown the traditional way, intercropped with other species. Second, many grow it as a cash crop, and therefore in larger extents than they would if it were solely for subsistence needs.

On the varietal level, the answer regarding the renaissance's conservation outcomes is mixed. At least in this initial stage, there is a positive effect on local varietal diversity by the new addition—farmers have one more variety from which to choose. However, since Tunkahuan now makes up over 40 percent of seed lots, at the same time as the amount of seed lots has been reduced, its entry has very probably reduced the extension of local landraces. If the new variety in future years pushes other landraces out of cultivation, the net conservation impact on varietal diversity will be negative.

Finally, on the genetic level, the answer reverberates with the preceding. The introduced variety is bred from landrace material from another Ecuadorian province, Carchi (Nieto et al. 1992) and thus brings new genetic diversity to Cotacachi. However, if the domination of the new variety leads to severe reductions in the extension of landraces, their populations may reach levels where genetic bottlenecks lead to loss of alleles. And if they are completely abandoned, their genetic composition will disappear from the repertoire of local farmers as well as more distant breeders.

Amid the excitement about the new seed and quinoa's shift into a cash crop, a few farmer voices question the trend. "Everyone grows quinoa now," doña María Dolores, a 55 year old farmer thoughtfully remarked, "but *our* quinoa was different." With this sentence, she neatly sums up the crop's current situation in Cotacachi; on one hand, it is gaining ground, but on the other, this gain is accompanied by an imminent, silent withdraw of local landraces along with former practices. Even if this withdraw was brewing from before, the forceful entry of the new variety and production system has likely fueled the process.

An eventual loss of Cotacachi's quinoa landraces would threaten the core of the crop's adaptive capacity. The survival of any of our crops over extended periods of time is dependent upon the maintenance of a broad genetic base, which enables the crop, aided by farmers and breeders, to adapt to changing conditions (FAO 2010; Hawkes 1983). Some of this function can be secured by the storage of collected samples of crop diversity in gene banks *ex situ*, but during the past decades, it has become increasingly clear that for various reasons such *ex situ* storage alone is not a secure way of conserving crop diversity; it must be accompanied by *in situ* cultivation of a broad suit of varieties on farms and in gardens (Brush 1999; Fowler 2013; Maxted, Ford-Lloyd, and Hawkes 1997). In this respect, the cultivation of landraces is particularly important because they are typically characterized by less uniformity and broader genetic variation than formally bred varieties (Brown 1999). Thus, because quinoa's landraces potentially carry a genetic base for the crop's adaptation to changing environments, their potential loss in Cotacachi and other Andean rural areas undermines quinoa's future cultivation. If one considers the agroecological sustainability of the new quinoa production system in a broader perspective, an additional concern arises from the shift from intercropping to monocropping, in combination with the reduction in quinoa's saponine content. Since both varietal diversity, intercropping, and saponine protect crops against pests, the new production system as a whole may be less resilient than that which it replaces (see Altieri 1999).

Several factors propel farmers' interest in participating in the quinoa renaissance. The new quinoa's popularity among farmers is in particular related to the income generation opportunity it offers and its cooking quality and appearance.

First, mishki kinuwa has good market acceptance in relation to the local quinoa landraces and sells for a high price, thus presenting a chance to earn extra income. Through participation in any of the local quinoa projects, farmers are provided a secure market outlet for their Tunkahuan grain; the projects only work with this variety. The market popularity and relatively high price level of the grain also makes it a better bet than many other locally grown crops.

In addition to market acceptance, the qualities that have made Tunkahuan so popular in the market—its low saponine content and light color—are also factors that favor the variety as a choice for home use among Cotacachi's farmers. The lack of saponine in particular thrills women, as it significantly reduces the amount of labor needed to prepare a pot of soup. Its white color is also appreciated; many consider it "purer" and more tantalizing than the reddish and brownish landraces.

Whether Cotacachi's quinoa landraces eventually will be completely displaced or not, of course, still stands to see. Previous analyses have shown that the introduction of formally bred varieties into a farming system does not necessarily lead to full abandonment of landraces (Brush, Taylor, and Bellon 1992; Perales, Brush, and Qualset 2003). This is also the situation for several other crops in Cotacachi; for instance, formally bred varieties of maize and beans have been incorporated into smallholder seed portfolios, while many landraces are maintained (Skarbø 2014). Yet, as shown above, the situation is quite distinct in the case of quinoa, where one newly introduced formally bred variety has rapidly gained a dominant role among the area's farms.

There may be several reasons behind this differential development. Importantly, in contrast to maize and beans, where Cotacachi's smallholders typically grow several varieties with different agronomic and culinary qualities, most quinoa growers plant only one variety. The adoption of Tunkahuan thus means a direct displacement of formerly grown landraces on many farms. Most of those who have begun to grow quinoa as a cash crop in monoculture have discontinued adding rows of the seed to their maize/bean intercropped fields, saving the labor it takes to grow and harvest it separately. Even though there are differences between the properties of the local quinoa landraces, there is, in contrast to what is the case for many other crops, not a clear differentiation into varietal suitability for different dishes. If landraces are to be maintained, farmers must value their other qualities or encounter alternative reasons to grow them.

Conclusion

The perceived loss of quinoa has led to concerted recuperation efforts involving a broad crew of actors. In Ecuador and Cotacachi, many are now jumping on the quinoa bandwagon, from researchers and institutions to farmers and restaurateurs. Eager to redress past neglect, researchers are drawn to the crop's fine adaptation to the region's harsh conditions as well as its nutritive and functional properties. Quinoa presents itself as a perfect alternative for rural development projects; it is a healthy product with a high price and thus promises to improve farm families' nutrition as well as increase their earnings while at the same time contributing to crop conservation. Farmers are curious to participate, drawn by the new variety's ease of preparation and market fame. Chefs and café owners cook up new recipes and place the heritage crop on their menus. Although sparkling with positive spirits and success, the process of recuperation presents some important paradoxes worth noting. Quinoa was never completely lost from Cotacachi's farms and food culture, yet instead of stimulating the recuperation of local landraces and associated cultivation and culinary practices, recent projects to save and boost the crop have "returned" a formally bred variety that was never there in the first place. The development of this variety, along with its dissemination to farmers, is in many respects a major advancement. In particular, its low saponine content is a characteristic highly appreciated both in the market and among the women who cultivate and also cook the crop at home, as it reduces the labor involved

in processing the grain. The creative ways through which the crop's cultivation and use is promoted are commendable efforts that contribute to quinoa's continued popularity. The process has likely led to an overall expansion of the area under quinoa cultivation. But at the same time, this study indicates that the rapid and expansive entry of the new variety and cultivation system contributes toward displacing formerly present local landraces. If a similar development takes place over a broader area in the Andes, which is quinoa's center of crop origin and diversity, this displacement may have dismal consequences for the crop's future adaptive capacity. The need of a broad genetic base is underlined by the challenge of climatic change, which is projected to be especially severe in the Andean highlands (Bradley et al. 2006; Urrutia and Vuille 2009). The main paradox is thus that initiatives that grew out of an original concern about genetic erosion and awareness about a need to conserve run the risk of inadvertently accelerating the loss of genetic diversity.

These observations call for particular caution in the planning and execution of crop recuperation projects, including a constant reconsideration of the relationship between aims, means of action, and outcomes. When breeding and the spread of new formally bred varieties is involved, conservation-motivated projects should take care to also incorporate local landraces into their activities, promoting the cultivation of a broader diversity. Ethnobotanical and laboratory-based documentation of the properties of different landraces could be one such effort, which might increase the value of landrace material both for future commercial and subsistence-oriented production. On the commercial side, this might allow the development of different products based on different varieties or varietal mixes, again creating a demand for their production. If activities additionally focus on the potential value of the maintenance of landrace diversity, traditional knowledge, and cultivation practices for local agricultural sustainability and cuisine, this could enhance the chance that farmers find reasons to continue cultivating also "their" quinoa.

Notes

[1] A geographical-administrative unit roughly corresponding to a U.S. county.

[2] A *landrace* can be defined as "a dynamic population(s) of a cultivated plant that has a historical origin, distinct identity, and lacks formal crop improvement, as well as often being genetically diverse, locally adapted, and associated with traditional farming systems" (Camacho Villa et al. 2006:381). Landraces are often contrasted with *modern* or *formally bred varieties* that have been bred and released from professional plant breeders, synonymous with high yielding varieties and improved varieties. In this paper, I use the terms landrace and formally bred variety as referred to above, as well as the term *variety* as encompassing any or both.

[3] After completion of fieldwork in 2010, the NGO became part of Oxfam International and changed its name to Oxfam Italia.

[4] The quintal is a common unit for measuring agricultural harvest in Ecuador and corresponds to about 46 kg.

References Cited

Abbott, J. Anthony
  2005 Counting Beans: Agrobiodiversity, Indigeneity, and Agrarian Reform. The Professional Geographer 57(2):198-212.

Abugoch James, Lilian E.
  2009 Quinoa (*Chenopodium quinoa* Willd.): Composition, Chemistry, Nutritional, and Functional Properties. Advances in Food and Nutrition Research 58:1-31.

Altieri, Miguel A.
  1999 Applying Agroecology to Enhance the Productivity of Peasant Farming Systems in Latin America. Environment, Development, and Sustainability 1(3-4):197-217.

Banco Central de Ecuador (BCE)
  2013 Online Database. Website of Banco Central de Ecuador. URL:<http://www.bce.fin.ec> (August 28, 2013).

Bradley, Raymond S., Mathias Vuille, Henry F. Diaz, and Walter Vergara
  2006 Threats to Water Supplies in the Tropical Andes. Science 312(5781):1755-1756.

Brett, John
  2010 The Political-Economics of Developing Markets Versus Satisfying Food Needs. Food and Foodways 18(1-2):28-42.

Brown, Anthony H. D.
  1999 The Genetic Structure of Crop Landraces and the Challenge to Conserve them *In Situ* On Farms. *In* Genes in the Field: On-farm Conservation of Crop Diversity. S. B. Brush, ed. Pp. 29-48. Boca Raton, Fla.: Lewis Publishers; Ottawa, Canada: International Development Research Centre; Rome, Italy: International Plant Genetic Resources Institute.

Bruno, Maria C.
  2006 A Morphological Approach to Documenting the Domestication of Chenopodium in the Andes. *In* Documenting Domestication: New Genetic and Archaeological Paradigms. Melinda A. Zeder, Daniel Bradley, Eve Emshwiller, and Bruce D. Smith, eds. Pp. 32-45. Berkeley: University of California Press.

Brush, Stephen B., ed.
  1999 Genes in the Field: On-Farm Conservation of Crop Diversity. Boca Raton, Fla.: Lewis Publishers; Ottawa, Canada: International Development Research Centre; Rome, Italy: International Plant Genetic Resources Institute.

Brush, Stephen B., and Erica Meng
  1998 Farmers' Valuation and Conservation of Crop Genetic Resources. Genetic Resources and Crop Evolution 45(2):139-150.

Brush, Stephen B., J. Edward Taylor, and Mauricio R. Bellon
  1992 Technology Adoption and Biological Diversity in Andean Potato Agriculture. Journal of Development Economics 39(2):365-387.

Cereales Andinos
  2011 Nuestros Productos. Cereales Andinos Website. URL:<http://www.cerealesandinos.com> (June 16, 2014).

Camacho Villa, Tania Carolina, Nigel Maxted, Maria Scholten, and Brian Ford-Lloyd
  2006 Defining and Identifying Crop Landraces. Plant Genetic Resources 3(3):373-384.

Food and Agriculture Organization of the United Nations (FAO)
  2010 The Second Report on the State of the World's Plant Genetic Resources for Food and Agriculture. Rome, Italy: Commision on Genetic Resources for Food and Agriculture, Food and Agriculture Organization of the United Nations.

Food and Agriculture Organization of the United Nations Statistics Division (FAOSTAT)
  2013 FAOSTAT database. URL:<http://faostat.fao.org> (October 23, 2013).
  2014 FAOSTAT database. URL:<http://faostat3.fao.org> (November 28, 2014).

Fowler, Cary
  2013 Complimentarity and Conflict: *In situ* and *Ex situ* Approaches to Conserving Plant Genetic Resources. *In* Seeds of Resistance, Seeds of Hope: Place and Agency in the Conservation of Biodiversity. Virginia D. Nazarea, Robert E. Rhoades, and Jenna Andrews-Swann, eds. Pp.196-213. Tucson: University of Arizona Press.

Friedman-Rudovsky, Jean
  2012 For Bolivian Farmers, Quinoa Boom is Both Boon and Bane. Time Magazine. April 3, 2012.

Hernández Bermejo, J. Esteban, and Jorge León
  1994 Neglected Crops: 1492 from a Different Perspective. Rome: Food and Agriculture Organization of the United Nations.

Harlan, Jack R.
  1995 The Living Fields: Our Agricultural Heritage. Cambridge, United Kingdom: Cambridge University Press.

Hawkes, John G.
  1983 The Diversity of Crop Plants. Cambridge, Mass.: Harvard University Press.

Instituto Nacional de Estadisticas y Censos (INEC)
  2011 VII Censo de Población y VI de Vivienda. Quito, Ecuador: Instituto Nacional de Estadisticas y Censos.

Jacobsen, Sven-Erik, Cecilia Monteros, Luis J. Corcuera, León A. Bravo, Jørgen L. Christiansen, and Ángel Mujica
  2007 Frost Resistance Mechanisms in Quinoa (*Chenopodium quinoa* Willd.). European Journal of Agronomy 26(4):471-475.

Jacobsen, Sven-Erik, and Stephen Sherwood
  2002 Cultivos Andinos en Ecuador: Informe Sobre los Rubros Quinoa, Chocho y Amaranto. Quito, Ecuador: Food and Agriculture Organization of the United Nations, Centro Internacional de la Papa, Catholic Relief Services, and Ediciones Abya-Yala.

Louette, Dominique
  1999 Traditional Management of Seed and Genetic Diversity: What is a Landrace? *In* Genes in the Field: On-farm Conservation of Crop Diversity. Stephen B. Brush, ed. Pp. 109-142. Boca Raton, Fla.: Lewis Publishers; Ottawa, Canada: International Development Research Centre; Rome, Italy: International Plant Genetic Resources Institute.

Maxted, Nigel, Brian Ford-Lloyd, and John G. Hawkes
  1997 Plant Genetic Conservation: The *in situ* Approach. New York: Chapman and Hall.

McElhinny, Elaine, Eduardo Peralta, Nelson Mazón, Daniel L. Danial, Graham Thiele, and Pim Lindhout
  2007 Aspects of Participatory Plant Breeding in Marginal Areas in Ecuador. Euphytica 153(3):373-384.

McKnight Foundation
n.d. Project summary. Lupin/Quinoa. Grant no. 05-112. Sustainable Production Systems to Guarantee Food Security in Impoverished Communities in the Province of Cotopaxi, Ecuador. McKnight Foundation Collaborative Crop Research Program. URL:<http://ccrp.org.tripark.net/projects/lupinquinoa> (June 17, 2014).

Morris, Arthur
1999 The Agricultural Base of the Pre-Incan Andean Civilizations. The Geographical Journal 165(3):286-295.

Mujica, Ángel
1994 Andean Grains and Tubers. *In* Neglected Crops: 1492 from a Different Perspective. J. Esteban Hernandez Bermejo and Jorge León, eds. Pp. 131-148. Rome, Italy: Food and Agriculture Organization of the United Nations.

National Research Council (NRC)
1989 Lost Crops of the Incas: Little-Known Plants of the Andes with Promise for Worldwide Cultivation. Washington, D.C.: National Academy Press.

Nazarea, Virginia D.
1998 Cultural Memory and Biodiversity. Tucson: University of Arizona Press.

Nieto, Carlos
1990 Proyecto Producción de Quinua en Ecuador 3P-85-0138, Informe Final de Labores (1986-1990). Quito, Ecuador: Instututo Nacional de Investigaciones Agropecuarias and Centro Internacional de Investicationes para el Desarrollo.
1993 The Preservation of Foods Indigenous to the Ecuadorian Andes. Mountain Research and Development 13(2):185-188.

Nieto, Carlos, Carlos Vimos, Cecilia Monteros, Carlos Caicedo, and Marco Rivera
1992 INIAP-Ingapirca e INIAP-Tunkahuan. Dos Variedades de Quinua de Bajo Contenido de Saponina. Quito, Ecuador: INIAP.

Ofstehage, Andrew
2012 The Construction of an Alternative Quinoa Economy: Balancing Solidarity, Household Needs, and Profit in San Agustín, Bolivia. Agriculture and Human Values 29(4):441-454.

Pearsall, Deborah
2008 Plant Domestication and the Shift to Agriculture in the Andes. *In* Handbook of South American Archaeology. Helaine Silverman and William H. Isbell, eds. Pp. 105-120. New York: Springer.

Perales, Hugo, Stephen B. Brush, and Calvin O. Qualset
2003 Dynamic Management of Maize Landraces in Central Mexico. Economic Botany 57(1):21-34.

Peralta, Eduardo
1985 La Quinoa...Un Gran Alimento y su Utilización. Boletín Divulgatorio N° 175. Quito, Ecuador: Estación Experimental Santa Catalina, INIAP.

Peralta, Eduardo, Nelson Mazón, Ángel Murillo, Elena Villacrés, Marco Rivera, and Cristian Subía
2009 Catálogo de Variedades Mejoradas de Granos Andinos: Chocho, Quinua y Amaranto, para la Sierra Ecuatoriana. Publicación Miscelánea N° 151. Quito, Ecuador: Programa Nacional de Leguminosas y Granos Andinos. Estación Experimental Santa Catalina, INIAP.

Rana, Ram Badahur, Chris Garforth, Bhuwon Sthapit, and Devra Jarvis
2007 Influence of Socio-Economic and Cultural Factors in Rice Varietal Diversity Management On-Farm in Nepal. Agriculture and Human Values 24(4):461-472.

Repo-Carrasco, Ritva, Clara Espinoza, and Sven-Erik Jacobsen
2003 Nutritional Value and Use of the Andean Crops Quinoa (*Chenopodium quinoa*) and Kañiwa (*Chenopodium pallidicaule*). Food Reviews International 19(1&2):179-189.

Rojas, Wilfredo, Milton Pinto, and José Luis Soto
2010 Distribución Geográfica y Variabilidad Genética de los Granos Andinos. *In* Granos Andinos: Avances, Logros y Experiencias Desarrolladas en Quinua, Cañahua y Amaranto en Bolivia. Wilfredo Rojas, José Luis Soto, Milton Pinto, Matthias Jagger, and Stefano Padulosi, eds. Pp. 11-23. Rome, Italy: Bioversity International.

Skarbø, Kristine
2006 Living, Dwindling, Loosing, Finding: Status and Changes in Agrobiodiversity of Cotacachi. *In* Development with Identity: Community, Culture, and Sustainability in the Andes. R. E. Rhoades, ed. Pp. 123-139. Cambridge, Mass.: CABI Publishing.
2012 Reconfiguration of Andean Fields: Culture, Climate, and Agrobiodiversity. Ph.D. dissertation, University of Georgia, Athens.
2014 The Cooked is the Kept: Factors Shaping the Maintenance of Agro-biodiversity in the Andes. Human Ecology 42(5):711-726.

Tapia, Mario
1979 Historia y Distribuición Geográfica. *In* Quinua y Kañiwa: Cultivos Andinos. Mario Tapia, Humberto Gandarillas, Segundo Alandia, Armando Cardozo, and Ángel Mujica, eds. Pp. 11-19. Bogotá, Colombia: Centro Internacional de Investigaciones para el Desarrollo and Instituto Interamericano de Ciencias Agrícolas.

Tapia, Mario, Humberto Gandarillas, Segundo Alandia, Armando Cardozo, and Ángel Mujica, eds.
1979 Quinua y Kañiwa: Cultivos Andinos. Bogotá, Colombia: Centro Internacional de Investigaciones para el Desarrollo and Instituto Interamericano de Ciencias Agricolas.

Teddlie, Charles, and Fen Yu
2007 Mixed Methods Sampling: A Typology with Examples. Journal of Mixed Methods Research 1(1):77-100.

Unidad y Cooperación para el Desarrollo de los Pueblos (UCODEP)
2010 Programa Cultivos Olvidados y/o Subutilizados (NUS). Arezzo, Italy: Unidad y Cooperación para el Desarrollo de los Pueblos.

Unión de Organizaciones Campesinas e Indígenas de Cotacachi (UNORCAC)
2007 UNORCAC en Cifras. Cotacachi, Ecuador: Unión de Organizaciones Campesinas e Indígenas de Cotacachi.

United Nations General Assembly
2011 Resolution 66/221. Resolution Adopted by the General Assembly [On the Report of the Second Committee (A/66/446)] 66/221. International Year of Quinoa, 2013.

Urrutia, Rocío, and Mathias Vuille
2009 Climate Change Projections for the Tropical Andes Using a Regional Climate Model: Temperature and Precipitation Simulations for the End of the 21st Century. Journal of Geophysical Research 114(D2) <http://onlinelibrary.wiley.com/doi/10.1029/2008JD011021/full>.

Villacrés P., Elena, Eduardo Peralta I., Luís Egas A., and Nelson Mazón O.
    2011   Potencial Agroindustrial de la Quinua. Boletín Técnico N°
    146. Quito, Ecuador: Departamento de Nutrición y Calidad de
    los Alimentos. Estación Experimental Santa Catalina, Instituto
    Nacional de Investigaciones Agropecuarias.

Weismantel, Mary J.
    1988   Food, Gender, and Poverty in the Ecuadorian Andes.
    Philadelphia: University of Pennsylvania Press.

Winkel, Thierry, Jean-Paul Lhomme, Juan Peter Nina Laura, Claudia
Mamani Alcón, Carmen del Castillo, and Alain Rocheteau
    2009   Assessing the Protective Effect of Vertically Heterogeneous
    Canopies against Radiative Frost: The Case of Quinoa on
    the Andean Altiplano. Agricultural and Forest Meteorology
    149(10):1759-1768.

Zapata Ríos, X., R. E. Rhoades, M. C. Segovia, and F. Zehetner
    2006   Four Decades of Land Use Change in the Cotacachi Andes:
    1963-2000. *In* Development with Identity: Community, Culture,
    and Sustainability in the Andes. Robert E. Rhoades, ed. Pp. 46-63.
    Wallingford, United Kingdom: CABI Publishing.

Discussion Questions: From Lost Crop to Lucrative Commodity: Conservation Implications of the Quinoa Renaissance

1. Where is Quinoa native? What signs do we have that Quinoa was indigenous to a particular place? What are the signs for adaptation to the site of origin?
2. Why is crop diversity said to be important? What are the benefits and necessities for maintaining crop diversity?
3. Why is quinoa said to be nutritious? What does quinoa include or add to the diet?
4. How did the US contribute to farmers abandoning quinoa? What was promoted in its place and why would farmers change crops?

READING 12

Ode to a Chuño

Learning to Love Freeze-Dried Potatoes in Highland Bolivia

Clare A. Sammells

Biographical sketch. Clare Sammells first went to Bolivia during the summer of 1993 as an undergraduate to research the consumption of llama meat in the city of La Paz. After graduating with a degree in folklore and mythology from Harvard College and living for two years in Costa Rica, she began graduate school at the University of Chicago in 1997. She returned to rural highland Bolivia to conduct an anthropological study of tourism at Tiwanaku, that nation's most important archaeological site. She traveled to Bolivia again in 1998, 1999, 2000, 2007, and 2010 and lived there for two years from 2002 to 2004. She completed her Ph.D. in 2009 and is now an assistant professor at Bucknell University. She loves Bolivian food and misses her *comadre*'s amazing cooking when in the United States.

I like *chuño*.

This statement sometimes surprises highland Bolivians but surprises Americans[1] who know the region even more. The former find it pleasant that I like Bolivian food. But some North Americans believe that this is clear evidence that I will eat "anything"—something I certainly aspire to but cannot claim to have fully achieved.[2] Meanwhile, those who have never been to the Andes usually have no reaction at all. Chuño? It's just a potato, right?

Chuño is a freeze-dried potato, but tastes nothing like a fresh potato.[3] When cooked, it looks like a whole truffle: small, round and wrinkly, dark gray or black in color, and a little larger than a ping-pong ball although often flatter in shape. Generally it is eaten with the fingers (sometimes with a spoon) and breaks apart in sections radiating from the center. Its texture is firm, not mushy like a fresh potato. It is dense, a little mealy, and slightly bitter. It is very filling. It can be eaten with various sauces, such as *llajwa*, which is a sauce made of ground tomato, *locoto* (an Andean chili pepper), and *kirkiña* (a green herb). Breaking the chuño apart with one's fingers, one uses it to scoop the spicy sauce. Or chuño can be broken into smaller pieces and mixed with crushed peanuts or scrambled eggs and served as a side dish. Raw chuño can be ground into a flour to be used as a base for soups such as *chairo*. Chuño can form an essential part of a dish or be placed in a communal bowl for diners to complement their individual plates. It is a versatile staple, and in my time living in Tiwanaku (a rural highland village), it was included in one-third of all the meals I ate.[4]

In addition to being tasty, chuño is also a product of a pre-Colombian technology that allows potatoes to be stored for decades and transported easily. The Inca empire had an elaborate system of storehouses used to provision travelers and soldiers; among the items stocked there were chuño and other freeze-dried foods, such as *charq'e*, a form of dried llama meat (and, later, sheep or beef) for which our own jerky is named. These storehouses were so well-provisioned and operated so efficiently that in one area they continued to function and in some places provision the Spanish for twenty years after the conquest (D'Altroy 2002). Indigenous miners sent to work in the colonial-era mines of Potosí were fed with chuño produced elsewhere in the highlands, transported by llama caravans, and either sold in enormous markets or brought to workers directly by their communities. Many of the caravan llamas were then slaughtered and consumed in the burgeoning city (Mangan 2005).

Despite its usefulness, the Andean technology of creating chuño did not cross the Atlantic with the crop. Studies of the potato's introduction into Europe tend not to comment on the failure to transfer this knowledge (see Messer 1997; Salaman 1949; Walvin 1997; Zuckerman 1998). Awareness of this technology has fallen out of North Atlantic stories about their love affair with the tuber. These accounts also usually fail to return to the Andes to consider recent misguided efforts to introduce North Atlantic varieties of potatoes into the Andes. European and U.S. varieties of potatoes are considered by most highland Bolivians to be watery and tasteless, and wealthy Bolivians who had traveled to the United States told me in no uncertain terms that the potatoes they encountered in their travels were inferior.

HOW TO PLANT A CHUÑO

In Tiwanaku some locals tell variants of a tale about the Spanish conquista-dores who came to the highlands in the early colonial period. Impressed with chuño, they forced the local people to plant it on the assumption that it was a unique crop. When the locals balked at this ridiculous request, the Spanish accused them of laziness. Of course, it was the Spanish who were disappointed to discover that their fields of chuño did not sprout.

This story highlights the fact that from the point of view of those who eat Andean cuisine without participating in its production, chuño seems so com-pletely different from potatoes that it would be easy to assume they were from different plants altogether. This is not true in a biological sense, but it is true in a culinary sense. Socially and culinarily, chuño is not a potato at all.

In Bolivian cuisine, *papas* are specifically fresh potatoes; chuño is not included in that category by highland Bolivians. Nor are the two interchange-able in all dishes. Without chuño, some dishes cannot be properly made. For example, *chairo* is a soup that must be made with ground chuño. While other ingredients are expected in the soup (grains of wheat, carrots, and other items) these can be substituted or omitted without changing the identity of the soup. Likewise, the soup *jakonta* must include whole chuño—otherwise it is some-thing else. One cannot make chairo without chuño, just as one cannot make French fries without potatoes.

Papas, chuño, and other tubers can be substituted for each other in some dishes, similar to the way that side dishes can be substituted in U.S. cuisine. Unlike U.S. dishes, which tend to include only one staple carbohydrate, Bolivian dishes regularly contain two or more staples—such as rice and papas, or papas and chuño—especially in dishes that involve meat (such as beef, mutton, or guinea pig). Chuño is a common option, but it can be replaced with multi-ple varieties of fresh potatoes, *oca* (a sweeter, oblong orange-colored tuber), or *isaño* (resembling a large oca but with a tart taste, which is also sometimes turned in to a frozen ice-cream-like treat called *thayacha*). Non-tuber staples include rice, pasta, and less commonly maize, *quispiña* (steamed biscuits made from *quinua* flour), sweet potato, and plantain.[5]

MAKING CHUÑO

Bolivia has hundreds of varieties of potatoes with vastly different characteristics. Only certain varieties are appropriate to be freeze-dried. Chuño is created from bitter potato ("*papa amarga*"; for a description of potato varieties, see La Barre 1947; and for detailed descriptions of chuño processing, see Condori Cruz 1992; Mamani 1981). Potatoes are generally harvested in May. Those potatoes chosen for making chuño are picked on the basis of variety and size; medium-sized potatoes are preferred (slightly bigger than a golf ball) as very large potatoes may not freeze evenly. Also potatoes with many *gusanos*—large worms that tunnel into the potatoes and are removed by hand after cooking—are avoided.[6]

The potatoes selected for making chuño are placed outside in the month of June, which is the coldest month of the year. The potatoes freeze during the frosty nights and then thaw in the bright sunshine when temperatures rise above freezing. This alternation of freezing and thawing is essential to making chuño and may explain why this technology did not travel to Europe, where winter temperatures often remain below freezing even in the daytime.[7]

Once the potatoes have alternately frozen and thawed for three consecutive days, the water must be squeezed out of them. My first experience with this was unplanned. I was walking in the rural countryside with my *compadre*.[8] We had gone to his village in part to see the raised fields, called *suka kollus*, that were once a mainstay of the region's pre-Columbian agriculture and had been restored in the 1980s (Kolata 1993, 1996). Nothing was growing at the time, because it was winter (June). But on the way back, we happened on two of his relatives who were in the process of making chuño.

The chuño they were making had already been left to freeze and thaw for three days and nights, and they were stepping on the tubers to remove the liquid. They invited me to join them. I am not sure they expected me to actually do so, but I happily sat down and took off my shoes and socks. They showed me how to gather the potatoes into small piles with my bare feet and then "dance" (*bailar*) on top of them. Here the Spanish verb meaning "to dance" describes the movement, although there is no music or imposition of rhythm. Each person steps on the potatoes while removing the potato skins with their feet (although the process is incomplete and is continued by hand after the tubers have dried and then finished when they are soaked in water before cooking). One alternates between stepping on the chuño and gathering them back together in a pile, using only the feet.

I found that the potatoes were firm but spongy. A cool, dark-purple liquid squirted through my toes and onto the hard ground as I tried to keep the slippery tubers in a compact pile so they did not scatter everywhere when stepped on. The ground was hard-packed with only very short grass on it, as is typical in the dry, cold Andean winter, and this grass stuck to our feet as we worked. They insisted I had the hang of it, but I suspect—as was the case with the majority of agricultural labor I helped with in Bolivia—that I was far slower than a woman my age should have been at such a task. Nevertheless, we had a great time, and they insisted on photos to commemorate the event. That moment was remembered fondly when I saw them even years later.

Once the liquid is removed and the chuño is dried, it is light, easy to move, and can be stored for years. I have visited houses of farmers who had rooms with bags of chuño from floor to ceiling, some of which were more than a decade old. This ability to store food is important in a region were periodic droughts can destroy a year's crop; chuño provides the food needed to survive.

In its dried form, chuño feels like Styrofoam packing peanuts. To cook it, it must be soaked overnight in water. The chuño is then boiled and served either in soup, as a side dish, or in a *fiambre* (explained in the following section).

Two other varieties of freeze-dried potatoes deserve mention. One is *chuño fresca*, which is only consumed in June, when chuño is made. Lighter in color, this is prepared by stopping the preparation process before the tubers are stepped on. Having undergone the freezing and thawing process for three days, they are immediately boiled and served, and thus they are only eaten a few times a year. The other is *tunta*, where the tubers are placed in a body of water or stream for a month after the freezing and thawing process. The tuber is then dried out and can be stored like chuño. Tunta is white in color, has a different taste, and is generally more highly prized. Much as a chuño is not a potato, a tunta is not culinarily a chuño. There are dishes that require tunta to be properly made and are assumed to include it even though the name of the dish does not mention the tuber (such as *sajta de pollo*).

THE BEGINNING OF A LOVE AFFAIR WITH A NOT-EXACTLY POTATO

When I moved to the rural village of Tiwanaku in 2002 (having already lived there for three months in 2000), I lived in a house with my *compadres*. I soon learned—through experience and the grapevine—that my *comadre* was an excellent cook. I miss her soups when in the United States. She told me that sometimes others would ask her what she had to cook for me—and when she replied that I ate what everyone else did, they were surprised. Apparently, some assumed that foreigners would require, or perhaps insist on, specific kinds of foods or preparations. But given my comadre's and her daughters' culinary skills—which I tried, unsuccessfully, to learn—it is hardly shocking that I found little to be picky about.[9]

At first I did have to get used to chuño being a much larger part of the diet than it had been for me during my previous time in urban Bolivia. On these visits, which ranged from one to three months in 1993, 1994, 1998, and 1999, I lived in the capital city of La Paz with middle-class Bolivian families or other foreigners and often ate in *pensiones*. While my research in marketplaces often led me to eat market food, which included chuño, I encountered it infrequently in other parts of the city. Chuño was eaten and enjoyed throughout the highlands by Bolivians of all social and economic classes, but it was eaten far more frequently by rural highland peasants and the indigenous urban poor. Members of the urban middle and upper classes tended to eat chuño less often, although they still enjoyed it and considered it an important part of their cuisine. Among Bolivians living in the United States, for example, chuño was important for recreating a taste of home while abroad (Katherine McGurn Centellas, personal communication). My own interviews with upper-class residents of La Paz in 1994 revealed that many of them found potatoes in the United States disappointing and bland compared to their more flavorful counterparts in Bolivia; the lack of chuño was part of their observations.

There was a turning point in my relationship with chuño. My compadres had hired a tractor that fateful day in mid-November 2002 in order to plant a large piece of land. The tractor picked us up at their house near the village—my compadres, their children and other relatives, the resident anthropologist, and heavy bags of seed potatoes—for transport to their field in a nearby rural community. There were few seats on the tractor so many of us rode hanging on—I clung to the outside of the driver's door, hands slippery with forty-five-plus sunscreen to protect myself from the tropical sun at more than 13,000 feet (4,000 meters) in elevation, and holding my three-year-old goddaughter in her seat as we bounced along the uneven dirt track. A few of the men came behind on bicycles, taking some of the smaller children with them.

Reaching the field, I discovered that planting with a tractor is faster than with ox-pulled plows, but also far more intense. The religious ceremonies associated with potato planting were hurriedly performed. Four women quickly ran to plant seed potatoes in the furrows created by the tractor before it turned around at the end of the field and came back to bury what they had just planted and open new furrows for planting. *Choq' siwa*! became a constant refrain—"Potatoes, she says!" as the women demanded that the men bring them more potatoes to plant (Figure 6.1).

Women plant potatoes (although in rare instances, if no women are available, men will do so). I was clearly the slowest planter in the group, which was acceptable for planting behind an ox-plow, but not for keeping up with the pace of a tractor. So I was sent to help the men cut larger potatoes in half before planting so the seed would go farther. We did this in between rushing out to give the women more potatoes for planting, pouring the seed out from textiles wrapped around our shoulders for easier carrying. The planting was finished in a mere forty-five minutes—quite a feat for a half-hectare field.

My compadres had assumed that we would have our *fiambre* at the field and then walk the two hours back to their house. They had brought the fiambre, already cooked and wrapped in a large textile bundle. But it turned out that the tractor was going most of the way back to the village. Since there was leftover seed that would be heavy to carry, we decided to take advantage of the tractor to return. The tractor left us and the potatoes at the junction with the

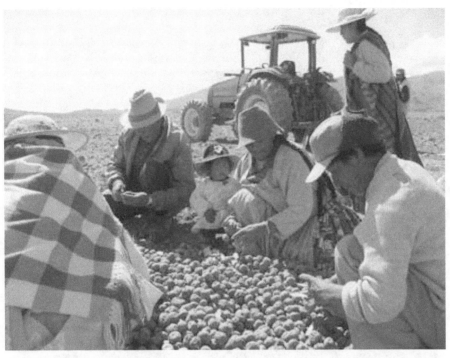

6.1. Preparing to plant potatoes on the Bolivian altiplano, November 2002. (PHOTO BY CLARE SAMMELLS)

highway, still a mile from the house. We waited for a passing public minivan to take us the remainder of the way.

Finally, back at their house, we were ready for lunch, a fiambre. Fiambres (also called *meriendas*) are meals where a common pile of food is placed on a blanket on the ground. They can include any combination of mixed tubers (potatoes of various varieties, chuño, tunta, oca, isaño, sweet potato), *fideo* (cooked pasta), rice, *mote* (maize kernels), *choclo* (maize on the cob), *quispiña* (a salty steamed *quinua* biscuit), and *postre* (boiled plantains sliced into thick circles with their skins, which are removed by the eater). During fiambres, each person is expected to eat the section closest to them in a wedge pattern, like a slice of pizza. Only fingers are used. Late in the meal the remaining food may be redistributed by one of the older women if it is clear that a particular individual is not eating as much. Allowances are made for young children who are still learning proper etiquette; small children sometimes raid preferred foods, such as sweet postre, from outside their areas. Foreigners can discretely avoid those tubers they dislike (Figure 6.2).

Fiambres can be planned events, such as when a family gathers friends, extended relatives, and "fictive kin" (such as compadres, godparents, or god-

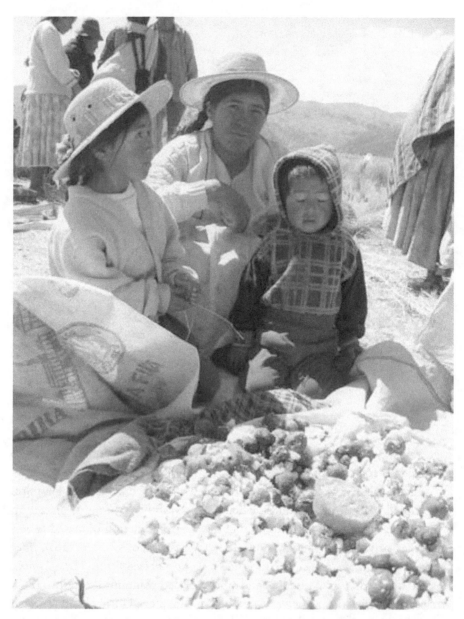

6.2. A woman and her two children dine with other family members at a *fiambre* with *chuño, papa, mote*, and a spicy sauce in the center, November 2003. (PHOTO BY CLARE SAMMELLS)

children) to help with planting, harvesting, or building a house. But they can also be more spontaneous—for example, when a group of vendors who sell in a marketplace gather at midday and collect together what each woman brought for lunch, or when unexpected relatives visit around lunchtime and soup is made to go farther by adding a blanket of tubers, sometimes brought by the visitors themselves.

During a fiambre, one woman generally gives out portions of non-staple foods to the diners to eat with the staples. These are foods with higher status and protein and fat content, including locally made "country cheese" (*queso de campo*), fried eggs, portions of cooked meat (commonly beef or mutton, but occasionally guinea pig, chicken, or more rarely high-status pork), and fried or boiled lake fish, such as carachi or ispi. Also included in this category are *tortillas* (not to be confused with Mexican *tortillas*), which consist of a dough of wheat flour, eggs, and onions fried into thick patties. These non-staple foods are categorized into one word in Aymara, *irxata*, which covers the non-staples eaten in a fiambre that give flavor to the staples.

During impromptu meals, the staples each person has brought are mixed together on a single textile on the ground. One woman may be given all the non-staples to divide between those present, or each woman may distribute what she brought herself. In fiambres that take place in the home where the cooking occurred, soup may also be served, ladled from a large pot into individual bowls. People eat from the fiambre while soup is served to each in turn. Soup is served roughly in order of status, with men, visitors, godparents, and older people served first, and women and then children last. This order is extremely flexible, however, depending on the circumstances. For example, a particularly hungry and fussy young child might be served sooner if there is the threat of a tantrum. Likewise, if one of the older men is washing his hands when the soup is being served, the women will serve others first, fitting him in when he arrives. Often there are not enough bowls for everyone, so those served first eat relatively quickly and hand the bowls back so that others can be served. No liquids other than soup are consumed until the end of the fiambre, when soda or *refresco* (a non-carbonated drink) is sometimes served, again roughly in order of status. As with bowls, there are fewer cups than people—sometimes only one—so each person quickly pours a small amount on the ground as a libation for Pachamama (the Earth Goddess), drinks, and returns the cup to be filled for the next person.

On this particular day, after our exhausting planting session, there was no soup, no plantains, no cheese. And there was no leeway for pickiness, since the blanket we gathered around was piled high with chuño with only a few fresh potatoes scattered among them. A dish of sauce was placed in the center to give the tubers flavor; it was made with chopped hard-boiled egg and *aji*, an Andean chili pepper that is commonly used to spice foods. The sauce was delicious and reminiscent of deviled eggs. My compadre had quickly bicycled into town and returned with a tin of Lydita-brand sardines in tomato sauce, which his daughter mixed with chopped onions to make a second sauce. I was very, very hungry, and I ate more chuño that day than I ever had before. My love of chuño was sealed. I now often prefer it to fresh potatoes.

CHUÑO-LESS TOURISTS

When my partner (now husband) first visited Bolivia in 2000, I wanted to share chuño with him as part of the Bolivian experience that he was signing up for. But, remarkably, he spent a week in Bolivia without ever trying chuño, despite my best attempts to put one on his plate. When he visited Tiwanaku for a day, my comadre made a local specialty for him that did not involve chuño—*pesq'e*, a quinua porridge served with milk or cheese, which he has been fond of ever since. Once traveling on the tourist circuit, we ate in places accustomed to serving foreigners in Copacabana and the Isla del Sol on Lake Titicaca. Chuño simply was not on the menu or even, as became apparent once I started asking specifically for it, in the kitchen.

Chuño was almost never offered to tourists because it was assumed they would not like it. One tourist restaurant owner in La Paz whom I spoke with in 2000 had even removed chuño from the menu because of the negative reactions of clients. This situation was not immutable, however. In my own field site, two of the restaurants began in 2004 to offer buffets to tour groups that included chuño. Neither put chuño on the individual plates ordered by tourists; it was served as a culinary curiosity rather than as a standard side dish. By 2004 some tourist-oriented restaurants in Copacabana had begun to offer chuño as well (Elayne Zorn, personal communication, 2005).

Despite the importance of chuño in the local diet, the tour books that influenced so many travelers in Bolivia often warned their readers away from experiencing it. Of course, descriptions of food in these guides are extremely brief and focus on guiding the visitor toward understanding the unfamiliar, finding the palatable, and experiencing the *típico* (a term that we can gloss in the Bolivian context as "authentic"). These books give tourists a food vocabulary that allows them to negotiate menus and advertisements, ensuring that readers know what they are getting into when confronted by unfamiliar foods.

Many of these books offered ambivalent descriptions of chuño, such as "[f]ew foreigners find them [chuño or tunta] particularly appealing, mainly because they have the appearance and consistency of polystyrene when dry and are tough and tasteless when cooked" (Swaney 1996:108; see also Swaney 1988, 2001; Swaney and Strauss 1992), or described the tubers as "gnarled looking and tasting, though some people love them" (Gorry et al. 2002; Lyon et al. 2000).[10] One even made the unusual comment that chuño "is rumored to be used by Bolivian women to suppress their husbands' sexual desires"

(Murphy 2000), a rumor I never heard elsewhere (although Coe [1994] provides evidence that this effect was attributed to the tuber isaño in the colonial period). A more generous description tells us that "these dehydrated potatoes have an unusual texture and a distinctive, nutty flavor that takes some getting used to. They're often boiled and served instead of (or as well as) fresh potatoes" (Read 2002). Descriptions are often repeated, verbatim, in reprintings of guides. Most guidebooks mentioned chuño as integral to dishes such as chairo, while others mentioned it only in passing (Cramer 1996). But none presented chuño as an integral and essential part of Bolivian cuisine that *must* be tried by the visitor.[11]

So why is it that chuño was so central to the highland Bolivian diet and yet so neglected by those trying to explain Bolivian cuisine to the foreign tourist market? Most Bolivians and North Americans seem to agree that the unfamiliar taste of chuño was the primary reason why it did not appear in Bolivian tourist cuisine—simply put, tourists did not usually like it.

I do not find this to be a complete explanation, however. Restaurants make money from what is ordered, not from what tourists discover that they like to eat. Touristic cuisine is constantly being re-presented to new diners who are at least partly willing to try unfamiliar local specialties, even if they are unconvinced they might enjoy them. Additionally, serving food to tourists is not entirely about money: most people take pride in their own region's food and want visitors to try, appreciate, and respect their cuisine.

Tourists, in short, do not single-handedly determine what they eat while traveling. They are limited, in large part, to the offerings of the establishments they visit. These establishments may be chosen by tour guides, recommended by tour books, or chosen by tourists on the basis of location, availability of menus in their language, appearance, or any number of other factors. Additionally, because of the networks of their travels, tourists often do not have the opportunity to eat in locals' homes or cook for themselves.

Touristic cuisines are predetermined by negotiations that occur on multiple levels of interlaced perceptions, such as what locals think are their tastiest dishes and those most appropriate to serve in a restaurant context; the seasonality, availability, and price of ingredients; what restaurant owners think tourists want to eat; what restaurant cooks think their employers want them to cook as well as what they think tourists want to eat; and what tourists think are the best choices available to them based on a variety of criteria (taste, freshness, exoticness, price, perceived sanitation, and the advice of tour books and guides). Tourists are sometimes served foods that they may not readily like (e.g., *poi* in Hawaii) because these foods are locally meaningful and presented as part of a local experience that tourists should participate in. But for tourists to try a particular dish, it must first and foremost be on the table.

Instead of focusing purely on taste, we must consider seriously the structures in place that reinforce chuño's neglect in tourist cuisine. In the touristic context—and every other eating context—there are different ways in which foods can be palatable. To make this point, I will compare chuño to llama meat, another Andean food I have researched (Sammells 1998, 1999; Sammells and Markowitz 1995), on three levels: the sensory experience of what is considered "good to eat," the cognitive aspects of what is "good to think" about these foods for both tourists and those who feed them, and finally what tourists find "good to relate" about their dining experiences once they return home.

Despite emphasis on the touristic search for the "authentic," the fact that some foods are locally produced or consumed is not sufficient to make them "good to think" or "good to relate" for visitors. Both chuño and llama meat were local to Bolivia. Both foods are indigenous to the pre-Columbian Andean highlands, currently produced locally, and served in few places outside the Andes. Llama was consumed less than other "non-native" (but still locally produced) meats, such as beef and mutton. Chuño, on the other hand, was ubiquitous. Nevertheless (and perhaps because of this discrepancy), llama garnered touristic attention in ways that chuño did not.

Since 1997, llama meat became an important authentic highland Bolivian dish served to tourists (Sammells 1999), even though many Bolivians (especially urban Bolivians) ate llama on rare occasions, if at all. This situation might seem counterintuitive. Llama meat was more highly marked as a food of the poor (especially the rural indigenous poor) than chuño. Despite the prejudices against its consumption, it underwent an incredible transformation into a meat lauded by expensive tourist-oriented restaurants.

Why has llama meat become widely popular in tourist cuisine since 1997, even though chuño—which was more widely consumed throughout Bolivian society than llama meat—has not? Llama captured the imagination in multiple ways. As a live animal it was depicted and photographed everywhere, appearing on tourist postcards as well as the Bolivian coat of arms. As meat it made a tasty dish lauded for its low fat and high protein. It was "good to eat" in that it was similar to red meats that North Atlantic visitors were familiar with. It was also "good to think" because of the position of llamas in both Bolivian cultures and touristic imaginaries. And llama meat was "good to relate" once tourists returned home to share tales of their culinary adventures in places where llamas were exotic animals and potatoes were boringly quotidian.

GOOD TO EAT

We should start with Mintz's (1996:93) warnings about ignoring the experiential aspects of food. We cannot ignore that tourists are seeking something that is "good to eat" within a cuisine that has both familiar and unfamiliar elements. The amount of space in tour books and other tourist literatures dedicated to describing, explaining, and promoting food and the large proportion of tourist budgets spent on dining indicate how important eating is to travelers' overall experiences.

In this respect, llama meat was "good to eat." While it is a common joke in the United States that all unknown meats "taste like chicken," llama actually tastes like beef or mutton—so much so, in fact, that stories abounded of llama being added clandestinely to street food, sausages, and hamburgers (Sammells 1998). As a steak, llama meat is slightly paler in color but similar in taste to other red meats. For a North Atlantic tourist, and even for many Bolivians, the difference would be difficult to detect. For tourists who like beef, llama tastes familiar.

In contrast, chuño could never be substituted secretly for potatoes. It is a completely different sensory experience from a potato in both taste and texture. In highland Bolivian cuisine, where tubers are eaten at least twice a day, these differences among fresh potatoes, chuño, tunta, oca, isaño, *papaliza, remolacha*, and other tubers are prized and relished. But what made chuño prized among Bolivians—the fact that it does not taste like a potato—was what made it difficult for some foreigners to appreciate. Tourists who were in Bolivia for a relatively short time might not become accustomed to the taste or texture of chuño.

GOOD TO THINK

Foods are not just "good (or not) to eat" but also "good to think," as famously stated by structural anthropologist Claude Levi-Strauss. The understanding that foods have social meanings beyond the purely nutritional, and that these meanings interact with social structures in other parts of society, has been elegantly demonstrated by Levi-Strauss (1963, 1969, 1978 [1968]) and Mary Douglas (1966, 1972, 1983 [1977]). Tambiah's work on food and incest taboos (1969) showed how animals can have related meanings in the realms of sex and edibility. All these authors discuss how foods are eaten or avoided for reasons that are not entirely based on how they taste. Food is part of a coherent system of meanings, interwoven with the other ways that people make sense of their lives and relationships.

Llama is "good to think" for tourists in part because it is a meat and therefore forms the centerpiece of meals where it is included. The now-outdated airline-food joke "chicken or beef?" highlights the emphasis we put on meat as the identifying feature of a meal, the key item on which decisions of edibility and preference depend. To give an example that may be familiar to some readers, in

U.S. holiday meals such as Thanksgiving, the turkey is an essential part of the meal. Even vegetarians are pressured to replace it with something turkey-like, such as tofurky. Other Thanksgiving dishes can be modified or substituted to suit individual taste or preserve ethnic traditions; one can serve either corn or wheat bread, baked or sweet potatoes, pumpkin pie or English trifle. Even in quotidian meals, staple foods—the everyday carbohydrates that make up our daily bread, such as wheat, maize, rice, manioc, millet, and potatoes—tend to play second fiddle to the more glamorous meats that flavor them.

This explains why meats are the focus of more food taboos than vegetables or grains (Douglas 1966; Fiddes 1991).[12] When Americans think about strange food experiences, they often focus on meats. They tend to be easily disturbed by meat products and the processes (especially industrialized ones) that create them (Sinclair 1906). I am not immune from this cultural bias. I, like many of my fellow Americans, was unaccustomed to consuming organ meats and preferred muscle; offering delicacies such as sheep's head to me was a source of mirth for Bolivians who found it amusing to watch me squirm (although I did eat it the first time). This focus on meat as potentially more upsetting to travelers often sidelines the importance of staples. In this sense, chuño is less "good to think" for tourists, who are more likely to choose their meals on the basis of the meat rather than the side dishes served with it.

Of course, llama was "good to think" for tourists precisely because it was unfamiliar to them. Llama had pseudo-pet status in the North Atlantic (similar to horses), and some North Americans reacted to the idea of eating it with pseudo-cannibalistic horror. My thoughts on this are informed by the reactions I received from U.S. residents when describing my undergraduate thesis research on the consumption of llama meat in La Paz (Sammells 1998). This topic quickly broke the ice at any party. Many would ask if llama meat tasted like horse meat—not because they had eaten either animal but because the two animals had similar social positions in the United States as four-legged luxury pets. (As I have not tried horse meat, I am forced to make more mundane comparisons.) Interviews I conducted with U.S. llama herders indicated they had mixed feelings about the possibility of consuming the animals. One who did occasionally slaughter camelids asked not to be identified for fear of negative reactions from peers. This concern was not misplaced; the editors of a U.S.-based llama magazine sent me a nasty letter rejecting a short article I wrote for them on the topic of eating llamas in Bolivia, even though I had first queried and they had indicated their interest. Clearly the topic was a sensitive one for the editors.

Llama meat may be transgressive for tourists, but urban Bolivians avoided eating it for completely different reasons. Middle- and upper-class residents of La Paz (whom I interviewed in 1993–1994) assumed that llama was something eaten by poor, rural, and indigenous peoples. They avoided llama meat and even places that served it—although few establishments did.[13] Llama meat was nevertheless sold in large quantities in the street markets of La Paz, where it quietly found its way into ground-meat products. Urban La Paz residents often denounced cheap, no-brand processed meats sold in street markets—sausages, hamburgers, and the like—as being made of llama or even stray dog. Stories abounded about cheap locales that would surreptitiously serve llama instead of beef to unsuspecting customers. Many that I spoke with believed that despite their best attempts to avoid it, they might have consumed llama unknowingly. Others were convinced that they had eaten llama disguised as beef, only later realizing the truth. These stories invariably placed suspicion on meals eaten while traveling in rural areas or on street food.

Despite these prejudices on the part of some urban Bolivians, llama meat had become integral to Bolivian touristic cuisine by 1997. Peña Huari in La Paz began offering llama meat to tourists and the local upper class in 1997—one of the first restaurants to successfully do so.[14] Located on Sagarnaga Street in the center of the tourist district, an area that sported colorful artisan stalls, tour operators, and backpacker hotels, the restaurant offered a nightly two-hour *peña* show of folkloric dances and music from all regions of Bolivia. The restaurant's walls and tables were decorated with masks, ceramics, and other contemporary Bolivian art, all of which the menu declared to be for sale. Llama meat was first on the list of house specialties on what was, by Bolivian standards, a very pricey menu. The owner, who was from the city of Oruro (where llama meat was more accepted restaurant fare than in La Paz), estimated in 1999 that 65 percent of his foreign clients ordered llama rather than beef, lamb, chicken, or Lake Titicaca trout.[15]

In the rural touristic village of Tiwanaku, home to that nation's most important archaeological site, llama meat had entered the menus of several tourist restaurants by 2002. Ironically, while urban La Paz residents often associated llama meat with rural cuisine, in this particular part of the altiplano there were few llamas—thus the meat was imported from La Paz to be served to tourists. Locals in my field site almost never ate llama meat themselves, although they valued it. For these Aymara people, eating llama meat was associated with strength. One man correlated the success of a neighboring village's soccer team with the fact that they had large llama herds and thus ate the meat frequently.

Despite the taboo against their meat among some, llamas have long been an undisputed symbol of Andean authenticity. Llamas appeared on the Bolivian national emblem and on many of the national currencies. This was neither contradictory nor coincidental. Trouillot (1991) has provided us with the useful concept of the "savage slot": while the content of the meanings attached to "othered" concepts and objects—and foods—may change, their position of alterity does not.[16] It was precisely because the llama was so marked—that is, as a rural and indigenous animal, to the point where it was even questionably edible to some Bolivians—that it also became a national symbol and useful as a representation of a national cuisine to present to outsiders.

Despite llamas' symbolic importance, consumption of llama meat had declined precipitously since the colonial era, corresponding to similar declines in the consumption of other native foods. Today rural Aymara purchase imported and processed foods, such as cooking oil, rice, bread, and cookies, and often view the cuisine of the past with nostalgia. Many in Tiwanaku agreed that their ancestors' better health and longer life spans were the result of eating llama and other traditional foods, including chuño. *Quinua, cañahua, p'itu,*[17] and other native grains are now eaten far less often than bread, pasta, and heavily sugared *mates* (herbal infusions). Rural Bolivians told me that their current dietary patterns were less healthy. They and their children consumed far more sugar, pasta, and bread than their grandparents, which had a negative impact on their health, strength, and life expectancy. The increasing incorporation of Western-style foods into rural Bolivian cuisine and an accompanying decrease in nutrition have been noted in rural Bolivia and elsewhere in the Andes (Orlove 1987; Weismantel 1988). Llama and guinea pig are now far less common in the highland cuisine than mutton and beef (although individual diets depend on the region, and there are areas where llamas are still the dominant meat source).

Llama meat is generally higher in protein and lower in fat than beef or mutton, however, and the animal is less damaging to the highland environment. This motivated several groups to make efforts to promote its consumption both within Bolivia and as a foreign export in the hopes that this would result in increased incomes for llama herders, better nutrition for the rural and urban Bolivian poor, and less damage to the environment (McCorkle 1990; Sammells and Markowitz 1995; Valdivia 1992). At the same time, there is a small but growing movement by Bolivians to promote llama as both a healthier meat and a source of national pride.

In short, llama meat is local and "authentic." It is neglected, yet available; promoted as both traditional and healthy for the future, but under-consumed in the present. MacCannell (1976) observed that tourists often take particular interest in things perceived to be part of the disappearing, premodern world. While Andean peoples are not premodern in any sense, tourist literature tends to present them as both descendents and members of ancient Andean cultures, always on the brink of suffering the consequences of incorporation into a global capitalist economy. (In reality, Andeans have been participating in that system for centuries.) The llama, as the animal most closely associated with this pre-Columbian past and the indigenous present, therefore takes on special meaning in these touristic narratives.

There are many accounts of locally denigrated foods becoming part of national cuisines or touristic fare (e.g., Wilk 1999, 2006). Llama meat's transformation from undesirable meat to authentic Bolivian cuisine is not at all surprising. Its clear association with the poor and indigenous was exactly what made it interesting to tourists—it served as a truly authentic representation of the "indigenous culture" that many came to highland Bolivia to see. In the touristic imagination, "Bolivianess" is intimately connected to indigenousness, with representations of Bolivians ranging from the "real" indigenous people who line the market streets of the city (who, despite being touristic attractions, receive little benefit from this industry) to those who play and dance to folkloric music at peñas.

In contrast to llama meat, potatoes and chuño are staples for all highland Bolivians (albeit in different proportions). Because chuño is eaten by all social classes, it was never clearly associated with only the poor or indigenous. Thus, it never became emblematic of "Bolivianess" (meaning, indigenous Bolivian) in the touristic imaginary in quite the same way. Chuño was part of an only loosely hierarchical arrangement of staples (in order from lowest ranked to highest ranked, chuño, *tunta*, potato, rice). However, this hierarchy was not stable; certain dishes and contexts required specific staples and granted them higher values. Chuño was not marked enough to keep on tourist plates and therefore was easily replaced with higher-status staples more familiar to tourists and more appropriate to their economic status in the Bolivian context. This suggests a self-reinforcing effect. Those who wrote tour books and marketing brochures did not write about chuño (or said little that was positive or interesting about it), perhaps in part because it was not offered. Thus, tourists who visited Bolivia did not think to seek it out.

GOOD TO RELATE

I argue that there is another reason why chuño has not been fully incorporated into Bolivian touristic cuisine. Chuño was also not "good to relate" in the sense that the tuber did not serve as an emblematic marker of travels in Bolivia specifically. In North Atlantic countries, the potato is a quotidian part of diets and national histories. It is common knowledge that the potato's nutritional and agricultural qualities led it to be adopted as a staple peasant food and later incorporated into several national cuisines (Salaman 1949). Whether we consider the spread of McDonald's French fries or the devastation of the Irish Potato Famine, the potato has been omnipresent in North Atlantic history for more than two centuries. Tourists were often told about the incredible variety of potatoes in the highlands but were less well-informed about the extraordinary qualities of chuño.

Potatoes are integral to the diet of the "modern" world and thus are generally ignored in the touristic imaginary. The potato is not disappearing—on the contrary, it is an important part of North Atlantic diets. The potato is Andean, but mentioning this fact in touristic marketing does little to distinguish "local" cuisine from what North Atlantic tourists believe they have already experienced. The chuño was not "good to think" or "good to relate" because tourists categorized it as a kind of potato—which, as I have argued, it is not.

Llama meat, in contrast, was "good to relate" for a number of reasons. When tourists talk about their experiences after returning home, their audiences probably know what a llama is but have rarely eaten one—if the idea has occurred to them at all. Eating llama has a certain shock value that adds to the value of the tourist's tale. For North Americans, eating llama was transgressive, much like the tales of eating guinea pig discussed by Goldstein (this volume). That made such tales all the more captivating.

Eating while traveling—whether as a tourist or an anthropologist—is not only about eating what is familiar. Travelers generally want to experience foods with unfamiliar tastes that will be interesting to talk about later. The popularity of cooking magazines and TV shows like *Iron Chef* demonstrates that we love to read about, hear about, and watch others eat unusual things, even when we are not in a position to replicate the dishes we see or even imagine what they taste like. In fact, this is one of the premises that underlies this book. Nothing I write here will allow you to taste chuño or any of the other foods described by my coauthors. Nevertheless, here we are—we as authors trying to create a taste in your mouth that we often cannot even recreate in our own kitchens at home, and you as readers trying to imagine these dishes and wondering if you can trust our assertions that you might like them.

TOURISTIC CUISINES

This comparison of llama meat and chuño brings me to my final point, one that I think can be expanded to an examination of touristic cuisines more generally. Bolivian touristic cuisine—meaning, the cuisine served to tourists in Bolivia—is not a watered-down, bland version of local food. Nor is it an attempt to cater to North Atlantic desires for McDonald's (which is itself not a uniform monolith; see Watson 1997) or other familiar dishes. Touristic cuisines have their own logics, ingredients, spices, styles of presentation, and dining contexts that derive from the cultural situations in which these dishes are cooked and served—specifically, the structured interactions between locals and visitors within a touristic context. The status that foods have within both Bolivian and North Atlantic societies entered into the cuisine that one prepared for the other, and ingredients and dishes were transformed by a distinct culinary logic that emerged from a touristic encounter fraught with inequalities and anxieties as well as steeped in cosmopolitan sophistication and entrepreneurial acumen.

Bolivian touristic cuisine is certainly different from the highland Bolivian cuisine typically consumed by locals. This is true of touristic cuisine in most places—the claim may be made that it is authentic, *tipico*, or local, but what is served in tourist restaurants is usually not the same as what people cook in their own homes. Some travelers might see this as an obstacle to be overcome in the search for the "real" or the "authentic." Some anthropologists might even consider their knowledge of local home cooking to be part of what separates them from tourists (Crick 1995). I prefer to see this division as part of regional culinary diversity; in other words, touristic cuisine is one part of the diverse culinary knowledges and practices that make up local cuisines rather than one that is external to them.

There is a long debate on how to best define the word "tourist" (for examples, see Boorstin 1961; Chambers 2000; MacCannell 1976; Nash 1996; Smith 1989 [1977]; Urry 1990). Any universal definition of this term is inherently unsatisfying precisely because this word takes on meaning through specific local interactions. These encounters are not limited to "host and guests" but include infrastructures that facilitate exchanges of currencies, images, goods, literatures, and services. An important part of these interactions is culinary.

In the context of Bolivian touristic cuisine, restaurants catered to a clientele that was not only foreign but also seen as upper-class. The word *turista*—which did not apply to all leisure travelers within that nation—carried the connotations of a short-term, foreign visitor (usually European, U.S., or Canadian but also those seen as racially "white" from other nations, including Latin America). This term also had class connotations, as turistas had substantial economic resources compared to most Bolivians (Sammells 2009:84–97). In this context, where turistas were not defined solely by the activity of travel but also by their race, nationality, and economic position, llama and chuño acquired very different meanings.

Thus, llama meat served with rice, a common dish in Bolivian touristic cuisine, combines ingredients with different class associations for Bolivians into a tourist cuisine with its own culinary logic. Llama is presented proudly as the truly Andean, quietly accompanied by rice and perhaps potatoes, both higher-status staples. Chuño and tunta generally go unmentioned and unserved in this context.

So, if you go to Bolivia, try the chuño. But wherever you go, recognize that it is not just your head and heart entering into a relationship with the people you visit, but also your stomach.

Acknowledgments. My deep thanks to Helen Haines and my fellow contributors to this volume, who gave many helpful suggestions, feedback, and food for thought. Conversations with members of the Gringo Tambo, including Maria Bruno, Stephen Scott, and Katherine McGurn Centellas, and comments specifically on this paper from Alison Kohn have been indispensable. I also thank Michel-Rolph Trouillot, Alan Kolata, Manuela Carneiro da Cunha, and John Kelly for their support and comments. I thank my compadres Paulina and Anaclo for making sure I was so well fed in Bolivia and for all the wonderful conversations we had in their kitchen. This research was supported by the Fulbright-Hays Doctoral Dissertation Research Abroad Program, the Tinker Foundation, the Orin Williams Fund, and the University of Chicago Center for Latin American Studies.

NOTES

1. By "American" I mean people from the United States of America. It is a misnomer, since "American" should rightly apply to people from the entire hemisphere. But this term is far more elegant in English, which lacks an alternative word such as *estadounidense* to describe those from the United States more specifically. My apologies to those who might be offended.

2. For example, I strongly dislike olives. This is a matter of some amusement among my friends.

3. I should note that *chuño* was the word applied to the raw product by Aymara speakers. If cooked and served whole (such as a side to a meal, or in a *fiambre*), it was referred to as *phuti* (also written *p'uti*). Phuti also referred to cooked *tunta*. In this essay, I will use the term "chuño" to refer to both the raw and the cooked product for the simplicity of those readers who do not speak Aymara and also to distinguish it from tunta.

4. I kept a detailed food diary for twelve months while conducting dissertation research. The one-third figure includes midday and dinner meals in Tiwanaku but excludes *tecito*, which usually consisted of only a hot drink and bread and was served twice a day, at breakfast and in the early evening.

5. In rural areas, the exact proportions of consumption of each staple depended on the climate and agriculture of the region. Regions that grow maize or *quinua* will obviously consume more of those grains. This paper shows my own bias in having done research in La Paz and Tiwanaku, but I recognize that cuisine can change radically even over short distances. For example, communities on Lake Titicaca eat far more lake fish and have a microclimate conducive to growing maize, whereas Tiwanaku, a mere ten miles (seventeen kilometers) from the lake, grows little maize, and residents tend to eat fish only on Sundays when it is sold at the weekly market.

6. One particular type of potato, *pitikilla*, was actually more delicious when it had worms. The worms were not eaten—they were removed while eating—but as a result of the worms, the potato's flavor resembled that of chestnuts. It was generally agreed that while the worms are troublesome to remove, the flavor was superior.

7. Informants in Tiwanaku often found it strange that although Chicago was colder in the winter than the altiplano and Chicagoans ate potatoes, no one made chuño. My description of bitter cold even during the day, high snowbanks, and short daylight hours seemed odd to them indeed (as did my description of the long daylight hours of summer). When I brought them a photograph of a Hyde Park, Chicago, street in winter, they were as interested in the parked cars lining the street—a clear sign of widespread wealth—as in the thick layer of snow covering them.

8. A *compadre* is a "fictive kin" relationship where two unrelated individuals are linked through one being the godparent—for the baptism, wedding, high-school graduation, or other kind of sponsorship—of the other's child. I had a number of *compadres* in Tiwanaku.

9. Again, this is not to claim that I ate everything with equal relish. I did try everything, but it quickly became clear to those who knew me well that there were certain dishes I was less fond of. My *comadre* did not insist I eat these things, because that meant there was more for everyone else. Fried liver (fresh from a slaughtered sheep) was a particular treat that I ate conspicuously less of than everyone else, but the children were happy to divide up whatever I did not want.

10. The 2002 edition of Lonely Planet's *South America on a Shoestring* displayed on its cover a photo of two of the artisans of Tiwanaku, Bolivia, playing soccer. When I contacted the publisher, they sent a complementary copy of the book for each of them.

11. Compare written guides' treatment of chuño to that paid to *salteñas*, a meat-filled pastry, which almost always received high praise and a detailed description.

12. I do not wish to suggest that all food taboos involve meats. In Bolivia, there were food taboos involving non-meat foods in particular contexts, such as in the diets of postpartum women.

13. No La Paz establishments offered llama meat openly during that time, although in the city of Oruro dishes made of llama meat, such as *charquekan*, were sold as specialties and very popular.

14. In addition to Peña Huari, another La Paz restaurant aimed at tourists also began serving llama meat around this time, although it had closed by 1998.

15. Trout from Lake Titicaca was another mainstay of Bolivian touristic cuisine that was rarely eaten by Bolivians, who tended to consume smaller native species of fish. The trout are not native to the region and were often farmed.

16. In fact, from the perspective of North Atlantic nations, Bolivia itself could be seen as squarely within the "savage slot"—as an underdeveloped, poor, "Third World" nation—or, as postcards and tourist brochures declared, as the "Folklore Capital of South America" that drew foreigners to see its vibrant indigenous culture and unspoiled natural landscapes.

17. *P'itu* is a preparation that can be made from *quinua*, *cañahua*, wheat, or fava beans. It involves toasting the grains and then grinding them into a powder. The powder is then served in a bowl with a mug of a sugared hot drink (usually an herbal tea). The drink is poured into the powder and then mixed to form a porridge. This was usually served for breakfast but has been largely replaced with bread. When made more watery, p'itu can also be served as a *refresco*, or beverage. P'itu falls somewhere between a food and a drink.

REFERENCES

Boorstin, Daniel J.
  1961   *The Image: A Guide to Pseudo-Events in America*. Vintage Books, New York.

Chambers, Erve
  2000   *Native Tours: The Anthropology of Travel and Tourism*. Waveland Press, Prospect Heights, IL.

Coe, Sophie D.
  1994   *America's First Cuisines*. University of Texas Press, Austin.

Condori Cruz, Dionisio
  1992   Tecnología del chuño. *Boletín del IDEA* (Puno, Peru) 2:70–97.

Cramer, Mark
  1996   *Culture Shock! Bolivia: A Guide to Customs and Etiquette*. Graphic Arts Center Publishing Company, Portland, OR.

Crick, Malcolm
  1995   The Anthropologist as Tourist: An Identity in Question. In *International Tourism: Identity and Change*, ed. Marie-Françoise Lanfant, John B. Allcock, and Edward M. Bruner, 205–223. Sage Publications, London.

D'Altroy, Terence N.
  2002   *The Incas*. Blackwell Publishing, Malden, MA.

Douglas, Mary
  1966   *Purity and Danger*. Routledge, London.
  1972   Deciphering a Meal. *Daedalus* 101:61–81.
  1983   Culture and Food. In *The Pleasures of Anthropology*, ed. Morris Freilich,
  [1977] 74–102. Mentor, New York, and Scarborough, Ontario.

Fiddes, Nick
  1991   *Meat: A Natural Symbol*. Routledge, London.

Gorry, C., F. Adams, S. Boa, V. Boone, K. Dydynski, P. Hellander, C. Hubbard, J. Noble, D. Palmerlee, and R. Rachowiecki (editors)
  2002   *South America on a Shoestring*. Lonely Planet Publications, Melbourne.

Kolata, Alan L.
  1993   *The Tiwanaku: Portrait of an Andean Civilization*. Blackwell Publishers, Cambridge, MA.

Kolata, Alan L. (editor)
  1996   *Tiwanaku and Its Hinterland: Archaeology and Paleoecology of an Andean Civilization*. Smithsonian Institution Press, Washington, DC.

La Barre, Weston
  1947   Potato Taxonomy among the Aymara Indians of Bolivia. *Acta Americana: Review of the Inter-American Society of Anthropology and Geography* 5:83–103.

Levi-Strauss, Claude

1963   *Totemism*. Beacon Press, Boston.

1969   *The Raw and the Cooked: Introduction to a Science of Mythology*, Vol. 1. Harper and Row Publishers, New York.

1978   *The Origin of Table Manners: Mythologiques*, Vol. 3. Harper and Row Pub-
[1968] lishers, New York.

Lyon, James, Wayne Bernhardson, Robyn Jones, Andrew Draffen, Leonardo Pinheiro, Krzysztof Dydynski, Maria Massolo, Conner Gorry, and Mark Plotkin (editors)

2000   *South America on a Shoestring*. Lonely Planet, Melbourne.

MacCannell, Dean

1976   *The Tourist: A New Theory of the Leisure Class*. Schocken Books, New York.

Mamani, Mauricio

1981   El Chuño: Preparación, Uso Almacenamiento. In *La Tecnologia en el Mundo Andino: Runakunap Kawsayninkupaq Rurasqankunaqa*, ed. H. Lechtman and A. M. Soldi, 235–246. Universidad Nacional Autonoma de Mexico, Mexico D.F.

Mangan, Jane E.

2005   *Trading Roles: Gender, Ethnicity, and the Urban Economy in Colonial Potosí*. Duke University Press, Durham.

McCorkle, Constance M. (editor)

1990   *Improving Andean Sheep and Alpaca Production: Recommendations from a Decade of Research in Peru*. University of Missouri–Columbia Printing Services, Columbia.

Messer, Ellen

1997   Three Centuries of Changing European Tastes for the Potato. In *Food Preference and Taste: Continuity and Change*, ed. H. Macbeth. Berghahn Books, Oxford.

Mintz, Sidney W.

1996   *Tasting Food, Tasting Freedom: Excursions into Eating, Culture, and the Past*. Beacon Press Books, Boston.

Murphy, Alan

2000   *Footprint Bolivia Handbook*. Footprint Handbooks, Bath, UK.

Nash, Dennison

1996   *Anthropology of Tourism*. Elsevier Science, Oxford.

Orlove, Benjamin S.

1987   Stability and Change in Highland Andean Dietary Patterns. In *Food and Evolution: Toward a Theory of Human Food Habits*, ed. M. Harris and E. B. Ross. Temple University Press, Philadelphia.

Read, James
    2002   *The Rough Guide to Bolivia*. Rough Guides, London.

Salaman, Redcliffe N.
    1949   *The History and Social Influence of the Potato*. Cambridge University Press, Cambridge.

Sammells, Clare A.
    1998   Folklore, Food, and Seeking National Identity: Urban Legends of Llama Meat in La Paz, Bolivia. *Contemporary Legend* 1:21–54.
    1999   Making the World "Authentic" for Tourists: The Transformation of Llama Meat into Bolivian Food. Master's thesis. Department of Anthropology, University of Chicago, Chicago.
    2009   Touristic Narratives and Historical Networks: Politics and Authority in Tiwanaku, Bolivia. Ph.D. dissertation. Department of Anthropology, University of Chicago, Chicago.

Sammells, Clare A., and Lisa Markowitz
    1995   La carne de llama: Alta viabilidad, baja visibilidad. In *Waira Pampa: Un sistema pastoril camélidos-ovinos del altiplano árido boliviano*, ed. D. Genin, H.-J. Picht, R. Lizarazu, and T. Rodriguez. ORSTOM/IBTA, La Paz.

Sinclair, Upton
    1906   *The Jungle*. Grosset and Dunlap, New York.

Smith, Valene L. (editor)
    1989   *Hosts and Guests: The Anthropology of Tourism*, 2nd ed. University of
    [1977]   Pennsylvania Press, Philadelphia.

Swaney, Deanna
    1988   *Lonely Planet Bolivia: A Travel Survival Kit*. Lonely Planet Publications, South Yarra, Australia.
    1996   *Bolivia: A Lonely Planet Travel Survival Kit*. SNP Printing, Singapore.
    2001   *Lonely Planet Bolivia*. Lonely Planet Publications, Footscray, Australia.

Swaney, Deanna, and Robert Strauss
    1992   *Lonely Planet Bolivia: A Travel Survival Kit*. Lonely Planet Publications, Hawthorn, Australia.

Tambiah, S. J.
    1969   Animals Are Good to Think and Good to Prohibit. *Ethnology* 8(4):423–459.

Trouillot, Michel-Rolph
    1991   Anthropology and the Savage Slot: The Poetics and Politics of Otherness. In *Recapturing Anthropology: Working in the Present,* ed. R. G. Fox. School of American Research Press, Santa Fe, NM.

Urry, John
    1990   *The Tourist Gaze: Leisure and Travel in Contemporary Societies*. Sage Publications, London.

Valdivia, Corinne (editor)

    1992   *Sustainable Crop-Livestock Systems for the Bolivian Highlands: Proceedings of an SR-CRSP Workshop.* University of Missouri–Columbia Printing Services, Columbia.

Walvin, James

    1997   *Fruits of Empire: Exotic Produce and British Taste, 1660–1800.* New York University Press, Washington Square, New York.

Watson, James L. (editor)

    1997   *Golden Arches East: McDonald's in East Asia.* Stanford University Press, Stanford, CA.

Weismantel, Mary J.

    1988   *Food, Gender, and Poverty in the Ecuadorian Andes.* University of Pennsylvania Press, Philadelphia.

Wilk, Richard R.

    1999   "Real Belizean Food": Building Local Identity in the Transnational Caribbean. *American Anthropologist* 101:244–255.

    2006   *Home Cooking in the Global Village: Caribbean Food from Buccaneers to Ecotourists.* Berg, Oxford.

Zuckerman, Larry

    1998   *The Potato: How the Humble Spud Rescued the Western World.* North Point Press, New York.

Discussion Questions: Ode to a Chuño: Learning to Love Freeze-Dried Potatoes in Highland Bolivia

1. What is *chuño* and how is it made and consumed?
2. How are potatoes and *chuño* different in Andean cuisine? How are potatoes of the Andes and those consumed in the US and Europe different?
3. Why must one participate in the production of food to understand its meaning?
4. What are *fiambres* and how is food culture of the Andes illustrated with a *fiambres*?
5. Why do llamas feature prominently in Andes and how have tourists become associated with llamas?

Caribbean Food Plants

LAURA B. ROBERTS-NKRUMAH

The Caribbean is a relatively small region with a wide range of native food plants, several of which have become important staples and agricultural commodities internationally. This chapter provides an overview of the genetic heritage of food plants that were used by the first peoples of the Caribbean and the factors that resulted in the change to their status that started with European colonization. The current status and nutritional value of these crops, as well as the main dishes in which they are utilized, are described. The implications of neglect of this aspect of the Caribbean heritage are discussed within the context of food and nutrition security for the region.

Introduction

The Caribbean consists of an archipelago of islands extending from the Bahamas in the north, at 24° 5′ north, 76° west, to Trinidad in the south, at 11° north, 61° west. In spite of the dominating effect of the sea on the climate within this small tropical space, several different microclimates and a range of vegetation exist. The biodiversity of this flora has provided the region with many plant species suitable for human food; this variety was extended further by domesticated crop species introduced from Mexico and Central and South America by the early peoples who migrated from these circum-Caribbean areas to the Caribbean. This chapter focuses on indigenous food crops and those introduced through such migrations, mainly in the pre-Columbian era, as a genetic resource that is an integral aspect of Caribbean heritage. The status of their contribution to the food supply in the region from pre-Colombian times is outlined, and some important historical factors that influence current

179

levels of production and consumption are described. Finally, the relationship between the status of our food plant resources and of food security and human health within the region is discussed.

Food plants comprise a very valuable component of the genetic diversity of the flora of the Caribbean, both in terms of the number of genera and the number of species and intra-specific variations. Many of these food plants originated and were domesticated in different parts of this archipelago, while others were imported by the earliest peoples of the region (table 17.1). These plants, some of which were already being cultivated as crops before Europeans' arrival, constitute a significant food resource through their nutritional content, representation in every major food group, and suitability for a wide range of food uses in Caribbean cuisine as they include starchy crops, legumes, vegetables, fruits, industrial crops that are consumed only as processed products, beverage crops, and condiments and spices. The discussion that follows considers the status of these crops and the extent to which their food potential has been recognized and developed in the course of the region's history, and the implications for its food and nutrition security.

Historical Status of Indigenous Food Crops

Pre-Columbian Status

During the Archaic period, which extended from 5000 to 200 BCE, the first migrants and earliest Caribbean peoples, the Ortoroids and Casimiroids, though primarily hunter-gatherers, practised some forms of cultivation (Keegan 2000). Archaeological evidence exists that maize (*Zea mays*), manioc or cassava (*Manihot esculenta*), sweet potato (*Ipomoea batatas*) and beans (*Phaseolus* spp.) were processed (Pagán Jiménez and Rodríguez Ramos 2007; Reid 2009). The later Saladoid peoples, so named for their pottery with its characteristic red and white markings, migrated downstream along the banks of the Orinoco River in Venezuela and from the coastal areas of the Guianas, moving northward through the Lesser Antilles as far as Puerto Rico. They established inland riverine settlements and extensive gardens from which they harvested manioc, their main staple, and other crops. Remnants of griddles suggest that they processed the cassava (Keegan 2000). Cassava was important in the diet as a major source of carbohydrates for energy. Since its protein content is low, they relied on animals for that nutrient; they migrated to coastal areas and utilized marine animals when the terrestrial sources were depleted.

Table 17.1 Caribbean Food Plants: Nutritional Composition and Use

Names (Common, Scientific and Botanical Family); Origin[*]	Major Nutrients/100 g[**]	Major Dishes[***]
CEREAL CROPS Maize/corn (*Zea mays*, Graminaceae); origin: Mexico	Cornmeal – 353 kcal, carb. – 71.5 g, protein – 9.3 g, DF3 – 11 g	Boiled or roasted cobs, cornmeal porridge, dumplings, coo-coo, fungi, arepas, pastelles, jug-jug
ROOT CROPS Cassava/manioc/yuca (*Manihot esculenta*, Euphorbiceae); origin: Mexico and Central America (CA)	Fresh root, cooked – 120 kcal; carb.2 – 27g; potassium 690 mg	Farine, porridge, cassava bread/bammie, pone, cassareep
Sweet potato (*Ipomoea batatas*, Convulvulaceae); origin: Tropical America (TA)	Fresh tuber, cooked[3] – 103 kcal; carb. – 24.3 g; vitamin A – 2182 RE4	Pudding, pone, baked sweet potatoes, ingredient in soups, chips
Yams – Cush-cush (*Dioscorea. trifida*, Dioscoreaceae); origin: Northern SA	Fresh root, cooked – 116 kcal; carb. – 27.6 g; potassium – 670 mg	Roasted yam, grilled yam, ingredient in soups, riced yams, yam balls, foofoo, salad, pie
Tannia, yautia, cocoyam (*Xanthosoma sagittifolium*, Araceae); origin: TA.	Fresh root, raw – 133 kcal; carb. – 31 g	Fritters, pudding, riced, grilled or fried tannia, pie, ingredient in soups, salad
Arrowroot (*Maranta arundinacea*, Marantaceae); origin: Northern SA, Lesser Antilles	Flour – 340 kcal; carb. – 85 g	Porridge, blancmange, thickening agent in sauces, soups, ice cream
Topi tambu/lleren (*Calathea allouia*, Marantaceae); origin: West Indies and Northern SA		Boiled tubers served with a savoury dip, curried topi tambu, salad, ingredient in soup
LEGUMES Ground nuts, peanuts (*Arachis hypogaea*, Leguminosae); Origin: SA.	Raw seeds with skin, dried – 567 kcal; fat – 49.2 g; carb. – 16.2 g; protein – 25.7 g; potassium – 717 mg; niacin – 13.8 mg	Roasted nuts salted or unsalted, nut cake or peanut brittle, peanut punch

Table 17.1 continues

Table 17.1 Caribbean Food Plants: Nutritional Composition and Use (*cont'd*)

Names (Common, Scientific and Botanical Family); Origin[*]	Major Nutrients/100 g[**]	Major Dishes[***]
LEGUMES (*cont'd*) Common beans, red/kidney beans, black beans (*Phaseolus vulgaris*, Leguminosae); Lima beans (*P. lunatus*, Leguminosae); origin: Mexico and CA	Red/kidney beans whole seeds, dry, raw – 337 kcal; carb. – 61.3 g; protein – 22.5 g; DF – 10.4 g	Red peas and rice, red peas soup, lima bean and oxtail
VEGETABLES Vegetable amaranths, bhagi, callaloo, spinach (*Amaranthus* spp., Amaranthaceae); origin: CA and Mexico	Raw – protein – 2.5 g; calcium – 215 mg; potassium – 611 mg; iron – 2.3 mg; vitamin A – 292 RE	Steamed calaloo/bhagi, pepper-pot soup, bhagi and rice
Pumpkin (*Cucurbita maxima*, *C. moshata*, Cucurbitaceae); orign: TA.	Raw – potassium – 340 mg; vitamin A – 160 RE	Steamed pumpkin, curried pumpkin, pumpkin soup, pudding, custard, fritters
Heart of palm (cabbage palm – *Roystonea oleracea*; pewah, peach palm – *Bactris gasipaes*, Palmae/Arecaceae); origin: Trinidad, TA	47.6 kcal; carb. – 5.2 g; protein – 1.5 g; calcium – 42.4 mg; potassium – 193.6 mg	Heart of palm steamed, salad
FRUITS Grapefruit (*Citrus paradisi*, Rutaceae); origin: West Indies, probably Barbados	30 kcal; potassium – 129 mg; vitamin C – 38 mg	Concentrate, juice, drink, fresh fruit, fruit salad
Avocado (*Persea americana*, Lauraceae); origin: Mexico and CA	161 kcal; fat – 15.3 g; protein – 2.0 g; potassium – 599 mg	Salad, guacamole
Pineapple (*Ananas cosmosus*; Bromeliaceae); origin: SA	49 kcal; carb. – 12.4 g; potassium – 113 mg	Concentrate, juice, drink, pina colada, fresh fruit, fruit salad, pizza topping, pie filling, jams, jellies, ice cream

Table 17.1 continues

Table 17.1 Caribbean Food Plants: Nutritional Composition and Use (*cont'd*)

Names (Common, Scientific and Botanical Family); Origin[*]		Major Dishes[***]
FRUITS (*cont'd*)		
Papaya, pawpaw (*Carica papaya*, Caricaceae); origin: Mexico and CA	39 kcal; carb. – 9.8 g; potassium – 257 mg; vitamin A – 201 RE	Fruit salad, nectar, juice; immature fruit – steamed, pawpaw balls, pepper sauce
Passion fruit (*Passiflora edulis* var. *flavicarpa*, Barbadine; *P. quadrangularis*, Passifloraceae); origin: SA	97 kcal; carb. 23.4 g; protein – 2.2 g; potassium – 200 mg; vitamin A – 201 RE	Nectar, drink, ice cream
Guava (*Psidium guajava*; Myrtaceae); origin: TA.	51 kcal; carb. – 11.9 g; potassium – 284 mg; vitamin A – 79 RE; vitamin C – 184 mg	Jam, jelly, cheese, nectar, juice
West Indian/Barbados cherry (*Malphigia glabra*, Malphigiaceae); origin: West Indies, Northern SA	32 kcal; carb. – 7.7 g; potassium – 145 mg; vitamin A – 77 RE; vitamin C – 1677 mg	Nectar, drink
Cashew (*Anacardium occidentale*, Anacardiaceae); origin: TA	Apple – 46 kcal; carb. – 11.6 g; vitamin A – 40 RE; vitamin C – 219 mg	Jam, drink
	Whole seeds, dry – 561 kcal; fat – 45.7 g; carb. – 27.9 g; protein – 17.2 g; iron – 3.8 mg; potassium – 464 mg	Roasted nuts
Guinep (*Melicoccus bijugatus*, Sapindaceae); origin: TA.	59 kcal, carb. – 19.9 g	Fresh
Soursop (*Annona muricata*, Annonaceae)	66 kcal; carb. – 16.8 g; potassium – 278 mg	Punch, nectar, drink, ice cream
Sugar apple (*A. squamosa*, Annonaceae), custard apple (*A. reticulata*, Annonaceae); origin: CA, SA and West Indies.		Fresh fruit

Table 17.1 continues

Table 17.1 Caribbean Food Plants: Nutritional Composition and Use (*cont'd*)

Names (Common, Scientific and Botanical Family); Origin[*]	Major Nutrients/100 g[**]	Major Dishes[***]
FRUITS (*cont'd*) Sapodilla (*Manilkara achras*, Sapotaceae), balata (*M. bidentata*, Sapotaceae), caimite/starapple (*Chrysophyllum cainito*, Sapotaceae), mammy sapote (*Calocarpum sapota*, Sapotaceae); origin: CA, Mexico, Trinidad and SA	Sapodilla: 83 kcal; carb. – 20 g; potassium – 193 mg Caimite: 68 kcal; carb. 14.5	Fresh fruit
Mammey apple (*Mammea americana*, Guttiferae); origin: West Indies and TA	51 kcal, carb. – 12.5 g	Jam, jelly
Jamaica plum (*Spondias purpurea,* Anacardiaceae), chili plum (*S. lutea*, Anacardiaceae), hog plum (*S. mombin*, Anacardiaceae); origin: TA		Drink
INDUSTRIAL CROPS Cocoa (*Theobroma cacao*, Sterculiaceae); origin: CA, SA, Trinidad		Chocolate, cocoa/chocolate drinks
BEVERAGE CROPS Mauby (*Colubrina arborescens* or *C. elliptica*, Rhamnaceae); origin: West Indies and TA		Fresh drink, fermented drink
Seamoss (*Gracilaria* spp., Rhodophyta); origin: West Indies		Punch with milk, drink
CONDIMENTS AND SPICES Hot pepper (*Capsicum frutescens*, Solanaceae); origin: Peru, Mexico		Pepper sauce, condiment in jerk seasoning and chutney
Sweet pepper (*C. annum*, Solanaceae); origin: Peru, Mexico		Salads

Table 17.1 continues

Table 17.1 Caribbean Food Plants: Nutritional Composition and Use (*cont'd*)

Names (Common, Scientific and Botanical Family); Origin[*]	Major Nutrients/100 g[**]	Major Dishes[***]
CONDIMENTS AND SPICES		
Pimento (*Pimenta dioica*, Myrtaceae), bay (*P. racemosa*, Myrtaceae); origin: Jamaica		Used in pickles, escoveitch fish, ketchup, pimento dram
Roucou/annatto (*Bixa orellana*, Bixaceae); origin: West Indies and TA		Annatto oil
Vanilla (*Vanilla fragrans*, Orchidaceae); origin: CA and the West Indies		Essence used in baked goods, drinks, ice cream
Tonka bean (*Dipteryx odorata*, Leguminosae); origin: SA		Grated seed added to baked goods

Notes:
[1]DF = dietary fibre
[2]Carb. = carbohydrate
[3] Varieties with ddep yellow flesh, cooked in skin
[4]RE = retinol equivalents

Sources:
[*]   Purseglove 1974.
[**]   Caribbean Food and Nutrition Institute 1998.
[***]   Benghiat 1985; Ortiz 1995; Parkinson 1999; Wood 1973.

The Taínos, who evolved from earlier groups in the Caribbean and occupied the Greater Antilles, cultivated large gardens of 1 to 2 hectares which they called *conucos*, in which they planted cassava, sweet potatoes, yautia or tannia (*Xanthosoma sagittifolium*), topi tambo (*Calathea allouia*), beans, peanuts (*Arachis hypogaea*), cucurbits (*Cucurbita* spp.) and chile peppers (*Capsicum frutescens*). Fruit trees, including guava (*Psidium guajava*), soursop (*Annona muricata*), mammee apple (*Mammea americana*), chenette (*Meliococcus bijugatus*) and cocoplum (*Chrysobalanus icaco*), were also cultivated. Their production system was partly based on "slash and burn" agriculture, in which cultivated plots were abandoned when their fertility could no longer support the food needs of the group or family (Keegan 2000). After a fallow period of several years, during which fertility was restored, cultivation could be undertaken again.

Among the Taínos cassava was the main crop, with both the sweet and bitter types being grown. The tubers of the sweet types contain low levels of cyanogenic glycosides, which form toxic prussic acid; they must be harvested soon after maturity to prevent deterioration in eating quality. The bitter types contain higher levels of these toxins, which must be destroyed before consumption. This was achieved by exposing the flesh of the tubers to air, first by grating, then by squeezing to remove as much liquid as possible. The resulting cassava meal was then baked on a griddle to make a flatbread or toasted to make farine, in which form it could be stored for long periods. The liquid that was removed was called casareep, which was used as a preservative by boiling it over several days and adding meat to the pot at intervals; it was also used to make a beer. Processing bitter cassava and baking the meal on griddles seems to have been practised since the Archaic period. However, the main method of food preparation the Taínos used for roots and vegetables was boiling, while fruits were eaten fresh. Maize was of secondary importance at this time and was consumed mainly as roasted whole cobs (Keegan 2000).

European Influence on the Status of Indigenous Crops

When the Spanish arrived in the Caribbean in 1492, they found indigenous people whose diet was varied, with several plant sources of energy, protein, and other nutrients. Protein needs were supplemented further by hunting. Also, a mixture of crops with varying maturity periods ensured that there was a constant supply of food. The arrival of European colonists – first the Spanish, then the British, French and Dutch – brought far-reaching changes to both the economic and social landscape and to the flora and fauna of the Caribbean, which completely disrupted the lifestyles and the livelihoods of the Taínos.

Initially the Taínos supplied food and labour to the Spanish as tribute. But, with few exceptions, the indigenous crops were not sustained, because of serious decline of the Taíno population due to war, disease caused by new pathogens to which they had no resistance, and abuse of their labour in the search for gold by the Spanish. Also, the cattle and pigs imported as protein sources for the Europeans were allowed to roam freely to forage, and in so doing they destroyed many of the Taínos' gardens (Keegan 2000).

One of the few crops that became important to the colonists was cassava, the source of cassava bread. Keegan (2000) cites other authors who describe cassava bread as "the bread of conquest". This was not a new role for the food: cassava meal could be stored for long periods, and the bread made from it had facilitated long-distance travel and wars of expansion by the early natives. It similarly sustained the European colonists during their conquest of the Caribbean and Latin America. This was not necessarily by choice, but rather an acceptance of the reality that bread made from wheat was less suited to sustaining life during long expeditions in this part of the world. But although the Portuguese and Dutch during their colonization of Brazil adopted indigenous foods and subsistence systems, the British and French colonists in the Caribbean showed little similar inclination. Their preference for their own foods was so strong that they attempted to import temperate food plants to the Caribbean. Though most of these failed to thrive, it did not deter eventual transformation of the biodiversity of the region and assertion of a preference for foreign foods that ultimately relegated the indigenous food plants to the status of minor crops.

No other plant so affected the Caribbean landscape as sugarcane (*Saccharum officinarum*), which was imported from Asia to produce sugar to satisfy the growing demand in Western Europe. Many of the remaining Taínos were enslaved for production of this crop, and when their numbers dwindled, Africans were enslaved and imported to supply the needed labour. Therefore, from the sixteenth century onwards there was an acceleration of the steep decline in the production of indigenous food crops that had started earlier. Among the major contributing factors was the clearance of large tracts of forest and cultivated areas for sugarcane production. Among the British planters, especially those in the flatter islands of Barbados, Antigua and St Kitts, which were cultivated only for sugarcane, little thought was given to food production, even for maintaining the enslaved labour force. Instead, imported food supplies such as cornmeal, wheat flour and salted meat and fish from the American colonies and Britain were strongly preferred to local food production (Sheridan 1976). The importation of corn products is noteworthy because it indicates that corn was not an important crop locally.

Another factor was that in territories such as Jamaica and St Vincent, the

Africans were expected to supplement their meagre rations of imported food with food crops familiar to them. These were introduced from Africa and included yams (*Dioscorea alata, D. rotundata* and *D. cayanensis*), plantains (*Musa* spp.) and akee (*Blighia sapida*). The enslaved were allowed to cultivate these crops in hilly areas that were of marginal quality for sugarcane production. Besides cocoyam (*Xanthosoma sagittifolium*) and sweet potato, they also grew cassava, which they had learnt to process thorough contact with the Taínos. Higman (2008) cites early writers who indicated that even the English planters in Jamaica ate cassava as a bread during the seventeenth century; by the eighteenth century a cassava cake – a precursor to the bammy – was being sold at local markets by the enslaved Africans.

The cocoyam was said to be preferred to yam or cassava, even though the tubers were less palatable, because they produced a higher yield with less care, had edible leaves and offered the common advantage of extended harvest of the tubers, which were eaten boiled or roasted. According to Higman (2008), although it stored poorly, sweet potato was regarded favourably by the Europeans because it was perceived as having a superior taste, was easy to digest and nourishing and was thought to have aphrodisiacal properties. Thus the Africans became custodians of the indigenous crops through recognition of their food value and acquisition of knowledge of their agronomy, processing technologies and methods of use. As the Taínos had done before them, they cultivated these crops both in nearby kitchen gardens and in distant provision grounds.

Nevertheless, the planters' overall attitude to the provision grounds where some indigenous crops survived was negative, especially during periods when sugar prices were high. All labour had to be devoted to sugarcane production for the greatest profit. Only when it became uneconomical to purchase food for the labour force, or when it became almost impossible to obtain regular supplies of imported food, was local food production encouraged. Supplies of imported food were cut off during the American War of Independence; hurricanes and droughts during the 1770s and 1780s destroyed the provision grounds, thereby exacerbating the food shortage and contributing to tremendous loss of life. Increasing competition with other sugar producers led to declining prices, so even after trade resumed with the former North American colony and continuing into the early nineteenth century, it became increasingly uneconomical to purchase imported food for the labour force (Sheridan 1976). It was these circumstances that forced legislation requiring a portion of all plantations to be used for food-crop cultivation, partly to meet the prescribed standards for rations for the labour force (Tobin 1999).

Although the legal requirements were not always observed, the provision grounds continued to be cultivated and eventually became a significant domestic food source. The local white population also benefited from supplies from the provision grounds – which were sold at Sunday markets – since they were the only available fresh foods. Tobin (1999) cites Mrs. A.C. Carmichael, a sugarcane planter's wife who frequented the markets; she noted, among the produce on sale, the presence of the indigenous cassava, sweet potato, corn, pumpkin (*Cucurbita maxima*, *C. moshata*), vegetable amaranths (*Amaranthus* spp.), legumes, peppers, pineapples (*Ananas cosmosus*) and arrowroot (*Maranta arundinacea*) and cassava starches. Corn was also grown, to feed pigs and poultry which were sold at the market. Many of these items were ingredients in the "negro pot", as various soups were called that were frequently prepared for the planters' families. Nevertheless, provision grounds were not universally encouraged. Even when profits from sugarcane production were declining, it was still important to the planters to maintain control over the labour force, and some sought to do so by controlling the supply of food. The sense of importance and independence that the provision grounds and the Sunday markets gave the Africans must have challenged this advantage. Where provision grounds were encouraged by planters, they were used as evidence that slavery was not as bad as it was being made out to be by the abolitionists, because even the enslaved were thriving financially (Tobin 1999).

Another factor emerged which militated against the indigenous food crops' regaining their prominence. This was the importation of many plant species from colonies in Asia, Africa and the Pacific, especially during the eighteenth century, in the search for other crops of possible economic importance and also for an easy food source. Breadfruit (*Artocarpus altilis*) was imported to fill the latter role because of the previously described food crises of the 1770s and 1780s. Besides sugarcane, other transplanted crops that eventually gained significance in the Caribbean included banana (*Musa* spp.), coffee (*Coffea arabica*), citrus (*Citrus* spp.) and other fruit crops such as mango (*Mangifera indica*). While this was not a one-way flow of germplasm – the colonists also distributed the region's germplasm to other areas of the world (Powell 1976) – the net effect was diminution of the significance of indigenous biodiversity as a food source.

During this period, indigenous crops and food ways were also preserved by the small populations of Amerindian descendants that remained in some territories. Within the English-speaking Caribbean, they were represented by the Carib descendants of Dominica and the Garifuna, a mixed Carib and African ethnic group that originated in St Vincent and was later forced to migrate to Belize (then British Honduras) and Honduras. While both groups were exposed to the newly introduced crops, and to European and other influences on the preparation of indigenous foods, they also retained the practice of cultivating and methods of use of some of the native food plants.

The period after emancipation of the enslaved people was marked by two major developments that influenced the future status of indigenous crops in the Caribbean. In spite of the legacy of the previous period that had established social distinctions and, consequently, preferences for crops and foods, a peasantry consisting primarily of emancipated Africans emerged and expanded production of the crops grown on the provision grounds (Marshall 1985). This not only served the purpose of developing a local food-crop sector within the economy but also preserved the remaining indigenous crops as an integral part of the region's food system. This peasantry was critical to sustaining the local population as sugarcane production declined and new export crops developed (Marshall 1985). Officially, however, production of local food crops was still not supported because it drew labour away from sugarcane; it gained support from the colonial governments only during periods of food shortage, when campaigns were mounted to encourage food production. This interest was not sustained when better economic circumstances prevailed, because of the preference for foreign foods and the stigma attached to local foods, especially the root crops, or ground provisions, as they had come to be known. In his book *The Middle Passage*, V.S. Naipaul describes the contempt in which Trinidadians held Grenadians because they ate ground provisions.

The second major development was the emergence of cocoa (*Theobroma cacao*), a plant indigenous to tropical America, as a major export crop. According to Purseglove (1974) it was cultivated from ancient times by the Amerindians of Central America, who held it in high esteem as a food for the gods. This status may have arisen from its consumption by persons of higher rank, as a thick beverage made by mixing the roasted and pounded beans with maize and pepper. The Spanish, who preferred to consume the ground beans mixed with sugar and vanilla (*Vanilla fragrans*), made it into chocolate and initiated the trade to Europe. Cocoa germplasm initially consisted of two strains: Criollo, from Central America, and Forastero, from the Amazon region. Both were brought to Trinidad (Criollo first, by the Spanish in 1525), where they hybridized to produce Trinitario, a strain that combined the best characteristics of the two parent groups: fine flavour and hardiness (Purseglove 1974). This permitted development of the cocoa industry in Trinidad, which was a leading exporter up to 1920. Cocoa transformed the local society because it was cultivated on much smaller holdings than sugarcane, so many more producers were able to participate and earn wealth.

Cocoa was the first indigenous crop to enjoy serious research attention. The Imperial College of Tropical Agriculture (ICTA), the forerunner of the

Faculty of Agriculture at the University of the West Indies, was founded in 1922 in Trinidad and became the first and foremost institution in the world for cocoa research and postgraduate training in tropical agriculture. Also, a board was established to regulate the industry, including production and all aspects of marketing the beans, in the same manner as the boards for the sugar and banana industries; the cocoa industry is still controlled by a board today. New, improved cocoa material was distributed to other territories, such as Grenada and St Lucia, expanding cocoa production for export throughout the region.

The Current Status of Food Crops

Starchy Crops

The starchy crops include cereal grains, tubers and rhizomes that are grown to supply energy from carbohydrates, primarily starch. Maize is the third most important cereal internationally after wheat and rice and is comparable to both as a source of energy. It also supplies appreciable quantities of protein and minerals and surpasses wheat and rice in vitamin A content (CFNI 1998). Within the Caribbean, maize is second to rice in both production (538,342 tonnes)[1] and consumption (17.51 kg per capita per year),[2] with Cuba and Haiti being the major producers. It is available fresh, processed as cornmeal, corn flakes, canned whole kernels and creamed corn, and as cornstarch. Maize is consumed at all main meals and in a variety of favourite dishes (see table 17.1). Snack foods such as tortillas and corn curls are popular, although chili bibi, or sansam – a traditional African snack prepared by mixing roasted and pounded corn grains with sugar – is less well-known today. The main dishes reflect Amerindian, African, European and modern North American influences.

Cassava and sweet potatoes are the major root crops produced (893,184 and 538,671 tonnes, respectively) and consumed (18.98 and 16.64 kg per capita per year) in the Caribbean, and among tropical root crops they rank first and second in international production. Within the region, most production is undertaken on small farms, and fresh tubers are available at local markets. Cassava roots are prepared by boiling, or they may be grated and made into several traditional dishes (see table 17.1). More modern uses include tapioca starch, a food extender, and fried chips are more evident. Cassareep is still used to preserve cooked meat in the popular Guyanese dish pepperpot.

Yams (*Dioscorea* spp.) rank third in production among root crops internationally and in the Caribbean. However, cush-cush, the only yam species native to the New World, is not widely cultivated in the region, although its small (15 to 20 cm long) tubers with white, cream, yellow or purple flesh are appreciated for their sweet flavour and soft texture. Tannia is an aroid and related to dasheen (also called taro or cocoyam; *Colocasia esculenta* var. *esculenta*) and eddoes (*C. esculenta* var. *antiquorum*), which are also grown as starchy tubers in the region, but more tannia is produced (215,344 tonnes). Tannia is available as fresh tubers and is consumed boiled or fried. Another minor root crop is topi tambo, which is produced in a very few countries that include Trinidad and Tobago. The small (2 to 5 cm long) tubers grow in a clump; when cooked they have a crisp texture and nutty flavour. All the root crops with the exception of topi tambo are consumed at main meals. Boiling as a preparation method predominates, while the more time-consuming roasting and preparation of meal have declined.

The key factor that has determined the current status of starchy crops in the Caribbean, especially the root tubers, is that during the colonial era these crops were not important for export; therefore their cultivation and improvement were not encouraged. The situation was different for maize, which was being produced in North America for human and livestock consumption and on which international research was being conducted at the Centro internacional de mejoramiento de maíz y trigo (CIMMYT) in Mexico beginning in 1943 (Morris 2002). When the food potential of cassava and sweet potato was recognized elsewhere, similar internationally funded research began at the International Institute for Tropical Agriculture (IITA), which was established in 1967 in Nigeria (IITA 2007). Eventually research also began within the Caribbean, at ministries of agriculture and regional research institutions, to address constraints to availability and consumption. Improved production, post-harvest management and processing technologies were sought for problems such as low yields, seasonality, lack of convenience forms and the presence of anti-nutritional constituents such as cyanogenic glycosides (University of Puerto Rico 2002). These efforts have been directed mainly towards cassava, sweet potato, introduced yams and, to a much less extent, tannia. Cush-cush and topi tambo have not benefited from these improvements. Germplasm collections for cassava, sweet potato and yams, consisting of both traditional local selections and imported accessions, are held by the University of the West Indies at St Augustine, Trinidad and Tobago, but much larger collections exist in the Spanish-speaking countries. These crops are considered non-traditional or minor export crops.

In its rhizomes, or underground stems, the arrowroot plant produces a fine-grained, highly digestible starch that is very useful in the diets of infants and convalescents. Because of its high viscosity it is also widely used as an extender to thicken soups and in ketchup. Arrowroot starch was a major export of St Vincent from 1900 to 1965 (Purseglove 1974). The industry has since declined but is being revived, since the demand for high-quality starch remains. Although little research has been undertaken to improve production of this crop, its importance in St Vincent is recognized by an annual Arrow-root Festival, held during the May harvest period.

Legumes and Vegetables

Peanuts are not a major legume in the region, and consumption is heavily reliant on imports. Production is undertaken by small farmers, and the major producing countries are Haiti, Cuba and Jamaica. The highly nutritious shelled or baked-in-shell nuts are among the most popular snacks in the region, consumed daily as a rich source of protein, energy – because of their high fat content – and dietary fibre. Nutcakes and peanut brittle are traditional sweetmeats that were developed by the African population. Imported peanut butter is much consumed, and its use in stews and soups may be of both Amerindian and African origin (Parkinson 1999). Varietal trials have been undertaken to develop the region's peanut production (CARDI 2005).

A variety of common beans are consumed, ranging in colour from white to black. Black beans are highly favoured in the Spanish-speaking Caribbean and, along with rice, are the basis of the Cuban national dish, Moros y Cristianos. Red or kidney beans are more popular elsewhere; in Jamaica they are used in a very popular dish, rice and peas (Parkinson 1999). Beans are a relatively cheap source of protein and other important nutrients, and when combined with rice they provide a complete amino acid profile. They are consumed widely on a daily basis at main meals. While most dried beans are imported, both immature pods and dried beans are also produced locally. They are commonly small-farmer crops, and production is highest in Cuba, the Dominican Republic and Haiti. Significant research has been conducted on cultural aspects of bean production, its genetics and diseases throughout the region, especially in Cuba and Puerto Rico, where germplasm collections are held.

Vegetable amaranths (*Amaranthus* spp.), better known as bhagi, callaloo or spinach, are a highly appreciated and cheap source of important minerals, vitamins and proteins and are eaten at all main meals. They much exceed green leafy vegetables of temperate origin, such as lettuce, in nutritional value; however, because of their calcium oxalate crystal content, persons with health problems such as kidney stones should avoid consuming large quantities. Several types are available in the region, differing in plant height, leaf size and vein colour, degree of succulence, flavour and nutritional content. The fast-growing plant is cultivated by small farmers and is available year-round as fresh bundles of green shoots. Small quantities are exported outside the region. Research has been undertaken on varietal evaluation, agronomic assessment and pest control for improved production. Since the amaranths can also be weeds in other crops, investigations have been conducted on their allelopathic effects, their role as carriers of viruses and methods of control (Martin, Ruberté and Meitzner 1998).

Pumpkin remains an important vegetable crop in the region, and among all the vegetables in Puerto Rico it is the second highest in revenue generation. Selections of traditional varieties are cultivated by small farmers. The University of Puerto Rico has conducted research on several areas of improvement, including growth habit, and a semi-bushy type, 'Taina Dorada', has been developed. 'Bodles Globe', an improved type with good flesh colour and culinary properties, has been developed in Jamaica; it is favoured for the export market because of its shape (University of Puerto Rico 2002).

The original "heart of palm", a high-priced delicacy, is the enclosed apical bud of the cabbage palm tree (*Roystonea oleracea*). The tender bud is consumed steamed and in salads. The tree is destroyed during harvesting of the bud, so the pewah, or peach palm (*Bactris gasipaes*), which regenerates naturally by suckers, is a better species for commercial production, because younger trees or suckers replace the harvested ones. Production in the region is not widespread; traditionally, as in Trinidad, pewah trees are grown mainly for their starchy fruits, which are consumed as a snack. A major constraint to production are the long, sharp spines along the stems of the plants. Heart of palm is usually available as an imported canned product. Production was attempted in Jamaica during the 1980s, and currently it is a major non-traditional export crop from Guyana, a CARICOM country on the South American mainland.

It is clear that the indigenous legumes and vegetable crops possess considerable potential to contribute to regional food supply. The high nutritional value of cassava leaves and those of other root crops is virtually unexploited compared with elsewhere in the tropics. They remain largely underdeveloped because, in most of the Caribbean, the major impetus for development of these crops is their export potential.

Fruits

It is thought that grapefruit arose in the West Indies, possibly in Barbados, as a mutation from pumelo or from a hybrid of pumelo (*Citrus grandis*) and orange (*C. sinensis*), both being close relatives of Asian origin (Purseglove 1974). Grapefruit is second only to the orange in the international citrus fruit trade, and it is the most important Caribbean fruit. Cuba and the Dominican Republic are major producers and exporters. 'Ortanique' and 'Ugli', hybrids of orange and tangerine (*C. reticulata*) and grapefruit and tangerine, respectively, were developed in Jamaica (Higman 2008), which is also a major producer and exporter. Citrus fruits provide appreciable quantities of vitamin C and other important nutrients such as bioflavonoids. Production is undertaken by enterprises of all sizes, with the level of technology being higher on larger farms. Production, processing, marketing and research of these fruits are coordinated and controlled by citrus growers' associations and state organizations. Grapefruit, 'Ortanique' and 'Ugli' are available as fresh fruit, juices and concentrates. The major threat to production in the region is the citrus tristeza virus (CTV), and new orchards are being established on CTV-resistant rootstocks.

Avocado (*Persea americana*) germplasm consists of three races: Mexican, Guatemalan and West Indian (Purseglove 1974). Within the Caribbean it is mainly the West Indian race, which is well adapted to the prevailing high-temperature conditions of most of the region, that is grown, with the highest production in Cuba and the Dominican Republic. The fruit is a good energy source because of its fat content; traditionally it is consumed at meals more as a vegetable in salads than as a dessert or snack, as with other fruits. It is exported from several territories.

Pineapple (*Ananas cosmosus*) and papaya (*Carica papaya*) are also among the Caribbean fruits that have become well-established on the international market. Apart from the nutrients they supply, they are valued for their enzymatic properties, which are especially effective for protein digestion. Both crops are grown throughout the region on farms of various sizes. Most pineapple and papaya production occurs in the Dominican Republic, Cuba and Jamaica, and among the pineapple cultivars, 'Antigua Black' and 'Sugar Loaf' were developed in the Caribbean. These fruits are available fresh and are also processed into a range of value-added products (see table 17.1).

Of less commercial importance are fruits such as passion fruit (*Passiflora edulis* var. *flavicarpa*), barbadine (*P. quadrangularis*), guava, West Indian cherry (*Malphigia glabra*), cashew (*Anacardium occidentale*), genip or chenette, soursop and sapodilla (*Manilkara achras*). These all supply significant levels of nutrients, with some fruits being particularly outstanding; for example, the cashew nut, which is a true fruit, provides high levels of energy, protein and potassium, whereas West Indian cherry is one of the best natural sources of vitamin C. Exports of fresh fruit to regional markets is limited, and commercial production is small-scale. With the exception of passion fruit, guava, West Indian cherry and imported cashew nuts, processing is generally limited to the cottage level.

The Jamaica plum (*Spondias purpurea*) and chili-plum (*S. lutea*) are probably better known and more utilized than hog-plum (*S. mombin*), mammee apple, mamee-sapote (*Calocarpum sapota*), caimite (*Chrysophyllum cainito*) and balata (*Manilkara bidentata*) because the relatively small plum trees are easily accommodated in backyards, whereas the trees of the other fruits are much taller and tend to occur in forested areas. While limited quantities of fresh fruit are available for sale, commercial production and processing of this last group of indigenous fruits are uncommon. All these fruits are extensively appreciated for their unique flavours, but many young persons do not know them. This lack of familiarity and, apparently, lower levels of consumption than in the past are due largely to declining tree populations and hence availability, especially in residential areas.

The picture that emerges among the fruits is that, with the exception of grapefruit, introduced fruits such as banana and mango have assumed more importance in the Caribbean than the indigenous species or those of tropical American origin. Within the latter group, only those fruits that are exported internationally have been developed and have organized industries. Others considered to have this potential have been included in agricultural diversification efforts. Research effort is needed to remove production and utilization constraints, such as low supplies for processing, pests and inadequate post-harvest handling. A wide range of fruit germplasm is held in Costa Rica, but except for efforts in Cuba (with guava), the Dominican Republic (with avocado) and Martinique and Guadeloupe (with pineapples), relatively limited attention is paid to the critical area of germplasm conservation in the Caribbean.

Industrial Crops

Fine-flavoured cocoa based on the Trinitario clones is produced mainly in Trinidad and Tobago, and also in Grenada, St Lucia and Jamaica. The quality of Trinitario cocoa attracts the highest prices on the world market; it is used to manufacture expensive dark chocolates. The beans from the Forastero type, grown mainly in West Africa, produce the less expensive bulk cocoa that is processed into milk chocolates, cocoa butter and cocoa/chocolate drinks. These cheaper cocoa products, but not the dark chocolates, are available throughout the region, and chocolate balls or blocks from which the traditional hot chocolate drink is made can be found at local markets.

In all exporting countries of the Caribbean, the cocoa industry is regulated by a board which plays a key role in the production and marketing of the cocoa beans. Current production and exports from Trinidad and Tobago are a mere fraction of their 1920s levels because of disease and loss of the labour force required for cultivation and processing of quality cocoa. Small quantities of cocoa are also exported by other Caribbean countries. True to its imperial mandate, the ICTA facilitated the growth and development of cocoa industries in other parts of the British Empire that eventually became much larger cocoa producers and exporters than the Caribbean. One enduring legacy of that institution in the region, however, is that Trinidad and Tobago has been designated an international cocoa germplasm repository, and germplasm is distributed to support research on cocoa improvement worldwide. This is the result of significant efforts by the ICTA and one of its successors, the Cocoa Research Unit (CRU) of the University of the West Indies, in collaboration with the ministry of agriculture in Trinidad, in germplasm collection, breeding and selection of improved clonal material. The work at the CRU on developing germplasm descriptors, disease control and flavour quality is ongoing. Currently efforts are being made to revive the regional industry, with increased funding for research, better financial support and prices to boost production, new approaches to marketing to secure a better international market share and prices, and plans to embark upon chocolate manufacturing.

Beverage Crops

Mauby is a drink with a bitter aftertaste. It is made by boiling the bark of the tree *Colubrina arborescens* (*C. elliptica*) with spices to which sugar and essence – typically aniseed (*Pimpinella anisum*) – are added, and it is served cold. Dried bark, concentrated syrups to which only water has to be added, and a carbonated drink, Mauby Fizz, are locally available; limited amounts are exported. Mauby trees are not cultivated in commercial plots, so the bark is collected from trees growing on farms or in forested areas. Research has been conducted on the chemical constituents, fermentation and preservation of mauby (Graham and Chaparro 1982; Burke 1991).

Sea-moss or Irish moss (*Gracilaria* spp.) refers to both the dried sea plants and the drink made from them. Traditionally the plants are collected in shallow water at the coastline and dried until ready for use. The dried plants are boiled in water with spices until they dissolve into a gel. When cooled, sugar and milk (which are optional) are added; the resulting drink is highly regarded for its nutritional value. Sea-moss is available as dried plants, as a gel and as prepared drinks. Overharvesting of natural stocks has decreased supplies, but commercial production has been undertaken in both St Lucia and Barbados (Smith 1986; St Hill 1986). Haiti, however, is a larger and cheaper producer. While most sea-moss processing is small-scale, Benjo's is a medium-scale producer in Dominica that produces a range of sea-moss-based drinks for the local and regional markets. Unlike citrus and cocoa, which are major beverage crops, and in common with most of the minor crops, mauby and sea-moss are still consumed primarily by the local market and their potential is relatively untapped.

Condiments and Spices

Both hot and sweet pepper (*Capsicum frutescens, C. annum*) are major condiments in Caribbean cooking, with the hot pepper in particular being used to flavour many dishes, including jerked meats, curries and souse. Several different pepper varieties, varying in pungency, size, shape and colour, are recognized, including the 'Scotch Bonnet' variety of Jamaica and the 'West Indian Red'. Traditionally, hot and sweet peppers were cultivated commercially by small farmers for local markets; however, recently hot peppers have been promoted as a non-traditional export crop with much potential, and in several English-speaking Caribbean territories it is a priority crop for development. Accordingly, research has been conducted on the breeding and selection of superior types such as 'CARDI Red' and 'Caribbean CARDI Green', improvement of agronomic techniques and post-harvest management for export (CARDI 2008). In the Spanish-speaking countries there has been research on both hot and sweet peppers.

Pimento (*Pimenta dioica*) is associated mostly with Jamaican cuisine (see table 17.1). This flavouring, which is said to have the combined flavour of spice, clove and nutmeg, is the dried berries of the pimento tree that grows throughout the island. Dried pimento berries are sold locally. There is little information within the region on overseas markets for the berries, production levels or research to improve aspects of production and processing. The bay (*P. racemosa*), a related species, is grown for its aromatic leaves, especially in Dominica, where small farmers tend bay trees in pure stands or intercropped. Bay leaves have been used traditionally as a spice in hot drinks, and they are distilled to produce bay rum.

Roucou (*Bixa orellano*) is a traditional food flavouring and colourant throughout the Caribbean region. For example, it is used to impart a yellow colour to confectionery, cheese and butter, and it has also been used in butter made from buffalo milk in Cuba (Ortega Fleitas et al. 1996). The demand for roucou as a natural food additive is growing internationally. There is little evidence of research on this product in the region, in contrast to work being done in Latin America.

Vanilla is a very expensive food flavouring used for sweet dishes, baked products and drinks. The extract is derived from the pods of a vine that grows on trees. Because of its expense, it has been significantly replaced by synthetic substances. The seeds of the tonka bean (*Dipteryx odorata*) fruit, for example, yield an extract that is very similar to vanilla. The trees grow uncultivated in Trinidad, and very small quantities of seeds are usually available for sale locally. Generally, with the exception of pepper, and to a lesser extent pimento and bay, little is being done to develop the commercial potential of indigenous condiments and spices.

Implications for Food and Nutrition Security in the Caribbean

From the preceding discussion it is clear that, with few exceptions, the indigenous food crops of the Caribbean have been relatively neglected. With a food import bill of almost US$4 billion, the Caribbean is the most food-insecure region in tropical America. This situation is made even more pathetic by the region's natural endowment of food resources and points to the policies regarding agriculture and food that have shaped the region's development. The most glaring policy error is the disconnect between agriculture and food, which has ensured that agriculture has not become a vehicle for development, but rather for underdevelopment, through its dominant focus on production of primary products for international markets. This is a legacy of the colonial era that continues to persist, even though the need for a new paradigm has been underscored repeatedly by the region's several periods of economic downturn.

The critical lesson learnt by the Maroons of Jamaica and, elsewhere in the region, African proto-peasants and the small entrepreneurial farmers of the post-emancipation and World War periods, is that food security is the foundation of true independence, a concept which has not yet been fully appreciated. In the post-independence period, especially in the English-speaking Caribbean, levels of root crop consumption declined drastically, primarily because of a preference for imported white potatoes and cereals and the traditional stigma against root crops – referred to colloquially as "blue" (slave) food.

Since food prices began to increase in 2008, governments in the Caribbean have placed domestic agriculture higher on the national and regional agendas, and campaigns are being mounted to encourage the consumption of local foods. In some cases – for example, in Jamaica in 2010 – food import bills have been slashed; in that same year, the rate of inflation in Trinidad and Tobago reached its highest level in twenty-seven years, mostly because of food prices. There is grave concern throughout the region about the potential impact of both natural disasters and increasing demand from China and India on access to food and on food prices worldwide. Farmers are once again being encouraged to grow more root crops, especially cassava, and various value-added products are being explored and made available on the market. While these efforts are necessary and must be encouraged, they are often too late to be as effective as desired.

The inadequacy of research and development work to support expanded production and utilization is one major deficiency, while the issue of consumer tastes and preferences, particularly among youth, is another. In countries outside the region, to which several of these crops have been introduced and have thrived, research has been undertaken to address these issues. The information and insight gained from such research provide a valuable starting point for developing these crops to make a sustainable and substantial contribution to food security in the Caribbean.

The prevalence of nutrition-related diseases such as diabetes mellitus, hypertension, cancer and various allergies create an additional imperative for increasing the content of indigenous food crops in the diet of the Caribbean. During the period of slavery, malnutrition due to over-reliance on inadequate supplies of poor-quality imported food was a key contributor to ill health and death (Pilcher 2000). Furthermore, overconsumption of salt (used as a preservative) led to death from hypertension-related dropsy, and the food was often of no nutritional benefit because of its significant deterioration. Pilcher cites Kiple as noting

> shortages of most important vitamins, as well as calcium and iron. The most serious problems resulted from deficiencies of vitamin B_1 (thiamine) and B_3 (niacin). Slaves subsisting on white rice were at risk of developing beriberi, a thiamine-deficiency disease that takes two distinct forms. Both wet beriberi, with symptoms including swelling of the limbs and cardiac failure, and dry beriberi, characterized by muscular deterioration and paraplegia, were common to the Caribbean under the names "dropsy" and mal d'estomach. Corn rations, meanwhile, led to pellagra, a niacin-deficiency disease that caused dermatitis, dysentery, dementia, and death. (Pilcher 2000)

Kiple also reported the prevalence of night blindness due to vitamin A deficiency and scurvy and festering sores and wounds due to vitamin C deficiency, which were also related to calcium and iron deficiencies. The toll on infants was particularly severe, since they were frequently born underweight, and mortality rates were high because of poor nutrition.

On the other hand, it was noted that enslaved Africans who produced their own food had a better diet and were healthier, and in territories such as the Bahamas, where sugarcane production did not dominate, they were taller. Pilcher (2000) notes that in the Caribbean the population of enslaved Africans had to be maintained by regular importation of new labour because reproductive rates were low. This was in large measure because of poor nutrition, and doctors recommended to planters that they encourage provision grounds for the cultivation of food crops, including indigenous crops, to increase the birth rate among enslaved women.

In the post-emancipation era, nutrition-related diseases still prevailed, primarily because of continued reliance on imported food, much of it in highly processed forms that came to be preferred to freshly prepared food. Even though most territories have become independent, nutrition-related lifestyle diseases continue to debilitate a high percentage of the population, affecting their productivity, quality of life and longevity. Naipaul notes in *The Middle Passage*, "To be modern is to ignore local products and to use those advertised in American magazines" (1978, 48). The more powerful and pervasive television and Internet advertising now available have undoubtedly reinforced this centuries-old psychological disposition towards foreign tastes. But perhaps it might also prove a crucial ally in changing people's taste patterns.

Conclusion

The Caribbean's rich biodiversity in food plants made major contributions to the diets of the indigenous people, early settlers and migrants to the region, and through their distribution they play a similar role, providing agricultural incomes in many parts of the tropical world. This contribution has been especially strong in the case of the starchy crops, cocoa and some of the fruits. In the Greater Antilles, while land and population size account for higher levels of production and consumption of these crops, research and germplasm conservation activities suggest that they generally enjoy a higher status than elsewhere in the region. Within the English-speaking Caribbean, the only species that are still considered important are primarily those that have secured extra-regional export markets. Most food plants are underutilized even though they offer significant potential for future development based on their nutritional value and adaptation to prevailing environmental conditions. However, there is need for improved consumer awareness of these benefits in order to create market demand, and for research to develop appropriate production systems and value-added products. Urgent attention to these issues is required, without which the indigenous food plants – an important Caribbean heritage and a critical resource for development of the region – could be lost.

Notes

1. FAO production data for 2006.
2. FAO consumption data for 2003.

References

Benghiat, N. 1985. *Traditional Jamaican Cookery*. Middlesex, UK: Penguin Books.

Burke, M.A. L. 1991. *Preliminary Studies on the Extraction of Water-Soluble Components from the Bark of the Tree* Colubrina arborescens *(or* Colubrina elliptica*)"*. MPhil thesis, University of the West Indies, St Augustine, Trinidad and Tobago.

CARDI (Caribbean Agricultural Research and Development Institute). 2008. *Annual Report 2005*. http://www.cardi.org/publications/annualreports/2005/2005annualreport.pdf (accessed 1 July 2008).

CFNI (Caribbean Food and Nutrition Institute). 1998. *Food Composition Tables for Use in the English-Speaking Caribbean*. 2nd ed. Kingston: Caribbean Food and Nutrition Institute and Pan American Health Organization.

FAO (United Nations Food and Agriculture Organization). 2011. FAOSTAT: "Crops". http://faostat.fao.org/site/567/default.aspx#ancor (accessed 1 July 2008).

———. 2011. FAOSTAT: "Food Balance Sheets". http://faostat.fao.org/site/368/default.aspx#ancor (accessed 1 July 2008).

Graham, H.D., and M. Chaparro. 1982. "Preservation of Mabi by Chemical and Physical Means (Fermented Drink Made from the Bark of the Mabi Tree, *Colubrina elliptica*, Pasteurization, Sodium Benzoate)". *Journal of Agriculture of the University of Puerto Rico* 66, no. 2: 89–98.

Higman, B.W. 2008. *Jamaican Food: History, Biology, Culture*. Kingston: University of the West Indies Press.

Inter-American Institute for Cooperation on Agriculture. 1996. "Potential Development of Minor Fruit Crops of Trinidad and Tobago". Workshop held at University of the West Indies, St Augustine, Trinidad, 25–26 October 1995. Port of Spain: Inter-American Institute for Cooperation on Agriculture.

IITA (International Institute for Tropical Agriculture). 2007. *Annual Report*. http://www.iita.org (accessed 1 July 2008).

Janick, J., and R.E. Paull, eds. 2008. *Encyclopedia of Fruits and Nuts*. Oxfordshire, UK: CAB International.

Keegan, W.F. 2000. "The Caribbean, Including Northern South America and Lowland Central America: Early History". In *The Cambridge World History of Food*, edited by K.F. Kiple and K.C. Ornelas. Cambridge: Cambridge University Press. http://www.credoreference.com/entry/cupfood/v_d_3_the_caribbean_including_northern_south_america_and_lowland_central_america_early_history (accessed 8 October 2010).

Marshall, W.K. 1985. "Peasant Development in the West Indies since 1838". In *Rural Development in the Caribbean*, edited by P.I. Gomes. Kingston: Heinemann Educational (Caribbean).

Martin, F.W., R.M. Ruberté and L.S. Meitzner. 1998. *Edible Leaves of the Tropics*. 3rd ed. North Fort Myers, FL: Education Concern for Hunger Organization.

Morris, M.L. 2002. *Impacts of International Maize Breeding Research in Developing Countries, 1966–1998*. Mexico: Centro internacional de mejoramiento de maíz y trigo.

Naipaul, V.S. 1978. *The Middle Passage: Impressions of Five Societies – British, French and Dutch – in the West Indies and South America*. Harmondsworth, UK: Penguin.

Ortega Fleitas, O., J. Camejo Corrales, M. Otero and M. Fonseca. 1996. "Colourants in Buffalo Butter Processing 1: Use of *Bixa orellana*". *Alimentaria (España)* 34, no. 273: 47–49.

Ortiz, E.L. 1995. *The Complete Book of Caribbean Cooking*. Edison, NJ: Castle Books.

Pagán Jiménez, J.R., and R. Rodríguez Ramos. 2007. "Sobre el origen de la agricultura en Las Antillas". In *Proceedings of the Twenty-first Congress of the International Association for Caribbean Archaeology*, edited by B. Reid, H.P.J. Roget and A. Curet, vol. 1, 252–59. St Augustine: School of Continuing Studies, University of the West Indies.

Parkinson, R. 1999. *Culinaria: The Caribbean, a Culinary Discovery*. Köln, Germany: Könemann.

Pilcher, J.M. 2000. "The Caribbean from 1492 to the Present". In *The Cambridge World History of Food*, edited by K.F. Kiple and K.C. Ornelas. Cambridge: Cambridge University Press. http://www.credoreference.com/entry/cupfood/v_d_4_the_caribbean_from_1492_to_the_present (accessed 8 October 2010).

Powell, D. 1977. "The Voyage of the Plant Nursery H.M.S. *Providence*, 1791–1793". *Economic Botany* 31: 387–431.

Purseglove, J.W. 1974. *Tropical Crops: Monocotyledons*. London: Longman Group, ELBS.

Reid, B.A. 2009. *Myths and Realities of Caribbean History*. Tuscaloosa: University of Alabama Press.

Sheridan, R.B. 1976. "The Crisis of Slave Subsistence in the British West Indies during and after the American Revolution". *William and Mary Quarterly*, 3rd ser., 33, no. 4: 615–41.

Smith, A., 1986. "Seamoss Farming in St. Lucia: From Myth to Reality". *Caribbean Conservation News (Barbados)* 4, no. 6: 7–8.

St Hill, C.A. 1986. *Mariculture of Seamoss in Barbados*. MPhil thesis, University of the West Indies, Cave Hill, Barbados.

Tobin, B.F. 1999. " 'And There Raise Yams': Slaves' Gardens in the Writings of West Indian Plantocrats". *Eighteenth-Century Life* 23, no. 2: 164–79.

University of Puerto Rico. 2002. *Annual Report of Accomplishments and Results*. Mayaguez: Agricultural Experiment Station, College of Agricultural Sciences. http://www.reeis.usda.gov/web/areera/AES.PR.report.2002.pdf (accessed 1 July 2008).

Wood, B. 1973. *Caribbean Fruits and Vegetables: Selected Recipes*. London: Longman Caribbean.

Discussion Questions: Caribbean Food Plants

1. What does archaeological evidence suggest was processed early on in the Caribbean and in what time period? What food preparation utensils or vessels were found in archaeological sites and what foods were suggested to be processed on them?
2. What makes cassava difficult to consume and how did early populations overcome barriers to consumption?
3. How did European colonization of the Caribbean alter the indigenous food systems once in place? Which change had the biggest impact on the people and their food production?
4. Why would it be important now to increase the consumption of indigenous crops in the diet of those in the Caribbean?

Tomatoes

Immigration and the Global Food Supply

Kimberly A. Weir

Tomatoes are a ubiquitous food item, eaten raw or cooked, grown in gardens and hothouses, and integral in cuisines as diverse as Italian and Indian. In a lot of ways, tomatoes are taken for granted. Order a salad in the United States or Europe in the middle of winter, and you will find fresh tomatoes, thanks to production in Florida, imports from Mexico and North Africa, and lots of greenhouses. The "locavore" movement and concerns for "food miles," however, have increased demand for locally produced, organic tomatoes, pushing Americans and Europeans to eschew not only imports but tomatoes that are not locally grown. The "Think global, eat local" approach to food selection has become popular, often in response to social and environmental concerns. Arguably, however, it does a disservice to farmers in developing countries.

Domestic production and the perishable nature of tomatoes limit cash crop exports to only those global south (GS) countries within close proximity to global north (GN) countries. Mexico is the top exporter to the United States, whereas African and Middle Eastern countries bordering the Mediterranean are top exporters to Europe. Because fewer GS countries have opportunities to exploit tomatoes as a cash crop export, the two prominent international issues that arise between the GN and GS countries regarding tomatoes are trade policies and reliance on immigrant labor.

GS countries have a difficult time competing with GN production due to trade policies. These include tariffs, in the form of taxes on imports, and subsidization through government support of domestic tomato industries. Tariffs on tomato imports entering the United States and European Union, supplemented by nontariff barrier policies such as regulations on environmental and sanitary production conditions, minimize foreign competition with domestic tomatoes. Food-security measures developed after World War II to ensure adequate food supplies at home and abroad, as well as Cold War strategies aimed at fortifying alliances, led to American and European farm support policies. Dismantling these outdated programs has proven difficult, despite World Trade Organization (WTO) rulings in favor of countries seeking recourse against the United States and European Union for unfair trade policies.

Reliance on immigrant labor has resulted in worker abuses in the American and European tomato industries. Although labor conditions in the global south tend to attract the most media coverage, GN consumers are far less aware of worker abuses and even labor trafficking in their own backyards. Years of activism by a small group of migrant workers in a Florida community finally drew enough attention to worker conditions to give the group sufficient leverage to effect change in the United States. An Italian labor union has also worked diligently to draw attention to farmhand abuses, eventually making headway in 2011 with passage of a law criminalizing exploitation of migrant labor. National attention thus far has been the most successful means of ensuring rights for immigrant farmworkers, as international efforts have been largely forestalled. And unlike with the push for fair trade in the cocoa and coffee industries, little attention has been given to the tomato industry because fair trade most often focuses on farmers in developing countries and not the farmhands working on GN farms. Abuse of GS workers, coupled with discriminatory competition, serves to exploit and undermine development.

Understanding the issues that have grown up around the tomato industry requires getting a sense of its origins. The tomato has an interesting history, having traveled around the globe to become an ingredient in almost every cuisine. The overwhelming majority of tomatoes in the world are produced for domestic consumption, but the trade in tomatoes—especially the hothouse variety—allows unexpected countries like the Netherlands to be a top exporter. Production of tomatoes for canning and processed foods offers some interesting twists, such as the relationship between Italy and China. A few key issues plague the tomato industry. Pricing demands put pressure on growers. One hot topic involving consumer concerns about how tomatoes are produced has given rise to a number of food movements. And probably the biggest dirty little secret of the tomato industry is the treatment of its laborers.

INTRODUCING *SOLANUM LYCOPERSICUM*

More than four hundred varieties of tomatoes have developed and been bred over the centuries. Red is the most common color, though the spectrum ranges from white to deep purple. The yellow variety, however, is likely closer to the first tomatoes that existed. Tomatoes rarely cross-pollinate, but several hundred specially developed "heirloom" or "heritage" varieties exist and of late have regained popularity, most likely due to Michelle Obama's gardening interests and the locavore movement.

Growing up to ten feet in height, plants stems need to be staked for support, lest they end up sprawling on the ground. The tomato plant developed a toxin over time to help protect against insects and vermin, though some have developed resistance; chipmunks have been known to wipe out an entire garden in no time. Although toxic to bugs, the chemical is not harmful to humans, though it may cause an allergic reaction in some people. Tomatoes vary in size and shape, from the elongated, ovular, bite-size grape tomato to the round, squat softball-size beefsteak variety. Specific varieties lend themselves well to different products. Roma tomatoes make better sauces and pastes, whereas slicing varieties, such as the beefsteak, are better on sandwiches, and cherry tomatoes are best in salads.

Tomatoes are a versatile food item that can be eaten raw or cooked, except for unripe green tomatoes, which must be cooked before consumption. Although related to tomatillos, which can be eaten raw, tomatoes belong to a different genus, making them more closely related to gooseberries. Popular ways to prepare tomatoes include sun drying, stewing, juicing, and cooking them into sauces, condiments, and soups. Tomatoes pair well with any number of grains, pastas, meats, vegetables, herbs, and spices, so they appear in many dishes. Very low in calories, tomatoes are a primary source of vitamins A and C, potassium, and fiber. This nutritionally packed food

New-to-You Food: Jicama

Infusion cuisine—that is, the melding of two cultures' cooking—has begun to increase the popularity of jicama (pronounced HEE-ka-ma), so that this root vegetable is more commonly appearing in restaurants, recipes, and grocery stores in the United States and Europe. As they did tomatoes, the Spaniards came across jicama when they colonized Central and South America. When Spanish traders introduced it to in Southeast Asia, it took root because the plant thrives in tropical areas. Today jicama is a staple food in Thai, Malay, and Indonesian cuisine.

The taste and texture of jicama resembles a cross between a water chestnut and a potato. The Aztecs domesticated jicama, which aptly means "edible roots," since this root vegetable can grow to weigh as much as forty pounds. The vines that grow above ground bear attractive, though toxic, blue or white flowers. Like cassava, yucca, and yams, which are staple foods in many developing countries, jicama is fairly inexpensive, available year-round, and extremely nutritious, with a long shelf life. This vegetable is also very versatile as it can be eaten raw, baked, steamed, braised, deep-fried, or boiled. The commonly used food thickener, arrowroot, is the powered form of jicama.

Demand in the United States is in large part due to migration. Latino influence in southwestern cuisine and Asian influence in the Pacific Northwest encouraged grocers serving these immigrant communities to stock jicama. Being very low in calories yet packed with nutrients, jicama quickly caught on with the health-food crowd, making it even more widely used. Due to globalization, jicama is widely available across the United States. Ironically, it is just now gaining interest in Spain, the country responsible for its spread across the globe.

---

also contains an abundance of lycopene, a phytochemical deemed to have disease-fighting properties.

The perennial question of whether tomatoes are vegetables or fruits is largely the result of a legal decision by the US Supreme Court. Tomatoes are the ripened ovaries of a flower, making them a fruit botanically, though legally they are considered vegetables. The confusion results from the 1893 ruling in *Nix v. Hedden*, in which the Court classified tomatoes as vegetables in order to tax sales through customs regulations. At that time, fruit was not subject to tariffs. The popularity of tomatoes encouraged benefitting from taxing trade, so for legal purposes, they became vegetables. Justice Horace Gray makes an interesting argument in his opinion, observing that even though botanically tomatoes are a fruit, people don't eat them as such; because they are treated as vegetables, they should be taxed as vegetables. Outside the United States, however, tomatoes are more often than not considered fruit.

Commercial seeds and plants used in agribusiness or sold by catalog or at gardening centers are hybrid strains. Seed companies and corporations that use a lot of tomatoes in their products have developed varieties for particular conditions and purposes. Tomatoes destined for canning, for instance, have been bred to be oblong for machine harvesting and have fewer seeds and less water content. These crops go from fields to cans within a matter of days— and sometimes even hours. This streamlined process allows the tomatoes to remain in the fields until they reach peak ripeness, making them much more flavorful than commercially grown tomatoes. Those destined for grocery store shelves not only have longer distances to travel to market but also spend time on the produce shelf and at home before being used.

Tomatoes are also bred to better withstand cold weather, resist insects and vermin, and even grow for specific durations to allow for a steadier harvest throughout a season for home gardeners and smaller commercial outdoor farmers. Although they grow year-round in warmer places, tomatoes are usually planted annually, as they cannot survive through winter freezes. Sometimes tomato plants "voluntarily" grow a second season in areas where the plants die in winter. This happens when seeds from the previous year's crop fall into the soil, then germinate the next year.

Tomatoes do not refrigerate well as the flesh turns mealy. Ripened produce is highly perishable, needing to be stored at between fifty-four and eighty degrees Fahrenheit and out of direct sunlight. When fresh tomatoes will be shipped, the destination determines how long the produce can be vine ripened. Most often, chemicals are used in commercial tomato production to extend their shelf life before they reach the point of sale. Ethylene is an organic compound used to make green tomatoes appear ripe. Mature tomatoes would rot before reaching grocery stores. In order for the highly perishable tomato to be picked, boxed, shipped, and shelved, then purchased and eaten, fresh tomatoes are green tomatoes in disguise and might ripen a bit further.

A BRIEF HISTORY OF TOMATOES

Think of tomatoes, and, without a doubt, Italy comes to mind, with images of pizza and pasta. The plant, however, is not native to Europe. The tomato's roots have been traced back to the Andes region of South America. The plant spread to Mexico through regional interaction, where European explorers encountered it in the late 1400s. The Aztecs first cultivated the *tomatl*, which influenced the Spanish name *tomate*. By the sixteenth century, tomatoes were commonly eaten in Spain and Italy. The tomato's reputation as an aphrodisiac was also carried back to Europe, where the French popularly referred to it as *pomme d'amour* (apple of love) through the seventeenth century until *la tomate* became a common food.

Like potatoes, eggplants, and tobacco, tomatoes belong to the nightshade family, so their poisonous leaves initially discouraged people from eating them. In some areas of Europe, particularly England, tomatoes were not eaten but grown only for observers to admire the flowers and fruit. The tomato, perhaps surprisingly, took a circuitous route to America and Canada via colonists who brought the ornamental plant with them, rather than spreading north from Mexico. By the eighteenth century, people had widely come to accept that tomatoes were not poisonous. As with other plants the Europeans found in the Americas, colonization spread tomatoes across the globe, integrating them into any number of cuisines, from the Philippines to Morocco.

The high acidity level of tomatoes lends well to preservation through canning, which is perhaps the reason that ketchup was popular before tomatoes appeared in salads. Campbell's introduced another popular canned product, cream of tomato soup, in the mid-nineteenth century, followed by Heinz Baked Beans, which became very popular in Britain later that century. Eventually tomatoes became appreciated as the versatile food they are, making their way out of the can and onto salad plates and eventually becoming a common sight year-round, thanks to hothouse production.

CONSUMPTION

The top consumers per capita of tomatoes in the world are in Egypt, Greece, Armenia, and Libya, with more than ninety kilograms eaten per person each year.[1] Not surprisingly, many Mediterranean countries top the list, with Americans eating their fair share, though US consumption is only about half that of the top countries. Year-round availability of tomatoes in the global north is due to the combination of outdoor and greenhouse production. In the United States, for example, California and Florida can produce tomatoes during most months of the year, with the remaining months filled by greenhouse suppliers and imports from Mexico. Much of Canada's supply is from greenhouse production since temperatures permit a limited outdoor growing season. Europeans are steadily supplied with outdoor tomatoes from the Mediterranean region and Africa, supplemented by hothouse production across Europe.

Fresh versus processed tomato consumption roughly correlates to a country's level of development, with GN countries tending toward processed consumption and GS countries toward fresh tomatoes. In the United States, almost 90 percent of all tomatoes produced are destined for processing,[2] versus the 98 percent eaten fresh in Central Asia.[3] Another interesting consumption pattern is that, although people in the African and most of the Middle Eastern countries bordering the Mediterranean consume very few processed tomatoes, fresh tomatoes are commonly used in cooked dishes. The European Mediterranean countries, however, consume about 20 percent more processed tomatoes, even though they are also big producers of fresh tomatoes.[4] Perhaps most notable is India, which ranks second in world production; Indians almost exclusively eat fresh tomatoes, with very few grown for processing.

When inflation hits developing countries, tomato prices can force poorer people to cut back on this staple food item. Political turmoil in 2011 caused tomato prices in Egypt to more than double.[5] Slowing economic growth and increased exports to Pakistan resulted in the doubling of tomato prices in India, where one kilogram (2.2 pounds) of tomatoes increased to twenty rupees.[6] Although this amount represents only about thirty-five US cents, it makes a huge dent in many pocketbooks in a country whose gross domestic product per capita is $1,400.[7] Because tomatoes are a staple in Indian diets, a person earning $1,400 a year who buys one kilo of tomatoes each day spends 9 percent of his yearly income just on tomatoes. Urban prices are even higher: a kilo sells for forty rupees, making an even bigger dent.[8] Translated into what this increase would mean in terms of US dollars, a kilo of tomatoes would cost $12 a day and $24 in the city.[9]

A regular concern with fresh produce consumption, particularly of lettuce, spinach, cucumbers, and tomatoes, is outbreaks of salmonella and *E. coli*; with sun-dried tomatoes, the concern is hepatitis A. Salmonella is a bacterium that infects produce. Before shipping, tomatoes are treated with chlorinated water to kill bacteria, but sometimes enough survives to cause infection. *E. coli* is a bacterium that causes infection and can lead to death, as evidenced by the thirty-one Germans who died in 2011 after eating tainted sprouts. During that scare, the government also cautioned consumers to avoid raw tomatoes, which might also have been affected. Sun-dried tomatoes contaminated with hepatitis A were sold in the Netherlands in 2010 and in the United Kingdom in 2011. Although hepatitis A is rarely life threatening, in people who are not immunized against the virus, infection may result in hospitalization. Lack of farm and packing plant inspections, intensive farming methods, and increasingly tainted water supplies account for increased food contamination. Anytime there is a scare, until the outbreak can be traced, tons and tons of produce rots in fields or gets tossed into supermarket Dumpsters. The European Union compensated farmers to the tune of US$306 million for produce that rotted in fields or went bad in warehouses due to the *E. coli* breakout.[10]

PRODUCTION

The top tomato producer in the world, by far, is China, which grew 41.9 million tons in 2010; the next biggest producers, the United States and India, grew only 40 percent of China's total.[11] Egypt, Turkey, and Italy round out the top six. In terms of imports and exports, tomato production is separated between fresh and processed tomatoes. The United States and Turkey are the only top-ranking producers that export fresh outdoor tomatoes, whereas hothouse production allows the Netherlands to be the global leader in fresh tomato exports.[12] Of the top twenty fresh tomato exporters, eight countries border the Mediterranean, giving an indication of not only the importance of tomatoes in those diets but also of the export value of the product. The top tomato importers, not surprisingly, are developed or emerging economies, as they have greater buying power.

Processed tomato exports differ primarily in that Italy is at the top, largely due to an interesting relationship with China. Domestic production in China is the result of Communist Party policies aimed at small-farm capitalist growth, initiated in the 1980s to achieve food self-sufficiency.[13] Families with small plots are financed to build greenhouses to grow fresh produce. These tomatoes are then processed in China before being exported to Italy, where they are reprocessed and exported. An Italian label attracts more consumer interest than pastes, canned tomatoes, and sauces from China, consequently exaggerating Italy's production numbers. Italy's domestic production and processing continue to be aided by government subsidies, as farmers and industries will receive US$230 million each year through 2015.[14] In 2009, Italy outpaced second-place Spain in processed-tomato production by more than eight hundred thousand tons.[15]

Figure 6.1 Tomato Production 2012 (Millions of Tons).

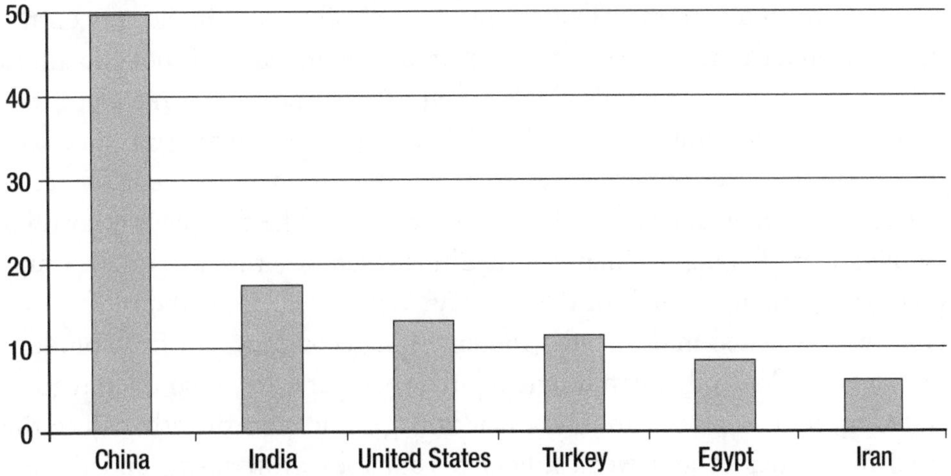

Source: FAOSTAT, 2012, Tomato Production.

The overwhelming percentage of tomatoes grown in developed countries are intended for processing, allowing for mechanized harvesting, which reduces the cost. As discussed below, fresh tomatoes are considerably more labor-intensive, requiring handpicking, which makes them comparatively more expensive than canned products. The H. J. Heinz Company uses more tomatoes than any other company worldwide, processing over 2 million tons that go into any number of its products, from its world-renowned ketchup to Smart Ones Angel Hair Marinara.[16] The company produces its own hybrid variety used by farmers who grow tomatoes solely for Heinz. More often than not, a corporation contracts with farmers to supply a specific variety of tomato for a particular purpose. Local conditions at times offer a bonus by producing a certain flavor. Corporations also strategize by using a tomato variety that is less demanding in terms of irrigation, fertilizers, and so on.

Developed and emerging economies increasingly rely on greenhouse farming to guarantee year-round fresh tomatoes and increased production for processing and export. In the United States, for example, shipping field-grown tomatoes south to north during the winter months means picking barely vine-ripened tomatoes, minimizing flavor and affecting texture. Greenhouse production may also require picking earlier than for those field-grown closer to market, but it allows for closer proximity to markets year-round. Canadian growers adopted this method in the 1990s, with the United States and Mexico following suit.[17] Although investment costs are considerably higher, agribusiness companies continue to invest in greenhouse tomatoes in developed and emerging economies because consumers are willing to pay for a regular supply of fresh tomatoes.[18] These tomatoes are often sold in clusters on the vine to lend a fresher appearance. Consumer demand alone is not enough to offset costs, so companies also look to sell to restaurants to make a profit.

The hothouse equivalent of industrial parks dot the Mediterranean coastline of Turkey, where greenhouses grow tomatoes to meet the huge domestic demand, as well as for export throughout Europe. The food supply corridor running from Beijing to Shanghai in China resembles that in Turkey,[19] supplying more than one-half of the country's tomatoes.[20] Greenhouse farming is increasingly used in developed and emerging economies for fresh produce production. Controlled conditions regulate temperature, guarantee regular watering, protect plants from weather damage, and significantly reduce the need for pesticides and weed killers.[21] Tomatoes grow faster under these conditions, taking at least one month less than those grown in the field, increasing the overall amount produced each year.[22] Tomatoes originated in the dry, hot, well-irrigated areas of the Andes, so they grow best in places that mimic those conditions. In regions with hot, humid seasons, such as Nigeria, which is the thirteenth biggest producer in the world, tomatoes are more susceptible to disease and pests. In some developing countries, such as Kenya, nongovernmental organizations (NGO) have funded growers to build hothouses for domestic production because during the wet season, tomatoes are more likely to get damaged, jacking up the price for people who depend on this staple food.

THE ISSUES

Tomato production for export is concentrated in the global north and a few GS countries. Because tomatoes are a key ingredient in most cuisines around the world, countries that can produce them do so to meet domestic demand. As previously mentioned, tomatoes are also highly perishable, reducing the number of miles they can travel before rotting. For both domestic and export production, pricing raises some issues. Growers are affected by prices set by retail grocers, weather conditions, political crises, and economic policies.

Consumers in GN countries are increasingly paying attention to how tomatoes and other foods are produced, under what environmental conditions, and how far goods have traveled. One aspect of food production particularly related to fresh produce that tends to slip under the radar of many consumers is who is involved in production. The most pressing issue in the tomato industry in the United States and Europe involves the use of immigrant laborers, who often migrate as seasons change, to pick produce.

Prices

Tomato production has provided a fairly stable income for farmers over time, though dependence on commodities (as seen in other chapters) puts farmers in a more vulnerable position in comparison to people in the manufacturing and service sectors. Leverage by retailers over price paid, as discussed in Chapter 1, has reduced farmer earnings in the United States by about 10 percent since the 1980s.[23] Global retail chains and multinational food companies have considerable bargaining power when contracting for products. The spread of big retail chains in developing countries has an effect not only on farmers, by influencing the price paid, but also on suppliers, by making more stringent demands. Walmart and Carrefour, two of the biggest retail grocers in the world, are moving into markets previously filled by small grocers, and multinational corporations (MNCs) are less tolerant of mediocre-quality produce and late deliveries.[24] To remain a chain supplier, farmers have to upgrade their service and product, or they will be replaced by another supplier willing to provide a constant, consistent flow of produce. Small farmers are often pushed out of the supply chain because they cannot compete with agribusinesses, as they are financially unable to accept below-production prices for their produce. One tomato farmer in India produces eight to ten tons of tomatoes each season, yet can barely make a living because, after investing $715 in seeds, pesticides, and fertilizer, he only earns about $1,000.[25]

Factors like weather conditions, strikes, conflict, and government policies also affect prices. In 2010, drought devastated tomato crops in northern India, and in 2012 floods damaged crops in Taiwan. Water shortages in 2012 in California resulted in extensive layoffs. Migrant farmhands in Italy protested work and living conditions by going on strike in 2011. Farmers in Syria, where tomatoes are the fourth biggest agricultural commodity, suffered losses from civil unrest.[26]

Tariffs, quotas, nontariff barriers, and subsidization policies give advantages to farmers in developed economies. Countries impose these measures to protect domestic production. The institution of the WTO allowed that organization to better address tariff and nontariff barriers than its predecessor, the General Agreement on Tariffs and Trade, which was not a formal organization but a set of multilateral trade policies. Because the WTO has the power to rule on disputes, countries are increasingly discouraged from implementing trade barriers. As discussed with sugar subsidies in Chapter 4, countries are more inclined to change their policies when a ruling by the WTO finds against them. Attempts to amend these policies, nevertheless, take time and often require a direct incentive to encourage implementation.

Under some circumstances, however, the WTO permits countries to retain tariffs. The European Union, for example, maintains tariffs to protect its wheat production, as well as pays out subsidies for produce under "special agricultural safeguard" arrangements.[27] GN producing countries are more likely to add seasonal tariffs, adopt health and safety restrictions, and set quotas to protect domestic produce sales from imports. The dumping of excess tomatoes from countries that subsidize tomatoes also affects farmers in developing countries, as they cannot compete with the cheaper prices.

Government subsidies impact market competitiveness, favoring the GN countries that can afford to earmark funds. As with soybeans and tuna, the United States and EU countries continue to support the agriculture and fishing industries, even though the threat of food shortages in the twentieth century that drove them to enact protective measures is no longer viable. Developing countries are particularly at a disadvantage because agricultural subsidies were largely eliminated as conditions for lending in the 1980s. Farmers in developing countries struggle to afford inputs such as fertilizers and seeds that were subsidized prior to restructuring. Farmers in sub-Saharan Africa have been particularly affected by these policies, where low input use has resulted in low food production.[28] Small farmers in GN countries are disadvantaged by subsidization as agribusiness averaged more than $1 million in funding under the US Farm Bill's federal crop-insurance program, whereas small farmers received about $40,000.[29] International pressures from countries filing subsidies disputes against the United States with the WTO encourages the US Congress to revise the Farm Bill, though, as explained in Chapter 4, subsidy reductions are complex and take years to accomplish.

Although the European Union has been actively working to reduce payouts in the tomato sector, developing countries find it difficult to compete. Tomato farmers in Italy, for example, earn an additional forty-one cents for every dollar of tomatoes sold, allowing them to undercut farmers in countries that do not subsidize the farming industry.[30] Due to its proximity to the EU market, Ghana is in a position to exploit its fresh tomato production as a cash crop export. Not surprisingly, Ghana has experienced difficulty breaking into the European market. EU subsidies and policies that limit competition with domestic tomatoes by claiming that production conditions do not meet EU standards have acted as a nontariff barrier on imports.[31]

Because Ghana was required to privatize state-owned processing factories under structural adjustment programs in the 1980s, farmers switched to tomato varieties bred for fresh consumption. Privatization opened the door to European canned tomatoes, which came to dominate the Ghanaian market.[32] Although the country is equipped to process tomatoes, farmers would have to shift production to canning tomatoes. They have little incentive, though, because of the stiff competition they would face from subsidized European imports.[33] With EU tomato processors receiving more than $300 million in subsidies annually, Ghanaian farmers have little chance to compete and lack bargaining power for getting their tomatoes processed.[34] Limited processing capacity leaves the country dependent on fresh produce instead of value-added goods.

On the heels of a rash of tomato farmer suicides in the late 2000s, the Ghanaian government set up a workshop in 2010 to strategize ways to improve tomato production and increase processing prospects. Competition from imports pushed down the price of tomatoes, burdening farmers with debt. Like the peppercorn farmers in India who were pushed to suicide when unable to repay their debts, Ghanaian farmers felt they had no other option but to end their lives.

"Think Global, Eat Local (and Organic)"

Competition has emerged in GN countries between the capitalist system that pushes for greater economy in production and the locavore movement. Local and regional produce have grown in popularity as better food because it is grown nearby by small farmers struggling against agribusiness to make ends meet. The locavore movement urges Americans and Europeans to save farmlands from ending up as paved parking lots for the next megamart. In reality, however, agribusiness is a far more efficient producer of food, leaving a smaller carbon footprint on the earth.

Despite arguments that opting for a locavore diet is better for the environment and more socially just, this thinking is considered a "local trap" that food activists and researchers fall into because they fail to acknowledge the greater implications of local-scale reliance.[35] Promoting national food independence by eating primarily locally produced foods has unintended consequences for people in the global south, as this small-scale strategy undermines development ecologically and socially. These "First-World fetishes," as one author calls them, push for farmers' markets and supermarkets to stock local produce, which often does not include genetically modified organisms (GMOs) and is organically grown.[36] These foods, however, are more expensive and thereby privilege wealthier people at the risk of providing less food locally and globally.

A "globavore" approach to eating is actually more energy efficient—even with transportation factored into the equation. GS farmers and the planet would be better served by farming on a large scale, growing GMO crops, and exporting food from places that can more sustainably produce it. Field-grown tomatoes shipped from Africa to Europe, for instance, require far less energy to grow and transport than those produced by hothouses in the Netherlands.

Recipe Box

Tomatoes Sprouting Gills

The public got wind in the 1990s that scientists were attempting to improve tomatoes' resistance to cold temperatures by splicing Atlantic cod genes into their DNA. Questions abounded about whether people with fish allergies would be allergic to the tomatoes, if vegetarians would be violating their pledge to avoid seafood if they unknowingly ate these tomatoes, and what Frankenfood would be next? Despite attempts to introduce a genome that would make tomatoes more impervious to the cold, the "fish tomato" never materialized. Yet the debate over the value of GMOs continues to pop up on political agendas, particularly in Europe, where protests against companies developing transgenic plants have provoked destruction of GMO crops.

A change in diet can address concerns about the impact of "food miles," or long-distance distribution of food, and better help the planet. Producing red meat and dairy actually contributes more to carbon emissions because of the methane produced by livestock, so moving away from these products and replacing them with chicken, fish, and eggs—or better yet, a plant-based diet—does more to save the planet than exclusively eating locally sourced food.[37] Although air transport of fresh foods is detrimental to the environment, shipping produce one thousand miles by sea uses less fuel per ton than driving it one hundred miles by truck.[38]

Reliance on organic foods, whose production rejects GMO seeds along with chemical fertilizers, herbicides, and pesticides, is also unnecessarily harsher on the planet. A joint university study found that organic methods are, on average, 25 percent less productive than conventional methods, particularly for staple foods.[39] In order to sustain current levels of crop production in the United States using only organic fertilizer, 5 to 6 billion more cows would have to be raised to supply enough manure.[40] Not using the herbicides that allow farmers to forego tilling fields before sowing seeds would cause a dust bowl equivalent of topsoil to erode.[41] GMO seeds also offer hope for producing tomatoes that not only require fewer pesticides but improve upon the dull

Recipe Box

Feeling Better about Food Choices

The adage "You are what you eat" might make us think twice before choosing a conventionally grown tomato over an organic one in the grocery store. To feel help us feel even better about ourselves, Dole began putting stickers on their organic produce so that consumers could see where their food is grown. On the Dole Organic website (http://www.doleorganic.com), consumers can input the number of the farm on their produce label for a virtual visit to that farm, where they can "meet" the farmers who grew their food. Despite the many disadvantages of organic farming for poorer people and the planet, one of its few benefits is that workers are not exposed to harmful pesticides and fertilizers used in the produce industry.

flavor of commercially grown tomatoes by developing a nonripening gene to extend the shelf-life of fresh tomatoes.[42]

The unfortunate outcome of growing produce—especially tomatoes—in locations like Florida where they do not thrive without excessive chemicals is that workers suffer. Reports of the chemicals used in field-grown tomato production and the harm spraying causes farmhands cause real concern for workers' lives. The sensationalized reports of possible health effects for consumers are unsubstantiated scare tactics used by the media to gain audiences. The need for chemicals comes from growing tomatoes in a place completely unsuitable for the plant. While California has reported health issues with pickers, the numbers are nowhere close to those in Florida, where producing unblemished tomatoes requires eight times the amount of chemicals.[43] Because the state is one of the few places in the United States where tomatoes can be grown in the winter months, entrepreneurial farmers figured out how to grow tomatoes in humid, soil-less conditions, so that Florida now supplies one-third of all fresh tomatoes in the country.[44] Because the land and climate are not suitable to growing tomatoes, an excess of chemicals are required for production, in turn exposing pickers to harmful work conditions. The spraying of fields when farmhands are harvesting has caused numerous health problems in the form of cancer, respiratory difficulties, and birth defects.

Organic farming has definite advantages. Farms benefit from raising diverse crops. Owners have greater autonomy from the big businesses that control GMO seeds and their necessary inputs, and workers are preserved from risk of exposure to chemical fertilizers and pesticides. Some plots have demonstrated yields comparable to conventionally grown crops. Consumers feel better about supporting these farms. Another concern about using GMOs is their effect on flora and fauna. Bee populations are at risk, and unwanted weeds are growing more resistance to chemicals. The unfortunate reality is that supporting the world's population—especially its future populations—through organic farming is not possible.

A number of factors make conventional farming that relies on GMO seeds more effective in terms of not only producing crops but protecting the environment. In most parts of the world, farmers lack the necessary inputs to reap yields comparable to conventionally produced foods. Insufficient development funds, coupled with the biological wall that evolution has hit for naturally grown plants, limit the possibility to match the pace of food demand with food production in most parts of the world.[45] With a steadily increasing global population, increasing reliance on locally grown organic foods is not practical. Another strike against organic farming is the amount of land necessary to support increases in the use of this method. Conventional farming was estimated to save an additional 750,000 square feet of new land from the plough in 2011[46]—the equivalent of the sea territory covered by the 1,225 Marshall Islands in the northern Pacific Ocean. Conventional farming also decreases reliance on fertilizers, pesticides, and other chemicals added to crops, since seeds are increasingly being programmed to be heartier, fight off pests, and yield greater output per plant.

Yet the locavore movement is growing traction. The unfortunate consequence of increased reliance on organic products is that, since yields are lower on organic farms, they require more land to meet increasing demand, pushing up the price on conventional foods for people who can't afford to indulge in "First-World fetishes." With an increasing number of MNCs, like Dole, jumping on the organic bandwagon to tap the wealth of those willing to pay extra for these products, more environmental damage will occur than through conventional production. The neoliberal economic model encourages these MNCs to meet the demands of GN desires at the risk of jeopardizing the food security of poorer people around the world.

Migration for Labor

A representative from the United Farm Workers of America (UFW) appeared on *The Colbert Report* in 2010 in an effort to raise awareness about rights for undocumented farm laborers with the "Take Our Jobs" campaign. The farmworkers invited Americans literally to take their jobs, since popular opinion holds that illegal immigrants steal American's jobs. The point of the campaign was to show that Americans are not really interested in filling these positions, so the country is dependent on immigrants. To underscore its point, the UFW invited workers to replace them in the fields, offering to help those interested connect with their employers. Of the eighty-six hundred people who expressed an interest in farmwork, only seven took jobs.[47] Not only is farm labor backbreaking, disrespected work, but farmhands have to migrate as crops ripen in different parts of the country to earn whatever money they can in a year.

When the House Judiciary Committee's Subcommittee on Immigration, Citizenship, Refugees, Border Security, and International Law raised the issue of immigrant farm labor in 2010, Stephen Colbert testified on behalf of the UFW. Responding, in character, to the subcommittee, he suggested that because "Americans are far too dependent on immigrant labor to pick fruits and vegetables … the obvious answer is for all of us to stop eating fruits and vegetables."[48] Although Colbert took a comedic approach to the subject, he was trying to draw attention to this serious matter, which is the same reason he spent a day in August working on a farm.

In most parts of the United States and Europe, crops are grown seasonally rather than year-round. Unlike hothouse tomatoes, field-grown crops rely heavily on migrant farmhands. Foreign-born laborers constitute 60 percent of agricultural workers in the United States.[49] Some of these laborers are in the country legally; many others are not. Of the illegal immigrants, some have been trafficked; they are trapped in involuntary servitude to farm owners until they pay off their debts. The issue is rooted in the desire for cheap labor. The problem is that people in the global north do not aspire to the mostly seasonal, backbreaking labor of picking tomatoes. Illegal immigrants willing to do the work do not have protection under the law; if they do, they may be unaware of their rights or unwilling to compromise the possibility of earning money to lodge a complaint. Workers endure harsh conditions and brutal treatment. Many emigrate to earn money to send to their families. Employers have leverage over laborers, threatening to report those who are illegal if they fail to comply. Field managers are likely to dock their pay if they complain. Traffickers have a business to protect and don't even hesitate to use death threats to keep workers in line. Without paperwork, illegal-entry and trafficked humans lack status, making them fear the law as much as their bosses.

Immigrant laborers in other developed countries face similar circumstances and conditions: poor living conditions, ridiculously high rent and food prices, no health care or benefits, and pay far below minimum wage. Employers are able to exploit pickers because of the questionable legality of their work status. Farm owners are able to distance themselves from culpability in using both illegal immigrants and trafficked humans, hiding behind layers of underlings who are directly responsible for the laborers. In cases where arrests have been made, prosecutors find it difficult to link owners to these activities.

Greed on the part of farm owners might seem like the obvious explanation for workers' conditions, but these owners are forced to find ways to cut costs to match the competition and face pressure from corporations to lower prices. Because agricultural inputs such as the price of land, fertilizers, seeds, and so on cannot be negotiated, wages are one of the few controls farmers have to improve their bottom lines. And for farms that sell fresh tomatoes, labor prices are a significant factor since the crop must be picked by hand. Of course, the situation does not excuse exploitation, but it explains why owners are inclined to pay as little as possible.

Migrant workers in the United States Reports of human trafficking, worker abuses, and poor living conditions for farmhands led workers in Florida to form a community group in 1993 to deal with their situation. Those workers were better able to organize because Florida is one of the few places where tomatoes are grown year-round, allowing the farmhands more permanent work and living conditions. Instead of earning a minimum wage, the more than thirty thousand tomato pickers in the state are paid by the number of bushels picked in a day. Because any number of factors can delay picking, and any amount of time spent on work-related activities is not compensated, farmhands earn $10,000 to $12,000 a year, though that number is distorted because field manager pay, which is slightly higher, is also included.[50] This pay does not include health-care benefits, sick leave, or retirement plans. Workers have to cover their own health- and dental-care costs, which many just cannot afford on such low wages. Below-poverty-level wages and poor work conditions led the community group to organize into the Coalition of Immokalee Workers (CIW), which has since made amazing strides in pushing national food and grocery store chains to sign onto its Campaign for Fair Food, now called the Fair Food Program, whereby they agree to pay an extra penny per pound for their tomatoes, with the extra money going directly to the pickers. If farm owners fail to pass the penny on to their workers, they lose their MNC contracts. CIW has also worked to raise awareness about human trafficking with its Modern-Day Slave Museum. Recreating a box truck used to imprison workers, the mobile museum travels up and down the East Coast of the United States to raise awareness about human trafficking and the squalid, confining conditions of the slaves.

After ferocious battles with the two biggest farms and the Florida Tomato Growers Exchange, the organization finally got the necessary support of the owners to implement the penny-per-pound system.[51] Although a penny might not seem like a lot, consider that just one bushel of tomatoes weighs between thirty-two and thirty-five pounds.[52] A worker in Florida earns forty to forty-five cents per bucket.[53] If the worker fills ten buckets an hour, each holding one bushel, and works for eight hours, at most, the farmhand makes $36 a day. An extra penny means that the farmhand can earn almost a dollar more a day. This supplement might not seem like much, but it represents a 2 percent increase in annual income.

CIW was also able to negotiate a number of additional supports to improve worker rights and conditions, which, along with the penny-per-pound agreement, promote increased transparency in the supply chain and reduce the risk of worker abuse and human trafficking. Although successful thus far in persuading the biggest restaurant chains, CIW has yet to garner support from supermarket chains. For several years, Whole Foods was the only grocery store to sign the agreement, though after fifteen years and much criticism, Trader Joe's finally agreed. These chains, however, only buy a small portion of the fresh Florida tomatoes sold throughout the United States, encouraging CIW to continue its mission. Progress made by the CIW encourages other grassroots groups to organize to push for change when the government's efforts and effectiveness are limited.

Migrant workers in Italy As in the United States, migrant workers are necessary to harvest fresh field tomatoes in Italy. Work and living conditions in the two countries mirror one another, as farmhands pay exorbitantly to live in slums and buy food, only to be abused by corrupt field managers to earn a pittance. Dubbed "Europe's tomato slaves," workers from North Africa and eastern Europe migrate in August to earn money to send home.[54] Reports of threats, beatings, and racial abuse by "gangmasters," who act as brokers between workers and farm owners, are not uncommon. Because the immigrants have no benefits, if injured they have to rely on mobile health clinics run by NGOs like Doctors without Borders. Farm owners rely on migrant labor primarily for two reasons. Like Americans, Italians feel the work is beneath them. To make ends meet, owners need to cut costs somewhere to compete for sales. As they cannot negotiate lower prices for agriculture inputs, paying lower wages is the only solution enabling small farmers to earn a living.

FLAI-CGIL, a food, farm, and hotel union formed to address workers' issues, has been pushing the Italian government to recognize the problem. With no response, the union promoted the *Oro Rosso*, or "Red Gold," campaign to raise awareness about migrant laborer abuses.[55] Although it was far less visible than the Campaign for Fair Food in the United States, its strategy differed in that the FLAI-CGIL went to fields and slums to distribute information to the workers, alerting them to their rights to unionize. Its next step was the national "Stop *Caporalato*," or "Stop Illegal Hiring," campaign, which gained support from political parties and trade unions to push a bill through the Italian senate in 2011 to criminalize "illicit brokering of labor based on the exploitation of the work," which affects 550,000 migrant workers every year.[56]

In addition to the illicit brokering of labor through human trafficking, exploitation includes workers' earning below minimum wage, resulting in pay between $25 and $38 a day.[57] If pickers put in an eight-hour workday, they earn between $3.25 and $4.75 an hour. The need for income and competition to keep their positions make them more amenable to working longer hours, meaning an eight-hour workday is a very conservative estimate during harvest time. Although pressure by the union demonstrates that governments can be pushed to address migrant labor issues, the extent to which implementing the law will change work and living conditions remains to be seen. Perhaps the survey conducted by the government in 2012 not only shows progress but also indicates its intention to follow up on migrant labor issues.[58]

Laborers may risk losing work if they push for higher pay and benefits. Farm owners will upgrade as soon as investing in mechanized harvesting equipment proves more cost-effective than paying pickers. Because the Coalition of Immokalee Workers targeted restaurant and grocery chains to pay the additional penny per pound, farm owners did not incur any additional wage burden. The extent to which the Italian law is enforced may push tomato farmers to invest in harvesters and forego manual laborers. Increased labor costs in Italy may also result in increased competition from neighboring exporters with lower standards.

Globally regulating labor standards has proven difficult. Although GS countries should seemingly favor setting universal standards, they argue that the low cost of labor is one of their few comparative advantages in the global economy. This position has prevented the WTO from implementing international labor regulations.[59] As an agency of the United Nations, the International Labor Organization is only as effective as member countries allow it to be, as the cocoa labor situation, discussed in Chapter 4, demonstrates. GS states are in the precarious situation of needing to use their labor to their competitive advantage, making it more difficult to institute laws if they are not uniform across all developing countries. Even when they want to set standards, developing countries are in less of a position to adopt, implement, and enforce laws, given that they have limited resources and struggle against corruption. Businesses are the key to effecting change, though they need an economic incentive to implement minimum standards.

CONCLUSION

Concern for human rights abuses in the tomato and other industries gave rise to the fair trade movement in the 1980s.[60] One of the biggest driving factors behind its conception was ensuring that workers in developing countries were not exploited. MNCs and NGOs operate companies that set standards for fair trade. The only qualification to earn a fair trade label is a guaranteed minimum wage. Labels otherwise vary in stringency for qualifications, with Fairtrade International having the highest standards.

Fair trade goods are not synonymous with organically produced products. Fair trade focuses on the labor behind the produce, while organics focus on the product. Although fair trade–certified tomatoes are often also organic, the reverse is not necessarily the case. The biggest difference is that workers may not receive the livable minimum wage guaranteed by the fair trade process even though the tomatoes are grown organically. Because the use of chemicals can be detrimental to the health of workers, fair trade production may encourage growing organic produce. Organic farming presents a number of barriers. This type of farming offers lower crop yields, while at the same time requiring more land, water, and natural fertilizers, pesticides, and herbicides. These factors also make farming organic products more labor-intensive. The small demand for products that are both fair trade and organic is likely to dissuade struggling families in developing countries from selling certified produce.

Exposés of picking conditions in the United States and Europe have encouraged a push for fair trade tomatoes. Although the Coalition of Immokalee Workers is not a fair trade organization, ground gained by its Campaign for Fair Food has helped farmhands earn a more livable wage with the additional penny per pound MNCs were willing to pay for tomatoes. Fair trade tomatoes are late coming, as worker conditions in the tomato industry have received less attention in comparison to those in the coffee and cocoa industries. Perhaps one reason for the lack of publicity is that, unlike imported commodities, tomatoes are produced domestically, so consumers are more inclined to turn a blind eye to injustices happening at home. The low demand for fair trade tomatoes has thus far been another factor contributing to slow growth. Few farms grow fair trade–certified tomatoes in the United States and the European Union, which means that few companies sell certified processed tomatoes.

The Food Alliance, a collaborative project conceived in 1993 in the Pacific Northwest, is the only certified fair trade label for tomatoes in the United States, Canada, and Mexico, with over 320 certified farms.[61] Minimum requirements to earn certification focus on sustainable agricultural practices for humans and the environment. Farm conditions must promote safety, be nondiscriminatory, offer employee benefits, and pay the minimum wage. Farmers must use non-GMO seeds, minimize reliance on chemical pesticides and herbicides, and adopt water, soil, and wildlife habitat-conservation measures. Farms are subject to third-party inspection to ensure standards are implemented and upheld. Foods certified by the Food Alliance bear a fair trade–certified label.

The European Trade Union Institute, in reaction to treatment of migrant tomato pickers, is working toward devising a fair trade strategy to ensure minimum livable wages and humane conditions. FLAI-CGIL, the Italian union pushing for migrant labor rights, is pushing for an industry-wide fair trade certification program. Instituting a labeling scheme would increase awareness and improve conditions for pickers. Getting the country's senate to pass such a bill would be monumental, though the implementation of such regulation would be costly and undoubtedly meet with great resistance.

Examining tomatoes offers insight into other perishable food commodities. A number of vegetables (green beans, asparagus, and lettuce) and the overwhelming majority of fruit (apples, oranges, grapes for raisins, and strawberries, to name a few) grown in developed countries have to be hand-picked. Labor costs burden farm owners, who have few options for cutting costs beyond wage reduction. Reliance on migrant workers has encouraged human trafficking and mistreatment of undocumented workers. GN farm policies and trade practices disadvantage developing countries. The push to eat locally, organically produced tomatoes in order to reduce food miles and protect the environment also serves to undermine opportunities for farmers in developing countries. Organized movements in the United States and European Union have helped to address worker injustices, though widespread produce-industry improvements remain necessary.

Discussion Questions: Tomatoes: Immigration and the Global Food Supply

1. What do tomatoes provide the consumer in terms of nutrition?
2. How is a Supreme Court case linked to describing tomatoes in the US? What was the case and what is the outcome?
3. What are some of the characteristics that have been favored in breeding?
4. Where are tomatoes indigenous and how did they end up as one of the most commonly consumed plants in the world?
5. Who is the top tomato producer in the world? Who is the second most common producer? Why are chemicals needed to produce tomatoes?

Nutrition and the Indigenous Body
A Genetic Concept of Food

ANDREA ZITTLAU

WHEN LOOKING FOR A CULINARY EXPERIENCE in Washington, D.C., Mitsitam, the café in the National Museum of the American Indian, located directly on the Mall, is no longer exclusively an insider's tip. The secret to its success is a menu inspired by the traditional cuisine of the Indigenous peoples of the Americas. Hungry customers can find anything from corn bread and freshly prepared salads to buffalo meat and prickly-pear ice cream. Reviews have praised the exotic range of the dishes, but have often reproved the café for its 'inauthentic' albeit creative food preparation and combinations. Tom Sietsema, the food critic for the *Washington Post*, found the food selections satisfying, although the menu, he wrote, included "a few silly exceptions":

> The Indian tacos from the Plains heap iceberg lettuce, grated cheddar cheese and chili on saucer-size fry bread, which doesn't bring to mind the prairies so much as it does a TGIF. And I seriously doubt any Indians traditionally finished their meals with fruit tarts or coconut macaroons, both of which are also available here. But the success stories prevail over the lapses.[1]

This perception of Indigenous cuisine is a prevalent one. Indigenous peoples have long been portrayed as belonging to the past, to vanished civilizations that were assumed to be inferior to those of the Western world. The twentieth century revolutionized this view in several arenas, including those of art, music, and the celebration of numerous festivals and rituals. The contempo-

---

[1] Tom Sietsema, "Mitsitam Café," *Washington Post Magazine* (16 October 2005).

rary expressions of these cultural practices, which have refused to be constricted or constrained by traditional notions of authenticity, contributed to the acknowledgment that today's Indigenous cultures are essential parts of modern society. An opposite move, however, can be observed concerning environmental issues, and food in particular. The concept of an authentic cuisine, which has over the centuries resisted all cultural influences, is a common one. And in the wake of claims of Indigenous identities based on genetics, food discourses have carved out a field all their own. The Indigenous body is perceived (by Natives as well as by non-Natives) as fundamentally different from that of the non-Native, thus requiring a special diet and particular kinds of physical activity. Often portrayed as hunter–gatherers, warriors, and shamans, and as masters of the wilderness, Indigenous people remain closely and stereotypically connected with discourses on food. And although Native communities are making their contemporary voices heard, the long shadow of the past continues to follow them into the future. This is an interesting phenomenon, one that relates to centuries-old debates, arguments that have tried to prove the Indigenous body unfit for Western civilization. The present essay seeks to explore a genetic concept of food in relation to diabetes resulting in a quest for authentic Indigenous ingredients, which then revive colonial constellations of Self and Other.

Decoding Diabetes

Contemporary civil society, as Janet Flammang summarizes it, is a fast-paced consumer culture driven by workaholics.[2] People's daily routines allow little time for diversified meals and food rituals. The market is dominated by processed and flavoured food that has been manufactured, not grown. The success of books like Jonathan Safran Foer's *Eating Animals* and Michael Pollan's *In Defense of Food* reflects a public concern with food production and careless consumption:

> Most of what we are consuming today is not food, and how we are
> consuming it – in the car, in front of the TV, and increasingly alone –
> is not really eating. Instead of food, we're consuming 'edible foodlike
> substances' – no longer the products of nature but of food science.[3]

---

[2] Janet Flammang, *The Taste of Civilization: Food, Politics, and Civil Society* (Chicago: U of Illinois P, 2009): 1.

[3] Michael Pollan, *In Defense of Food: An Eater's Manifesto* (New York: Penguin, 2008): blurb.

This element of artificiality is thought to cause numerous health problems, including allergies and diabetes. Formerly known as non-insulin-dependent diabetes mellitus (NIDDM), or adult-onset diabetes, it is currently one of the world's most serious health threats – some scholars even refer to it as an emerging global epidemic,[4] and *Indian Country Today* has called diabetes "an enemy that must be confronted."[5] Presently, at least 100 million people suffer from Type 2 diabetes worldwide (hereafter referred to as 'diabetes'), rising fastest in developing countries and among ethnic-minority groups, migrant populations, and disadvantaged communities in developed nations.[6] Native Americans have been described as a population particularly at risk for diabetes, the disease having surfaced in many Native communities after World War Two, increasing after the 1970s, and continuing to spread at alarmingly high rates.

Diabetes causes the body to either fail to produce enough insulin through the pancreas or to render it incapable of properly using the insulin it does produce. An essential hormone, insulin transports glucose, the body's basic fuel, to all its cells. When this function breaks down, it can lead to, among other things, infection and gangrene, and may further result in nerve damage, blindness, kidney failure, limb amputation, and ultimately death. There is, as yet, no cure for diabetes, because its causes remain unknown. The disease is controlled as much as possible through a variety of protocols that are known to prevent it from progressing, such as a change in diet and an increase in physical activity.

The supposition is that, in order to manifest itself, diabetes requires a certain genetic precondition, one that is found more routinely in Native Americans than in any other population:[7]

---

[4] See, for example, Paul Zimmet et al., "Epidemiology, Evidence for Prevention: Type 2 Diabetes," in *The Epidemiology of Diabetes Mellitus: An International Perspective*, ed. Jean–Marie Ekoé, Paul Zimmet & Rhys Williams (New York: John Wiley, 2001): 41.

[5] "Confronting Diabetes with Tradition," *Indian Country Today* (20 December 2000) in *America is Indian Country. Opinions and Perspectives from Indian Country Today*, ed. José Barreiro & Tim Johnson (Golden CO: Fulcrum, 2005): 236.

[6] See Daniel C. Benyshek, John F. Martin & Carol S. Johnston, "A Reconsideration of the Origins of the Type 2 Diabetes Epidemic among Native Americans and the Implications for Intervention Policy," *Medical Anthropology* 20.1 (2001): 25–26.

[7] Other sources mention the Australian Aboriginals and the Torres Strait Island people as the populations with the highest risk (Zimmer et al., "Epidemiology,

There are approximately 100,000 genes packed into 23 pairs of chromosomes in each person. Within a gene, chemicals form individual codes, like words, which tell the cells of the body what to do. It is the code within a gene that directs the body to [...] circulate blood and hormones such as adrenalin and insulin.

Some diseases are caused by bacteria or viruses that infect the body and make it sick. Others, such as diabetes, occur because a gene's code causes it to function differently under some circumstances. [...] A person can't choose his or her genes.[8]

This genetic argument can be traced back to the 'thrifty genotype' hypothesis, which was most prominently developed by James Neel in an article published in 1962 in the *American Journal of Human Genetics*. According to Neel, Native Americans faced difficult conditions on their way from Asia to North America thousands of years ago. They suffered through cycles of starvation that alternated with periods of an overabundance in food supplies. This situation favoured the survival of those whose bodies could "more readily convert blood sugar into stored fat when food was available."[9] Whereas Neel's 'thrifty genotype' hypothesis applies to all humans who undergo this starvation/overabundance cycle with food, a "population specific evolutionary model [...], the New World Syndrome, was proposed."[10] This syndrome was considered applicable to Indigenous populations and was thought to be related to the traditional ways in which they lived, ways that were believed to have been lost.[11] In contemporary society, the body's ability to effectively use all the energy sources it consumes has become a disadvantage, leading, in many

---

Evidence for Prevention: Type 2 Diabetes," 41). And Benyshek et al. call attention to the fact that urban Fijians of East Indian ancestry, the Chinese population of Mauritius, and Singaporean Malays have some of the highest rates of Type 2 diabetes in the world. Benyshek et al., "A Reconsideration of the Origins of the Type 2 Diabetes Epidemic among Native Americans and the Implications for Intervention Policy," 34–35.

[8] Jane DeMouy, "Genetic Research," *The Pima Indians: Pathfinders for Health*, http://diabetes.niddk.nih.gov/dm/pubs/pima/genetic/genetic.htm (accessed 23 September 2010).

[9] Benyshek et al., "A Reconsideration of the Origins of the Type 2 Diabetes Epidemic among Native Americans and the Implications for Intervention Policy," 30.

[10] Emőke J.E. Szathmáry, "Non-Insulin Dependent Diabetes Mellitus among Aboriginal North Americans," *Annual Review of Anthropology* 23 (1994): 465.

[11] Szathmáry, "Non-Insulin Dependent Diabetes Mellitus among Aboriginal North Americans," 465.

cases, to diabetes and obesity. Since the Indigenous body, according to the assumption of the New World Syndrome, processes food differently, it is more likely to succumb to diseases brought by Western civilization.

As a hypothesis, the genetic argument is now taken for granted, markedly influencing clinical studies on diabetes over the last five decades, with investigations of the disease continuing to focus on Native Americans and their food habits. Titles such as "Diabetes in Relation to Serum Levels of Polychlorinated Biphenyls and Chlorinated Pesticides in Adult Native Americans"[12] and "Mental Health Status and Diabetes among Whites and Native Americans: Is Race an Effect Modifier?"[13] are typical, confirming that Indigenous peoples have yet again become subjects of scientific surveys.[14] Whereas the pesticides study was carried out in a community identified as Mohawk, the examination of mental health in relation to diabetes makes no mention of tribal affiliations. In these two studies, as well as many others, because ethnicity was categorized not as a cultural phenomenon but as a biological factor that contributed significantly to the outbreak of the disease, chemical, biological, medical, and anthropological surveys of diabetes have most often been conducted among Indigenous communities.

One prominent example is the Strong Heart Study (SHS), which has been observing cardiovascular disease and its risk factors among Native Americans since 1988, and has become "the largest epidemiologic study of American Indians ever undertaken."[15] Thirteen American Indian tribes and communities situated in four states (Arizona, North and South Dakota, and Oklahoma) are participating in the long-term study, which in the course of its investigations

---

[12] Neculai Codru et al., "Diabetes in Relation to Serum Levels of Polychlorinated Biphenyls and Chlorinated Pesticides in Adult Native Americans," *Environmental Health Perspectives* 115.10 (October 2007): 1442–47.

[13] Abe E. Sahmoun, Mary J. Markland & Steven D. Helgerson, "Mental Health Status and Diabetes among Whites and Native Americans: Is Race an Effect Modifier?" *Journal of Health Care for the Poor and Underserved* 18.3 (August 2007): 599–608.

[14] The genetic argument has also been taken up in studies of other ethnicities – for example, "A Comparison Between Japanese-Americans Living in Hawaii and Los Angeles and Native Japanese," another study that presupposes genetic origins of diabetes Type 2. The participants were especially chosen because they were "genetically identical to native Japanese" and had not "intermarried with other races." Shigetada Nakanishi et al., *Biomedicine and Pharmacotherapy* 58.10 (December 2004): 571–77.

[15] *Strong Heart Study*, http://strongheart.ouhsc.edu/ (accessed 12 September 2010).

of heart disease, has identified age, parental diabetes, obesity, and "a higher degree of American Indian ancestry" as diabetes risk factors.[16]

Evidence of genetic susceptibility and diabetes, however, has yet to be found, and scholars have challenged the 'thrifty genotype' hypothesis. Beny-shek et al., for example, point out that there is no proof that hunter–gatherers suffered significant periods of starvation in the prehistoric past:

> In fact, the vast majority of archaeological and ethnographic evidence suggests that agricultural societies throughout time have been much more susceptible to severe, periodic famine than have hunters and gatherers.[17]

They also call attention to the fact that several Indigenous communities, including the Pueblo, have a long agricultural history and still experience a high rate of diabetes; according to the 'thrifty genotype' hypothesis, the opposite should be the case.[18] Gilbert Velho and Philippe Froguel offer the proposition that diabetes "seems to result from several combined gene defects,"[19] that "many different combinations of gene defects may exist among diabetic patients,"[20] and conclude that "complex interactions between genes and environment complicate the task of identifying any single genetic susceptibility factor."[21] Still, none of the extensive inquiries into the relationship between diabetes and genetics has met with success so far.[22]

---

[16] Lee et al., quoted in Yvette Roubideaux & Kelly Acton, "Diabetes in American Indians," in *Promises to Keep*, ed. Mim Dixon & Yvette Roubideaux (Washington DC: American Public Health Association, 2001): 195.

[17] Benyshek et al., "A Reconsideration of the Origins of the Type 2 Diabetes Epidemic among Native Americans and the Implications for Intervention Policy," 34.

[18] Benyshek et al. suggest a connection between undernutrition *in utero* and the appearance of Type 2 diabetes in later life. They point out that many Native Americans share a history of deprivation and forced relocations, which resulted in such conditions ("A Reconsideration of the Origins of the Type 2 Diabetes Epidemic among Native Americans and the Implications for Intervention Policy," 35–37).

[19] Gilbert Velho & Philippe Froguel, "Type 2 Diabetes: Genetic Factors," in *The Epidemiology of Diabetes Mellitus: An International Perspective*, ed. Jean–Marie Ekoé, Paul Zimmet & Rhys Williams (New York: John Wiley, 2001): 141.

[20] Velho & Froguel, "Type 2 Diabetes: Genetic Factors," 141.

[21] "Type 2 Diabetes: Genetic Factors," 141.

[22] However, it was proven that genetic factors play a significant role in some rare forms of diabetes, such as in the Maturity Onset Diabetes of the Young (MODY) from

These studies do suggest, however, that because of supposed genetic differences, Indigenous people process modern food differently from non-Native people. Less tolerant of processed food, according to this argument, Native populations should go back to traditional diets. This assertion has been made most prominently by Kerin O'Dea, who suggests a return to an archaic way of life. O'Dea himself supervised a project in 1980 in which "13 full-blood Aboriginal men and women"[23] participated. Together, they simulated the conditions on which Neel based his 'thrifty genotype' hypothesis: living as hunter–gatherers. The thirteen men and women spent three months "living a relatively traditional lifestyle"[24] which consisted mainly of hunting and gathering the food essential for their survival. Among the outcomes was the fact that all "Aboriginals [...] lost weight during the study,"[25] especially those overweight prior to the study, and their state of health improved significantly. O'Dea confirmed, as have many others, that a healthy diet minimizes the symptoms of diabetes and slows the progress of the disease. Healthy eating habits are also believed to reduce the risk of developing the disease in the first place. At the same time, his investigation illustrates the significance of the assumption that the Indigenous body is genetically different from the non-Native body. The simulation project considered no parameters (e.g., social, environmental, educational) other than ethnicity (perceived to be biologically determined), and it did not test other populations for their tolerance of culturally specific foods. Furthermore, the fabrication of an historical setting demonstrates both an imperialist nostalgia for a past that is impossible to recreate, and the revival of nineteenth-century discourses on indigenous peoples.

---

which only two percent of all Type 2 diabetes patients suffer (see Velho & Froguel, "Type 2 Diabetes: Genetic Factors," 142, and Benyshek et al., "A Reconsideration of the Origins of the Type 2 Diabetes Epidemic among Native Americans and the Implications for Intervention Policy," 32).

[23] Kerin O'Dea, "Traditional Diet and Food Preferences of Australian Aboriginal Hunter–Gatherers," *Philosophical Transactions: Biological Sciences* 334/1270 (November 1991): 233–41, quoted in Zimmet et al., "Epidemiology, Evidence for Prevention: Type 2 Diabetes," in *The Epidemiology of Diabetes Mellitus: An International Perspective*, 45.

[24] O'Dea, quoted in "Epidemiology, Evidence for Prevention: Type 2 Diabetes," 45.

[25] O'Dea, quoted in "Epidemiology, Evidence for Prevention: Type 2 Diabetes," 45.

The Desert Walk

The Centre for Indigenous Peoples' Nutrition and Environment (CINE) is an independent research institute concerned with environmental and cultural changes affecting the traditional food systems and nutrition of Indigenous peoples worldwide.[26] One of their goals is to conserve or re-establish traditional agricultural techniques and cultivate historical crops and plants judged to have escaped modern scientific manipulation. Whereas this can be seen as a counter-movement to the contemporary food industry, it has also been inspired by biological discourses on the Indigenous body. CINE's research activities include identifying nutritional deficiencies that have resulted "from discontinued use of traditional food resources altered by degradation of the environment" and have increased "chronic diseases such as diabetes, cancer and heart disease when people move away from traditional diet and activity patterns."[27] This approach presupposes that there exists an original cuisine that needs to be rediscovered. It also assumes that food cultures are stable cultural phenomena resistant to changes: there is only a 'before' European contact and an 'after,' but nothing in between.

Beginning in the seventeenth century, a diet that included fried potatoes, butter, rice, and coffee with sugar was introduced to Native Americans. These 'new' staples, however, did not immediately replace the traditional menu; rather, they were added to the traditional diet of game, fish, fruit, and vegetables. After World War Two, the diet of all Americans changed dramatically and cases of obesity and food-related diseases increased in all populations. For Native Americans, this process was clearly forced by the Bureau of Indian Affairs' Urban Relocation Program of the 1950s, during which the US government's promotion of acculturation and assimilation used, among other methods, the encouragement of 'American' food habits, which consisted of a high-calorie and high-fat diet. These efforts, Brooke Olson speculates, combined with several other factors, including the stress the programme caused in most of its participants, were a major cause of the massive outbreak of diabetes in Native American populations during the 1970s.[28] These food patterns

---

[26] *Centre for Indigenous People's Nutrition and Environment*, http://www.mcgill.ca/cine/ (accessed 13 October 2010).

[27] "Research Activities and Publications," *Centre for Indigenous People's Nutrition and Environment*, http://www.mcgill.ca/cine/research/ (accessed 13 October 2010).

[28] Brooke Olson, "Meeting the Challenges of American Indian Diabetes: Anthropological Perspectives on Prevention and Treatment," in *Medicine Ways: Disease,*

established themselves especially on reservations where the local food store controlled the community's food supply. It has only been hesitantly that initiatives have been launched to break this vicious circle between unhealthy living habits and diabetes. One recently established programme to promote healthier living is the Tohono O'odham Community Action, which includes a campaign to return to the consumption of supposed-to-be traditional foods.

The Tohono O'odham Nation is based in Arizona in the heart of the Sonoran Desert. In 1963, a survey of rheumatoid arthritis was taken in the Gila River area, during which a high rate of diabetes was discovered. Since then, the community has made itself available for an intensive long-term study of diabetes – of which they have the highest reported incidence in the world – by NIDDK, the National Institute of Diabetes and Digestive and Kidney Disease.[29] More than half of all community members suffer from diabetes, among them children as young as seven, which is particularly unusual for the disease. Scientists have conducted a number of tests within the community in order to gain some understanding of the causes of diabetes and its consequences. A key segment of the study is identifying the genes responsible for the disease and specific aspects of its behaviour. The idea is to break the genetic codes and determine as early as possible those individuals at risk, intervening before the disease has established itself.[30] Researchers have noted the "uniqueness of the community":[31] intermarriage with other ethnicities is rare and the same families have lived in the Gila River community for generations, both situations providing ideal conditions for carrying out genetic studies. Despite this hospitable environment, progress in detecting the particular genes responsible for diabetes remains at a standstill.

The Tohono O'odham, however, have drawn their own conclusions from the study and are in the process of reviving traditional diet and food rituals. On 10 March 2000, a group of about forty Tohono O'odham, Comcaac, and Yoeme Indians set out to walk 240 miles across the desert, following in the footsteps of their ancestors. Their journey lasted twelve days, during which

---

Health, and Survival among Native Americans, ed. Clifford E. Trafzer & Diane Weiner (New York, Toronto & Plymouth: AltaMira, 2001): 163–84, here 166.

[29] K.M. Venkat Narayan et al., "Non-Caucasian North American Populations: Native Americans," in *The Epidemiology of Diabetes Mellitus: An International Perspective,* 184.

[30] DeMouy, "Pathfinders for Health."

[31] "Pathfinders for Health."

they ate only foods of the desert and used only medicines made from Native plants. The idea was to call attention to the high rate of diabetes in the Tohono O'odham population and to promote a return to traditional foods and ways of living. Daniel Lopez, an elder who participated in the walk, says (referring to the traditional diet):

> These foods are low in fat and sugar but high in the complex carbo-hydrates and soluble fibers that studies among desert dwellers, both in Arizona and Australia, have shown to lower blood glucose, insulin and cholesterol. But their connection to desert tribes is more complex than the dance of biochemicals.[32]

He further observes that

> We were once healthy people who ran, walked, and worked in the fields. We didn't have TV, and didn't sit a lot. Now we have to do drastic things, like walk 240 miles in the desert, to make our people realize that today's illnesses come from not eating healthy. Our people have to get back to eating foods from the desert.[33]

Both of the above statements allude to the notion of the Indigenous body as manipulated by white Europeans. Once healthy and vital, the Indigenous body has been severely compromised by foreign influences and, along with that body, the culture in which it was placed. And while scientists have been unable to work their way through the genetic maze of diabetes, they have managed to prove that a healthy diet minimizes the risk of diabetes, as Lopez, the elder, understood. The Desert Walk highlighted the history of food and food loss and one of its main consequences for these communities – diabetes. The walk was seen as a first step, both toward better health and toward cultural revival.

One of the actions taken to foster the shift in Tohono O'odham eating habits was the opening in March 2009 of the Desert Rain Café, created by the Tohono O'odham Community Action (TOCA), a nonprofit organization dedicated to "creating a healthy, culturally vital and sustainable Tohono O'odham community."[34] The re-introduction of traditional food and a healthy diet

---

[32] Daniel Lopez, quoted in "Desert Walk," http://www.ausbcomp.com/redman/desert_walk.htm (accessed 5 October 2010).

[33] Daniel Lopez, Museum Label, National Museum of the American Indian, 2000.

[34] *Tohono O'odham Community Action*, http://www.tocaonline.org/www.tocaonline.org/Home.html (accessed 19 September 2010).

became one of TOCA's top priorities. The café offers fresh, organic, regional food, low in fat and high in fibre and vitamins. At its busiest during lunch time, Desert Rain has become a place of social contact and exchange. The menu includes dishes such as prickly-pear chicken sandwiches and tepary bean, wild rice, and quinoa salad. The tepary bean is a traditional ingredient of Tohono O'odham meals and also plays a role in several traditional stories. The prickly pear, fruit of the cactus, is both a sweet addition to many meals and a popular ingredient in many drinks. Once comprising the basics of life, traditional ingredients began disappearing from the local food market at the start of the twentieth century. Initially, it was water-rights disputes, forced migrant labour, Indian boarding schools, and relocation programmes that made it impossible to continue to practise traditional agriculture and hunting. But, as mentioned earlier, Indigenous food cultures were also dealt a heavy blow by the US government's introduction of processed food, which became easily available and slowly replaced the traditional diet.

The Perfect Medicine

> Christine Johnson heard her son, Tony, sing the songs she had nearly forgotten, after a feast of rabbit, venison, beans, giant tortillas and mesquite cookies at an O'odham community center in the settlement of Little Tucson. [...] [When she watched him leave for the Desert Walk] she ate a bowl of cholla cactus buds, which are full of the complex carbohydrates and soluble fibers that doctors now think can not only protect her from diabetes, but control the disease by regulating glucose and insulin levels. [...] Native foods, in other words, may be her best medicine.[35]

It sounds simple – in order to be healthy, just consume Indigenous foods moderately and avoid westernized meals. But health and well-being are culturally defined, which in turn leads to different understandings of the disease, its causes, treatment, and its control.

> The Sandy Lake community [studied by Gittelsohn et al.] identified 'bad diet' and eating too much 'white man's' food as causes of diabetes but did not link lack of physical activity and obesity directly with diabetes.[36]

---

[35] Lopez, "Desert Walk."

[36] Zimmet et al., "Epidemiology, Evidence for Prevention: Type 2 Diabetes," 46.

Being overweight or obese is, in fact, considered 'normal' in many communities,[37] and weight loss may even be negatively perceived among Indigenous community members, seen as representing a communal history of poverty, hunger, and illness.[38] As in most cultures throughout the world, food plays a major role among Native Americans, hence it should come as no surprise that it is considered impolite to reject offers of food from friends and family.[39] This attitude is accompanied by the belief that the Indigenous body is genetically programmed to fall prey to diabetes anyway. As the Native American Diabetes Project explains,

> Diabetes means your body has trouble using food for energy. Diabetes is in the genes you were born with, just like the color of your hair and eyes! Do not blame yourself for having diabetes, it is not your fault. You did not get diabetes because you did something wrong.[40]

Based on this explanation, one might conclude that any attempts to prevent the disease are pointless. Genetics are often interpreted by Indigenous people as a complex entanglement of biological, social, and cultural identity.[41] Whereas "notions of genes are perceived and presented by scientists and health professionals as 'culture-free facts'" to Native Americans, they appear to be "social constructs."[42] Consequently, the notion of the Indigenous body as essentially different from the non-Native body goes beyond a biological perception. As one elder explains, diabetes runs in families:

> You inherited it from your mother. Well, of course, you watched your mother cook and all the things she gave you to eat, and now you serve yourself that and the kids that. [...] Yes, it's inherited that way.[43]

---

[37] Roubideaux & Acton, "Diabetes in American Indians," 205.

[38] Olson, "Meeting the Challenges of American Indian Diabetes. Anthropological Perspectives on Prevention and Treatment," 172.

[39] Diane Weiner, "Interpreting Ideas about Diabetes, Genetics, and Inheritance," in *Medicine Ways: Disease, Health, and Survival among Native Americans*, ed. Clifford E. Trafzer & Diane Weiner (New York, Toronto & Plymouth: AltaMira, 2001): 120.

[40] "Meeting 1: Exercise More," *Native American Diabetes Project*, http://www .laplaza.org/health/dwc/nadp/mtg1.htm#diabetes (accessed 14 March 2011).

[41] Weiner, "Interpreting Ideas about Diabetes, Genetics, and Inheritance," 109.

[42] "Interpreting Ideas about Diabetes, Genetics, and Inheritance," 109.

[43] "Interpreting Ideas about Diabetes, Genetics, and Inheritance," 119.

In the Indigenous world-view, the body is inseparable from culture, whereas Western science identifies the body as an independent entity. Both notions view the Indigenous body as exceptional, with diabetes seen by the former as the consequence of a loss of cultural heritage, and by the latter as a biochemical reaction to cultural change. Consequently, to cure diabetes requires returning to the original cultural habits and practices, which also presumes that an original, uninfluenced cuisine exists. A nostalgic past is perceived to be the perfect medicine to cure the Indigenous body of the illnesses apparently imported by Western civilization.

Exotic Tastes

The Indigenous body is not the sole target of culinary revivals. Venues that promote Indigenous food are gaining popularity on a much broader scale. Whereas the Tohono O'odham Desert Rain Café functions primarily as a destination for its community members, similarly themed enterprises have become major tourist attractions. The Brambuk Living Cultural Centre near Budjy Budjy (Halls' Gap) in the Gariwerd, or Grampian region of Victoria, Australia, which opened in December 1990, consists of a permanent exhibition, a gift shop, a café, and a restaurant, elements that are characteristic of more conventional museums. Nevertheless, Brambuk regards itself as a "living cultural centre" and is especially recognized for its unique cuisine. In the Brambuk Café, visitors can experience contemporary interpretations of native dishes that use traditional ingredients, such as crocodile and kangaroo meat, wattle seed, and bunya nuts, which are in turn transformed into selections that include crocodile and emu sausages, roo burgers, and, instead of cappuccino, a drink dubbed "wattlechino."[44] Three nights a week the café becomes the Gugidjela Restaurant and serves dinner. Its menu features courses like *cumbungi djarj gadjin cress* (hearts of reed and water cress), *gdjin yabidj* (yabbies – similar to crayfish – with garlic, bush tomato concassé, and wild rice), and *midjun quandong* (kangaroo fillets pan-fried with wild peach and bush chutney relish).[45] These evenings in the Gugidjela Restaurant have become the Brambuk Living Cultural Centre's main attraction.

Mitsitam, the café at the Smithsonian Institution's National Museum of the American Indian has also earned praise and has become one of the most

---

[44] Moira Simpson, *Making Representations: Museums in the Post-Colonial Era* (New York: Routledge, 2001): 128.

[45] Simpson, *Making Representations: Museums in the Post-Colonial Era*, 128.

successful sections of the museum. Meaning 'Let's eat' in the Piscataway and Delaware languages, Mitsitam offers seasonal food from the Western Hemisphere. Five serving stations arranged in a semicircle represent five different regions: South America, Northern Woodlands, Great Plains, Mesoamerica, and the Northwest Coast. The food is freshly prepared every day and the ingredients are mostly organically grown and provided by Indigenous communities. Wild salmon is flown into Washington, D.C. several times a week from tribes in the western states, and buffalo comes from animals bred by members of the Intertribal Bison Cooperative.[46] Visitors are willing to wait in line – which can last up to almost an hour on busy days – to try the food. The menu includes buffalo burgers and fry-bread with cinnamon and honey, stewed Anasazi beans, hominy, smoked ancho chilies, and prickly-pear ice cream.

Although Mitsitam is highly popular, food critics and scholars have questioned the authenticity of its recipes. Deborah Duchon, a nutritional anthropologist and *Food Network* personality, is sceptical about the café's food selection. The prickly-pear ice cream, for example, is not traditionally Native American, she argues. The prickly pear is indeed an Indigenous fruit, but ice cream is not something Native Americans ate, since their traditional diet did not include dairy products.[47] Other items criticized on the menu include the buffalo burger (Native Americans traditionally did not grind meat) and salmon with a wild berry sauce (Native Americans did not cook with fancy sauces). Richard Hetzler, the executive chef at the Mititsam, admits to working with traditional ingredients in order to make them more accessible to the café's patrons. Traditional corn bread, for example, is very dense, not sweetened, and thus would not appeal to a wide audience.[48] Whereas Duchon's position on the café's food is informed by her disciplinary location: i.e. history, the ethnobotanist Gary Nabhan considers the food to be a great representative of contemporary Indigenous cuisine and praises the café's efforts.[49]

Reproaches such as Duchon's concerning the authenticity of food reveal a desire for the presence of static monocultures that are incapable of adapting to

---

[46] Donna Boss, "Mitsitam Native Foods Café at the National Museum of the American Indian in Washington, D.C.," *Foodservice Equipment and Supplies* 60.5 (2007): 44.

[47] Gabriella Boston, "American Indian Variations at Café," *Washington Times* (30 July 2008): B1.

[48] Boston, "American Indian Variations at Café," B1.

[49] "American Indian Variations at Café," B1.

globalized modernity. The two cafés and one restaurant discussed here constitute a strong statement against any kind of assumed 'cultural authenticity'. At the same time, they are perceived as exotic by a growing crowd of culinary tourists. In the age of processed and flavoured food and the promotion of multiculturalism, Indigenous cuisines claim their place on the food-arts stage by employing the natural and the unusual. In an age of artificial flavours, the desire for the natural, or the *original*, is reflected in new recipes and eating facilities.

Conclusion: The Cultural Memory of Food

The desire for the culinary exotic by "the agents of colonialism" reflects a yearning "for the very forms of life they intentionally altered or destroyed."[50] This ongoing imperialist nostalgia is shaping not only taste in the arts but the taste of the palate as well. But beyond influencing these cultural shifts, this nostalgic turn has taken up residence in the sciences, where, at least in some quarters, the Indigenous body is perceived as different from the non-Indigenous one, a stance that perpetuates a discourse of oppositions. Diabetes, a product of Western civilization, therefore seems to confirm the notion that the Indigenous body is better off in the wilderness, thus moving Indigenous people off the stage of modernity. And regardless of the lack of scientific proof, diabetes is seen as a genetically determined disease mainly affecting Indigenous populations. Taking a broader view, diabetes also appears to be more prevalent in African Americans, Latinos, Asian Americans, Native Hawaiians and other Pacific Islanders, as well as the aged population. This information opens the door to the possibility that diabetes may after all be a "'political disease' whose roots lie deep within the structural inequalities engendered through conquest, colonization, and capitalist 'development'."[51] Once more the Indigenous body proves to be out of sync with civilization, rejecting the modern high-calorie/high-fat/low-fibre diet. Genetically, Native Americans once more become a monoculture whose death rates far exceed those of the rest of the American population in several areas – diabetes (249%), pneumonia and influenza (71%), tuberculosis (533%), and alcohol-

---

[50] Renato Rosaldo, "Imperialist Nostalgia," *Representations* 26 (Spring 1989): 107–108.

[51] Benyshek et al., "A Reconsideration of the Origins of the Type 2 Diabetes Epidemic among Native Americans and the Implications for Intervention Policy," 52.

ism (627%).[52] The notion of genetic determination greatly influences pro-grammes aimed at the prevention and control of these serious health threats; the roots, however, might be located somewhere else.

During the sixth century, the Brahman period of Hindu medicine, diabetes was identified as "the disease of the rich and one that is brought about by the gluttonous overindulgence in oil, flour and sugar."[53] But whereas this is a de-scription of aspects of a privileged life-style in sixth-century India, the trend has by now reversed, and those affected are predominantly from socially dis-advantaged populations. Indigenous foods carry within them the cultural memory of their peoples' history, of destruction, starvation, and assimilation. They are fresh, organic, and rich in vitamins – a luxury in the age of artifici-ality, and a treat to any body.

WORKS CITED

Anon. "Confronting Diabetes with Tradition," *Indian Country Today* (20 December 2000), repr. in *America is Indian Country: Opinions and Perspectives from Indian Country Today*, ed. José Barreiro & Tim Johnson (Golden CO: Fulcrum, 2005): 236–38.

Benyshek, Daniel C., John F. Martin & Carol S. Johnston. "A Reconsideration of the Origins of the Type 2 Diabetes Epidemic among Native Americans and the Impli-cations for Intervention Policy," *Medical Anthropology* 20.1 (2001): 25–64.

Boss, Donna. "Mitsitam Native Foods Café at the National Museum of the American Indian in Washington, D.C.," *Foodservice Equipment and Supplies* 60.5 (2007): 44.

Boston, Gabriella. "American Indian Variations at Café," *Washington Times* (30 July 2008): B1.

Codru, Neculai et al. "Diabetes in Relation to Serum Levels of Polychlorinated Bi-phenyls and Chlorinated Pesticides in Adult Native Americans," *Environmental Health Perspectives* 115.10 (October 2007): 1442–47.

---

[52] Senator Ben Nighthorse Campbell, "Charting a New Course in Indian Health Care," *Indian Country Today* (24 January 2003) in *America is Indian Country: Opinions and Perspectives from Indian Country Today*, 45.

[53] Quoted in Tim Mann & Monika Toeller, "Type 2 Diabetes: Aetiology and En-vironmental Factors," in *The Epidemiology of Diabetes Mellitus: An International Per-spective*, 133.

DeMouy, Jane. "Genetic Research," *The Pima Indians: Pathfinders for Health*, http://diabetes.niddk.nih.gov/dm/pubs/pima/genetic/genetic.htm (accessed 23 September 2010).

Flammang, Janet A. *The Taste of Civilization: Food, Politics, and Civil Society* (Chicago: U of Illinois P, 2009).

Foer, Jonathan Safran. *Eating Animals* (New York: Penguin, 2009).

Mann, Jim, & Monika Toeller. "Type 2 Diabetes: Aetiology and Environmental Factors," in *The Epidemiology of Diabetes Mellitus. An International Perspective*, ed. Jean–Marie Ekoé, Paul Zimmet & Rhys Williams (New York: John Wiley, 2001): 133–40.

Nakanishi, Shigetada et al. "A Comparison Between Japanese-Americans Living in Hawaii and Los Angeles and Native Japanese: The Impact of Lifestyle Westernization on Diabetes Mellitus," *Biomedicine and Pharmacotherapy* 58.10 (December 2004): 571–77.

Narayan, K.M Venka et al. "Non-Caucasion North American Populations: Native Americans," in *The Epidemiology of Diabetes Mellitus: An International Perspective*, ed. Jean–Marie Ekoé, Paul Zimmet & Rhys Williams (New York: John Wiley 2001): 184–91.

Neel, James. "Diabetes Mellitus: A 'Thrifty' Genotype Rendered Detrimental By 'Progress'," *American Journal of Human Genetics* 14 (1962): 353–62.

Nighthorse Campbell, Ben. "Charting a New Course in Indian Health Care," *Indian Country Today* (24 January 2003), repr. in *America is Indian Country. Opinions and Perspectives from Indian Country Today*, ed. José Barreiro & Tim Johnson (Golden CO: Fulcrum, 2005): 44–49.

O'Dea, Kerin. "Traditional Diet and Food Preferences of Australian Aboriginal Hunter–Gatherers," *Philosophical Transactions: Biological Sciences* 334/1270 (November 1991): 233–41.

Olson, Brooke. "Meeting the Challenges of American Indian Diabetes: Anthropological Perspectives on Prevention and Treatment," in *Medicine Ways: Disease, Health, and Survival among Native Americans*, ed. Clifford E. Trafzer & Diane Weiner (New York, Toronto & Plymouth: AltaMira, 2001): 163–84.

Pollan, Michael. *In Defense of Food: An Eater's Manifesto* (New York: Penguin, 2008).

Rosaldo, Renato. "Imperialist Nostalgia," *Representations* 26 (Spring 1989): 107–22.

Roubideaux, Yvette, & Kelly Acton. "Diabetes in American Indians," in *Promises to Keep*, ed. Mim Dixon & Yvette Roubideaux (Washington DC: American Public Health Association, 2001): 193–208.

Sahmoun, Abe E., Mary J. Markland & Steven D. Helgerson. "Mental Health Status and Diabetes among Whites and Native Americans: Is Race an Effect Modifier?" *Journal of Health Care for the Poor and Underserved* 18.3 (August 2007): 599–608.

Sietsema, Tom. "Mitsitam Café," *Washington Post Magazine* (16 October 2005), http://www.washingtonpost.com/gog/restaurants/mitsitam-cafe,1113026/critic-review.html (accessed 22 October 2010).

Simpson, Moira. *Making Representations: Museums in the Post-Colonial Era* (New York: Routledge, 2001).

Szathmáry, Emöke J.E. "Non-Insulin Dependent Diabetes Mellitus among Aboriginal North Americans," *Annual Review of Anthropology* 23 (1994): 457–82.

Velho, Gilberto, & Philippe Froguel. "Type 2 Diabetes: Genetic Factors," in *The Epidemiology of Diabetes Mellitus: An International Perspective*, ed. Jean–Marie Ekoé, Paul Zimmet & Rhys Williams (New York: John Wiley, 2001): 141–53.

Weiner, Diane. "Interpreting Ideas about Diabetes, Genetics, and Inheritance," in *Medicine Ways: Disease, Health, and Survival among Native Americans*, ed. Clifford E. Trafzer & Diane Weiner (New York, Toronto & Plymouth: AltaMira, 2001): 108–33.

Zimmet, Paul et al. "Epidemiology, Evidence for Prevention: Type 2 Diabetes," in *The Epidemiology of Diabetes Mellitus: An International Perspective*, ed. Jean–Marie Ekoé, Paul Zimmet & Rhys Williams (New York: John Wiley, 2001): 41–49.

Websites

The Centre for Indigenous Peoples' Nutrition and Environment (CINE): http://www.mcgill.ca/cine/ (accessed 13 October 2010).

The Desert Walk: http://www.ausbcomp.com/redman/desert_walk.htm (accessed 5 October 2010).

The Native American Diabetes Project: http://www.laplaza.org/health/dwc/nadp/mtg1.htm#diabetes (accessed 14 March 2011).

The Strong Heart Study: http://strongheart.ouhsc.edu/ (accessed 12 September 2010).

Tohono O'odham Community Action: http://www.tocaonline.org/www.tocaonline.org/Home.html (accessed 19 September 2010).

⌘

ANDREA ZITTLAU works currently as a research assistant and lecturer in the department of North American Studies at the University of Rostock, Germany. Additionally, she coordinates the Graduate School "Cultural Encounters and Discourses of Scholarship," also at the University of Rostock. She has written about museums and the representation of Native Americans in exhibitions, and on issues of tourism. Her latest project is concerned with aspects of medical history and disability studies.

⌘

Discussion Questions: Nutrition & the Indigenous Body: A Genetic Concept of Food

1. Which populations around the world have the highest rates of diabetes? How has the disease been applied to indigenous peoples?
2. What is the 'thrifty genotype' hypothesis and how has it impacted the study of diabetes?
3. When did indigenous peoples of the US have their indigenous diet altered? What were they forced to eat? What foods were once part of their indigenous diet?
4. Who are the Tohono O'odham? Describe this population in terms of diabetes, traditional diets, and a return to a healthy lifestyle?

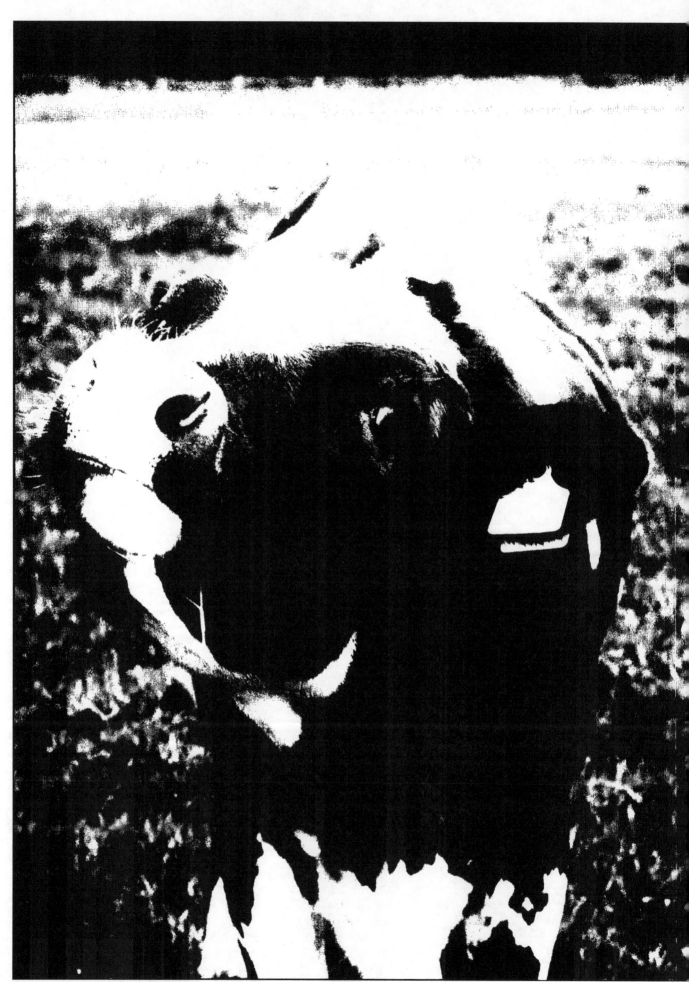

On Eating Animals

BY NAMIT ARORA

SOME YEARS ago in a Montana slaughterhouse, a Black Angus cow awaiting execution suddenly went berserk, jumped a five-foot fence, and escaped. She ran through the streets for hours, dodging cops, animal control officers, cars, trucks, and a train. Cornered near the Missouri river, the frightened animal jumped into its icy waters and made it across, where a tranquilizer gun brought her down. Her "daring escape" stole the hearts of the locals, some of whom had even cheered her on. The story got international media coverage. Telephone polls were held, calls demanding her freedom poured into local TV stations. Sensing the public mood, the slaughterhouse manager made a show of "granting clemency" to what he dubbed "the brave cow." Given a name, Molly, the cow was sent to a nearby farm to live out her days grazing under open skies—which warmed the cockles of many a heart.

Cattle trying to escape slaughterhouses are not uncommon. Few of their stories end happily though. Some years ago in Omaha, six cows escaped at once. Five were quickly recaptured; one kept running until Omaha police cornered her in an alley and pumped her with bullets. The cow, bellowing miserably and hobbling like a drunk for several seconds before collapsing, died on the street in a pool of blood. This brought howls of protest, some from folks who had witnessed the killing. They called the police's handling inhumane and needlessly cruel.

It's tempting to see these commiserating folks as animal lovers—and that's how they likely see themselves—until one remembers what they eat for dinner. A typical slaughterhouse in the United States kills over a thousand Mollys a day—lined up, shot in the head, and often cut open and bled while still conscious, an end no less cruel and full of bellowing—all because Americans keep buying neatly-packaged slices of their corpses in supermarkets. Raised unnaturally and inhumanely, over a million protesting birds and mammals are violently killed in the United States every hour (that's 300 per second). How is it unreasonable then to say that nearly all meat-eaters in America participate quite directly in a cycle of suffering and cruelty of staggering scale?

Yet the idea persists that Americans love animals, largely because of their love and concern for a class of animals called "pets" (and other "cute" animals like dolphins, polar bears, and pandas). Most Americans have had at least one pet at some point in their lives, and many see their pets as extensions of their families; they photograph their pets, swap stories about them, buy them gifts and treats, spend money on their illnesses, support taxes to build shelters for them, and mourn their deaths. Yet, the question continues to rankle, as Elizabeth Kolbert put it in a November 2009 *New Yorker* piece:

> How is it that Americans, so solicitous of the animals they keep as pets, are so indifferent toward the ones they cook for dinner? The answer cannot lie in the beasts themselves. Pigs, after all, are quite companionable, and dogs are said to be delicious.

What might explain this disjunction? From humankind's long community with farm animals, how has it come to this?

A Brief History of Farm Animals

For much of our settled history—and even today in parts of the world—most people lived in close proximity to farm animals. Animals fertilized our crops, shared our labors, and nourished our bodies, helping us enlarge our settled communities. Families commonly kept a few farm animals, gave them names, and saw them as individuals with distinct temperaments. Children grew up around them, related to them effortlessly, and came to know their cycles of birth, aging, and death. Our obligations to domestic animals arose in part from a sense of kinship, community, and mutual dependence; we saw in them our own instincts, physical vulnerabilities, and social-filial attachments. They frequently inhabited our myths and polytheistic beliefs. Each time we killed and ate one of them, we also silently paid the price, however small, of having known the animal in life and in its dying moments. Children were often saddened by the slaughter of an animal they knew, and missed the animal for a while. Ritual animal sacrifices occurred only on special occasions. Abuse of animals occurred too, but it was neither systematic nor centrally organized, and depended on the moral compasses of the owners. Like people, animals had their own luck in ending up with a severe human family or a gentler one.

In later millennia, urbanization, specialization, and new economic, religious, and humanistic ideas began altering our relations with farm animals. As Lesley J. Rogers explains in *Minds of their Own* (1998), ownership of farm animals became concentrated in fewer hands, and flocks and herds grew larger. As a result, the individuality of animals was lost to their owners and they began receding from most people's everyday lives. Over time, farm animals became yet another natural resource managed by specialists, who harvested their material value and transferred it to others via the market.

It would hardly be an exaggeration to say that a hallmark of our modernity is a drastic loss of first-hand knowledge and experience of nature's beats and rhythms, including knowledge of animal lives. Most people today have no experience with farm animals. Generations of us have grown up in urban housing, public parks, and city streets, and rarely around the animals we eat. From a young age, we socialize our children—rather indoctrinate them, for there is nothing natural about it—to dearly love and fuss over some domesticated animals while eating others without thought, not unlike eating carrots.

In the twentieth century, the inexorable logic of modern economics and the assembly line turned farm animals into number-tagged bodies to be fattened, disinfected, and processed as quickly and cheaply as possible. We found new uses for animal parts in plastics, detergents, tires, cosmetics, dyes, contraceptives, crayons, and more. This went hand-in-hand with our portrayals of them as "dumb animals," making it easier to overlook their abuse and ignore their manifold social and emotional lives. Only animal behaviors with an economic impact merited attention. For example, factories had to deal with the tendency of animals to injure others or themselves when forced to stand in cramped feedlots in ankle-deep excrement, or when packed in tiny cages.

To raise efficiency and cut costs, farm animals began to be engineered for abnormally rapid weight gain, fed unnatural corn-based diets that cause metabolic disorders and liver damage, and injected with pre-emptive antibiotics and growth hormones. To reduce fights and injuries due to overcrowding, animals began to be routinely mutilated—for instance, their beaks, horns, or tails might be chopped or burned off *without* anesthesia—and they were often confined in tiny crates in windowless rooms. All of these procedures are now standard and legal. As with so many aspects of our economy, the full cost of this enterprise, whether ethical, environmental, or health-wise, has never been factored in. The tragedy was complete when raising and killing animals for meat came to be seen as agriculture, which is why the U.S. Department of Agriculture regulates this industry.

> **Americans somehow don't realize that cruelty is the norm, not the exception, and is, in fact, infused into the very idea of factory farms; what makes meat cheap is the assembly-line processing of animals who essentially subsidize it with their suffering.**

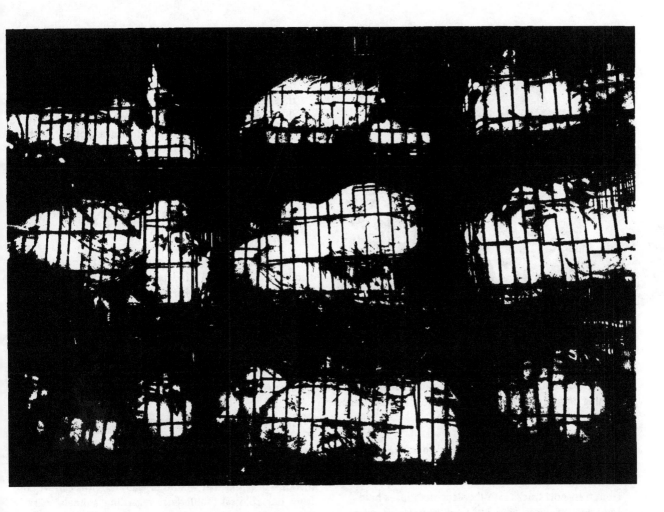

What might have arrested this decline in the fortunes of farm animals are big cultural ideas, both religious and secular, that for whatever reasons opposed killing animals. But those did not arise in the West as they did, for example, in India. Depending on whom you ask, Western monotheistic religions, while seeing humankind as God's special creation, ranged in attitude from passive disaffection to active malice towards animals. Christian doctrine has practically no injunctions against treating animals as a means to human ends, so no sin is committed when mistreating or killing animals. Rather, animals were declared vastly inferior, incapable of possessing souls, and created for the use of humans, who stood right below the angels. And so Western monotheisms have long seen animals as dispensable for human interests, desires, and whims. (This is also true for the "Confucian zone" of East Asia.)

In the modern age, even secular humanism, with its nearly exclusive focus on humans, has shown little regard for the treatment of animals. "In the West," writes Mary Midgley in *Animals and Why They Matter* (1998), "both the religious and the secular moral traditions have, till lately, scarcely attended to any non-human species." With notable exceptions like Jacques Rousseau, Jeremy Bentham, Arthur Schopenhauer, and contemporary animal welfare organiza-tions like the Society for the Prevention of Cruelty to Animals (SPCA), the dominant strands of Western culture have remained heavily invested in denying moral consideration to animals. Rather conveniently, animals are presumed to lack feelings, thoughts, emotions, memory, reason, intelligence, sense of time, language, consciousness, or autonomy. Until the 1980s scientists entertained the idea that animals do not feel pain. Such self-serving presumptions, enabled by our estrangement from farm animals, certainly made our consciences rest easier. This helps explain why the animal rights movement focuses so hard on demonstrating many of these capacities in animals (sometimes overstating their case). So tenacious can our habits of life and mind be that even today, despite everything we know and the genuine alternatives we have for a nutritious diet, less than 1 percent of U.S. adults have turned away from factory-farmed meat for ethical reasons.

The Modern Business of Killing

Slaughterhouses today operate behind closed doors, their violence increasingly concealed from society at large. Even their design tells a revealing story: careful division of labor, compartmentalized zones, non-unionized immigrant labor (especially on the kill floor), with few workers ever witness-

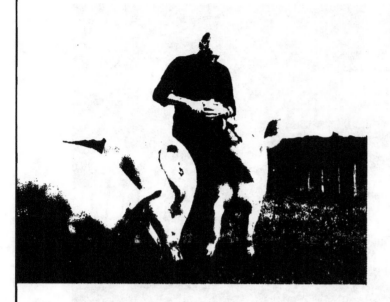

ing a killing despite working there for years. Language, too, cushions the psychological impact of the job, says Timothy Pachirat, an assistant professor of politics at The New School for Social Research. In an interview published last year at the group blog *Boing Boing*, Pachirat talked about his experience working undercover in a slaughterhouse.

> In addition to spatial and labor divisions, the use of language is another way of concealing the violence of killing. From the moment cattle are unloaded from transport trucks into the slaughterhouse's holding pens, managers and kill floor supervisors refer to them as "beef." Although they are living, breathing, sentient beings, they have already linguistically been reduced to inanimate flesh, to use-objects. Similarly, there is a slew of acronyms and technical language around the food safety inspection system that reduces the quality control worker's job to a bureaucratic, technical regime rather than one that is forced to confront the truly massive taking of life. Although the quality control worker has full physical movement throughout the kill floor and sees every aspect of the killing, her interpretive frame is interdicted by the technical and bureaucratic requirements of the job. Temperatures, hydraulic pressures, acid concentrations, bacterial counts, and knife sanitization become the primary focus, rather than the massive, unceasing taking of life.

In the United States, farm animals make up a whopping 98 percent of all birds and mammals humans use, the rest being pets, victims of research and sport, or those held in zoos. We can't ignore this 98 percent and still claim to be serious about animal welfare. According to David J. Wolfson and Mariann Sullivan, who contributed a chapter titled, "Foxes in the Hen House: Animals, Agribusiness, and the

Law," to the 2004 collection, *Animal Rights: Current Debates and New Directions,* the factory farming industry

has persuaded legislatures to amend criminal statutes that purport to protect farm animals from cruelty so that it cannot be prosecuted for any farming practice that the industry itself determines is acceptable, with no limit whatsoever on the pain caused by such practices. As a result, in most of the United States, prosecutors, judges, and juries no longer have the power to determine whether or not farm animals are treated in an acceptable manner. The industry alone defines the criminality of its own conduct.

Veterinarians who report abuses against farm animals risk liabilities. And in 2011 independent journalist Will Potter wrote: "the FBI Joint Terrorism Task Force has kept files on activists who expose animal welfare abuses on factory farms and recommended prosecuting them as terrorists." The FBI file, obtained through a Freedom of Information Act request, detailed activists' actions trespassing on farms to videotape abuses and suggested these actions violated the Animal Enterprise Terrorism Act.

"The Axe for the Frozen Sea Inside Us"

The above quote comes from Franz Kafka, who was writing about literature and contended that, "we ought to read only the kind of books that wound or stab us." How can we confront our colossal indifference regarding animals? Clearly, most people don't even know about the horror and pain we inflict on billions of birds and mammals in our meat factories. But there's no good excuse for this, is there? It's more likely that we don't want to know—*can't afford to know for our own sake*—so we turn a blind eye and trust the artifice of bucolic imagery on meat packaging. Some see parallels here with the German people's willful denial of the concentration camps that once operated around them, or call those who consume factory-farmed meat little Eichmanns. "For the animals, it is an eternal Treblinka," wrote Isaac Bashevis Singer (who also used to say he turned vegetarian "for health reasons—the health of the chicken").

Predictably enough, many others are offended by such comparisons. They say that comparing the industrialized abuse of animals with the industrialized abuse of humans trivializes the latter. There are indeed limits to such comparisons, though our current enterprise may be worse in at least one respect: it has no foreseeable end. We seem committed to raising billions of sentient beings year after year only to kill them after a short life of intense suffering. Furthermore, rather than take offense at polemical comparisons—as if others are obliged to be more judicious in their speech than we are in our silent deeds—why not reflect on our apathy instead? Criticizing vegetarians and vegans for being self-righteous—or being moral opportunists in having found a new way of affirming their decency to themselves—certainly doesn't absolve us from the need to face up to our role in perpetuating this cycle of violence and degradation.

Not long ago a Humane Society sting operation at a slaughterhouse in California caused a large public outrage and media hubbub. A cynic might say that the outrage was motivated less by the cruelty, and more by concerns about the nutritional safety of meat from downer cattle. But genuine disgust at the cruelty was also evident in the response and in the flurry of donations to animal welfare groups. So it's not that farm animals get no sympathy in the United States, only that Americans somehow don't realize that cruelty is the norm, not the exception, and is, in fact, infused into the very idea of factory farms; what makes meat cheap is the assembly-line processing of animals who essentially subsidize it with their suffering.

Treating animals humanely requires natural diets, open spaces for living, eliminating the use of hormones that explode body weight and mutilations like chopping off beaks, tongues, and tails, together with more stringent training for caretakers and inspectors, surveillance cameras, professionals who enforce laws and prosecute violators, and so on—all of which make meat more expensive. Our desire for cheap products is often at odds with our desire to be ethical and humane. Few things strike me as more absurd than calling oneself an animal lover while patronizing industrialized meat, though people will surely continue to deceive themselves and even offer various lame justifications to defend their habit (for example: many other animals also eat animals, humans are at the top of the food chain, people need meat protein to live, our traditions or religions sanction meat eating, and so on).

The modern animal rights movement has certainly impacted a range of concerns—such as reducing the use of animals for furs and cosmetics testing, and enforcing laws against wanton hunting and certain cruelties—but not quite factory farming, which seems a more difficult case. This may well be because the industry is tied up with big corporate interests and serves more widely entrenched cultural habits. Another reason may be that the rights movement has not fostered enough discussion on where animal rights come from. What's needed in my view are not theories of rights or liberty for animals, nor talk of "speciesism" or utilitarian optimization—at least not primarily—but narratives and experiences that reawaken us to a sense of kinship with farm animals, which is the ground upon which we build our obligations to them. (I can recommend the documentary film, *The Emotional World of Farm Animals*, as a place to begin.) There is no evidence that farm animals suffer any less than dogs or cats. They too are lovable, intelligent, and have individual personalities and social-emotional lives; many of them even bond with humans. They too have behaviors that in our pets we describe as fear, elation, loneliness, anxiety, playfulness, and so on. More of us rediscovering this may be a prerequisite to bringing greater dignity to their lives and deaths—and in doing so, greater dignity to our own.

With its dedication to affirm the inherent worth and dignity of each individual, the humanist movement is especially well positioned to deliver and exemplify such a message.

It's also possible that even if we really took the time to discover how we treat farm animals, most of us might in good faith still decide to patronize factory-farmed meat. We might conclude that the price we make animals pay, and the price we pay in sacrificing part of our humanity, are worth the benefits. Such honest deliberation would require that we make our meat factories open to the public—give them glass walls, so to speak—even visit them with our kids, so they too can decide for themselves. That might be a step towards a clear conscience. But meanwhile, how terribly dishonorable we look by averting our gaze and choosing ignorance, and—in a surreal twist—going sentimental for cows that escape while callously sponsoring the anguish and pain of billions of their fellow animals.

Recommended online video: "Farm to Fridge—The Truth Behind Meat Production," by Mercy for Animals; narrated by James Cromwell. Ⓗ

Namit Arora is a travel photographer, writer, and creator of *Shunya*, an online photo journal. After nearly twenty years in the San Francisco Bay Area, he recently relocated to Delhi. An omnivore in his youth, he turned vegetarian in his thirties for ethical reasons.

Discussion Questions: On Eating Animals

1. How does the author say that meat eaters are part of the cycle of suffering and cruelty for animals reared in the US for consumption?
2. How were animals raised for much of our history? How is animal production different today compared to the past?
3. What are traits that are promoted in cattle breeding?
4. What is required for humane animal treatment according to the author?

Topic VI: Food and Nutrition in Asia

In *Durian: The King of Fruits or an Acquired Taste?*, the reader is exposed to a food that is classified as a fruit and one that is indigenous to Southeast Asia. Nearly every world region has one or more fruits that are indigenous, and typically, we love those that we know from the place where we grow up. In this article, we have the opportunity to examine the idea of culture driving or guiding our notions of what is considered to be a 'good' food, or fruit, and the qualities that we expect to find within as it is consumed. This article reviews the origin, history, and cultural use of this now famous fruit. Often, there are nutritional benefits to eating fruits that derive from the plant or tree's protective mechanisms and we learn about some of those entities here.

Most populations around the world produce and consume fermented foods and beverages. In *Fermented Marine Food Products in Vietnam*, we discuss the reason why a particular food was eventually fermented, the history of this process in Vietnam, and how ecology affects the food and the related culture of place.

Across the globe, as income increases, so does the consumption of animal products, especially meat and dairy. Such consumption is often associated with wealth and progress. This is true in countries such as India, where meat has not been an important dietary component, mostly because of religious ideals. China provides another example—modest amounts of meat have always been part of the diet, but now those who are wealthier are consuming more animal-based protein. Economic changes alter food culture, and in *The Pink Revolution or How Asia is Getting Hooked on Meat, Fast*, China and India are used to illustrate changes in daily life now linked to increased meat consumption. This is significant given that at least 50% of the world's people live in one of these two countries.

Cheese and Culture: A History of Cheese and its Place in Western Civilization outlines for the reader the way in which cheese was first discovered in Southwest Asia. From the animals whose milk was tapped to create cheese, to the types of containers needed for storage, we learn about the thousands of years in cheese history.

READING 17

Durian

The King of Fruits or an Acquired Taste?

Maxine E. McBrinn

Biographical sketch. Maxine McBrinn is an anthropological archaeologist who specializes in the arid lands hunters and gatherers of the western United States. While she has no formal background in the anthropology of food, she is an enthusiastic experimentalist of new tastes and cuisines. Maxine found her reaction to durian to be as complex as the flavor of the famed fruit itself.

Taste is one of the many ways to experience a new place. Enthusiastic visitors, including myself, seek out new foods and new dishes as part of being somewhere new. In an ideal scenario, the intrepid traveler tries the local cuisines and is rewarded by delicious or intriguing tastes. In the real world, however, squeamish eaters and sometimes even accommodating diners will find foods that repel them for one reason or another. In this manner, taste can also be a visceral and immediate indication that, to borrow from the *Wizard of Oz*, "Toto, I've a feeling we're not in Kansas anymore!" Yet there is something oddly satisfying about finding a repulsive new food, as it confirms that there are significant differences in eating habits and choices across the world. It would be disappointing if everyone everywhere ate the same things and yearned for the same flavors. There are foods that are highly sought after in one place but arouse immediate disgust in diners from other places. For example, ripe European cheeses can also be viewed as clotted, rotting milk, a view held by many Asians, who would never think of nibbling on such a thing. In turnabout, Asian deli-cacies such as kimchi and the so-called thousand-year-old eggs may be refused by suspicious Westerners. Some people are immediately repulsed by the idea of eating familiar (or not so familiar) animals, such as horses, dogs, snakes, or snails—meats that are enjoyed elsewhere. Many of the foods that arouse such divergent views are from animal sources, such as meat or dairy foods (Harris 1985; Simoons 1994), but there are also plant foods that are unappreciated by some diners. Many people, for example, dislike okra because of its texture when completely cooked, which some malign as "slimy" and for which the for-mal term, mucilaginous, suggests a comparison to mucus. One of the risks and rewards to traveling is to try these foods for oneself.

The joy of being in a new place is to try as many local culinary favorites as possible. Much of what is available to eat day in and day out can get boring, but new foods and new spices may reawaken our enthusiasm. But more than this, food is a shortcut into experiencing new worlds and new lives. Food informs us about the environment, about the plants and animals that live in the area (Messer 1984, 1989; Mintz and Du Bois 2002). For example, while it is appro-priate to find fresh seafood near the ocean, catfish, trout, and other freshwater fish would be expected at inland locations. Cuisine also tells us a lot about the history of the place: about how and when nonnative foods arrived and how they became incorporated into the local customs (Sokolov 1991). In this way, local foods encapsulate the relationships among history, the environment, and outside influences. One of the surprises from a visit to Kenya was the frequency that cabbage and potatoes were offered, legacies of that country's colonial past. Food also informs us about economics and cultural training. For example, tortillas are portable and widely used when people travel to their workplace, whereas soups imply local diners. Woks use less energy to heat, for when fuel is scarce, and hot tea warms chilled bodies and cold fingers. Through food, through tastes and textures, visitors absorb some of that place into their bodies and make it a part of themselves.

Within any given society, some foods are considered to be especially suitable for men, or for women, for children, or for elders, for healthy young adults, or for invalids (Messer 1984, 1989; Mintz and Du Bois 2002; McKay 1980; Wilson 1975, 1980). There are foods that are considered bad for preg-nant women, and foods that will boost the immune system. Some foods will heighten sexual desire and others will encourage sleep. There are foods that are eaten in a homemade meal, others that are more often eaten in restaurants, snack foods suitable for popular leisure activities, and other foods that are consumed privately or even in secrecy. These food categories are culturally constructed although there is also a wide degree of individual choice in the foods actually consumed.

Food and our responses to it are complex, in part because food selection offers a unique window into many aspects of human societies. There is a large body of literature on the anthropology of food and a wide diversity of theoretical approaches that can be used (for good review articles, see Messer 1984, 1989; Mintz and Du Bois 2002). Individual food choice is affected by a wide range of physical and sociocultural factors, including local ecology, economic status, gender, age, class, personal health, religious belief, and so on. Accordingly, anthropologists can choose a similarly wide array of approaches to study the topic, including ecological, ethnographic, economic, biocultural, nutritional, and ethnoscientific studies (Messer 1989). Those factors that lead to people classifying foods as "edible" or "inedible" are particularly interesting for the diner confronted by a new food that challenges their previous conceptions, the topic that unites the chapters in this volume. Food preferences are influenced by both sensory and cultural factors, by the taste, smell, look, texture, and source of the food as well as by the meaning assigned to those attributes. In other words, our cultural training influences how we interpret a potential food. Durian, the subject of this chapter, is an excellent example of a food that is loved, even immoderately desired, by some, yet reviled by others.

DURIAN FACTS

Durian is the fruit of the durian tree (Figure 7.1), *Durio zibethinus*, thought to have originated in Borneo and now cultivated in much of Southeast Asia, including Malaysia, Indonesia, Thailand, and the Philippines (Morton 1987; Rolnick 2003; Veevers-Carter 1984) *Duri* in Malay means "spike," prominent features of the large fruit (Figure 7.2) (Dunne 2002). The term *zibethinus* is derived from the Italian word, *zibetto* (civet cat or skunk), and notes the similarity of the odor of the fruit to that of the cat (Soegeng-Reksodihardjo 1962).

While not all members of the *Durio* genus produce edible fruit, a number of species do (Kostermans 1992; Soegeng-Reksodihardjo 1962; Veevers-Carter 1984), although only *Durio zibethinus* is commonly commercially cultivated. Durian grows wild or semi-wild around established villages (Morton 1987) and can even be used as a marker of previous settlements (Peluso 2003). There are hundreds of durian varieties, with more than 300 named varieties in Thailand alone (Morton 1987). Of these, somewhat less than a dozen are grown commercially. Durian grows best in jungle conditions, requiring lots of water and consistent warmth, especially for young plants becoming established

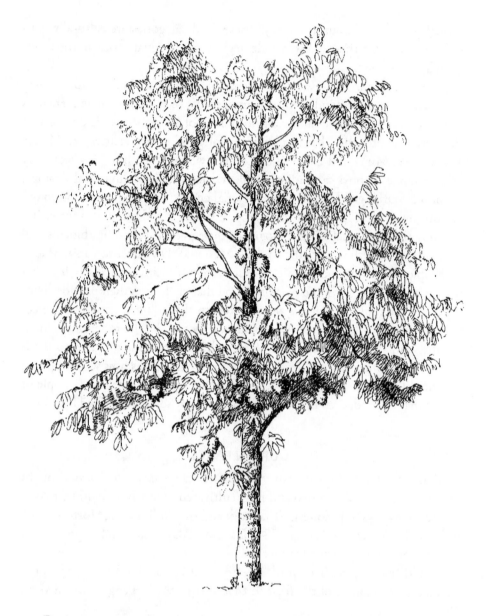

7.1. Durian tree. (DRAWING BY MAXINE MCBRINN)

(Morton 1987). Despite the fact that the trees do not fruit for five to ten years after being planted (Rolnick 2003), the amount of durian under cultivation has increased in at least some parts of Indonesia (Peluso 2003). New research on durian cultivars has focused on diminishing some of the characteristics that some find distasteful, including eliminating the odor (Fuller 2007; Sullivan 2007). Whether this will extend the appeal of the fruit to new markets remains to be seen.

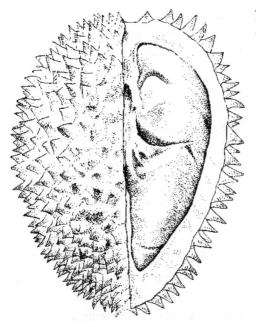

7.2. Durian fruit. (DRAWING BY MAXINE MCBRINN)

The durian fruit is also reputed to be prized by frugivorus animals. A Thai maxim says: "[T]he first to note the malodor is the elephant, which shakes the tree to bring down the fruit. After the elephant noses open the fruit with its tusks, the tiger fights the elephant for the fruit. Rhinoceros, wild pig, deer, tapir, monkey, beetle, and ant follow the tiger. The human must be very quick to get the durian" (Rolnick 2003). Perhaps to forestall not getting any fruit at all, villagers are reported to camp near trees with ripe fruit (Howell 1984:22; Morton 1987; Peluso 2003; Veevers-Carter 1984:42), ready to collect the harvest. Care must be taken, however, as the durian trees are tall, and the fruit heavy and covered by large, sharp spikes (Morton 1987; Wallace 1856). In some places, traps placed in the area add meat as well as durian to the diet by taking advantage of the game drawn by the durian scent (Morton 1987). The animal attraction for the scent of durian led E.H.J. Corner to posit his "Durian Theory," which states that the earliest fruiting trees used endozoochory (animals carrying seeds to new locations in their stomachs), rewarding the animals who dispersed the seeds with rich foods (Corner 1976; Veevers-Carter 1984:43–45). Corner believes that the durian is an outstanding example of a primitive fruiting tree.

VIEWS ON DURIAN

In Malay society, as in much of Southeast Asia, durian is highly esteemed. In fact, durian has been declared "The King of Fruits" (Dunne 2002; Rolnick

2003:541; Walsh 1999) and there are people who become fixated on all aspects of the fruit. Currently, there are large Web sites featuring many, many pages of discussion, advice, facts, photos, cartoons, recipes, and overall celebrations of durian.

Selling durian is a significant cash source for some groups, providing up to half their cash income (Peluso 2003:206–207). Southeast Asia has a number of aboriginal societies, some that traditionally focused on foraging (Brosius 1999; Endicott 1999a, 1999b; Howell 1984; Van der Sluys 1999) and others that have customarily cultivated swidden gardens of rice, maize, cassava, vegetables, fruit, and sometimes rubber trees (Dentan 1968; Peluso 2003:190). In Malaysia these groups are known collectively as the Orang Asli, which translates as "The First Peoples" (Endicott 1999b; Van der Sluys 1999).

At least one Orang Asli group, the Chewong, think so highly of durian that they move to live near the trees in harvesting season (Howell 1984:22). In addition, durian is one of the useful plants that are believed by the Chewong (Howell 1984:133) to have consciousness and a desire to help the people. In fact, durian has a starring role in the Chewong origin story, being the fruit stolen from Earth Six to feed the peoples of this earth (Howell 1984:74).

Among the Indonesian Dayak (Peluso 2003), durian also has an important economic role. Durian trees are long-lived, surviving perhaps up to seven human generations (Peluso 2003:191, 203–205). Once they have begun to fruit, they are individually named. Tree names most often honor the planter but sometimes refer to the quality of the fruit or some other distinctive attribute (Peluso 2003:184–185). Because of the high value of the fruit, once the planter and spouse have died, durian harvests are divided among the heirs according to how many generations removed they are from the planter (Peluso 2003:184–185), the heirs' residence, and other factors.

The Dayak (Peluso 2003:202), like many others, do not pick durian but rather wait for the fruit to fall naturally (also McCarthy 2005:69, but see Roseman 1998:110 for an example of durian being picked). This ensures that the fruit will be at its flavorful peak and that it will bring a good price if sold. Some towns and villages enforce this rule through social shame (McCarthy 2005:69) or fines (Peluso 2003:202) if residents pick underripe fruit, as this diminishes the value of all the fruit harvested in the community in the eyes of outsiders. A reputation for this practice could limit the price paid for future harvests.

Durian season lasts a couple of months, requiring an extended time when people must stay near the trees to collect the fruit and to keep animals and other people from taking it (Peluso 2003:202–203). Durian season, moreover, requires even greater logistical maneuvering. The fruit must be sold very soon after it falls and should be consumed within four or five days (Peluso 2003:202;

Soegeng-Reksodihardjo 1962; Wilson 1986), a challenge to people who live some distance from the roads or boats used to carry fruit to market.

Durian is considered a powerful aphrodisiac, as the Malay saying "When the durian falls, the sarong falls" (Rolnick 2003:542) implies. Perhaps love, or maybe just lust, follows, because when eating durian, the diner is reported to become heated and may start to sweat (Laderman 1981:474; 1983:44; Manderson 1986:132; Wilson 1986). Some of this heating effect may be caused by the high fat content of durian, second among fruits only to avocado, or perhaps by the similarity of durian's final chemical breakdown products to alcohol (Laderman 1981:474; Wilson 1986:264–265). This heating effect, and the resulting increase in attraction, may also explain why durian is considered an excellent make-up gift after marital discord. Instead of flowers or chocolates, Malay or other Southeast Asian men might choose to sweeten the relationship with durian.

The Malay belief that durian is heating reflects a complex ordering of food, drink, and medicine beyond classification as protein, fat, or carbohydrate or the commonly stated "good for me" or "bad for me." Like many Southeast Asians, Malaysians classify foods and other ingested substances as "hot" or "cold" (Laderman 1981, 1983:35–72; Manderson 1986; McKay 1980; Messer 1984, 1989; Wilson 1975, 1980, 1986). These terms signify intrinsic qualities that direct individual and group food use. The classifications are independent of temperature or spiciness and are linked to medicinal values and humoral conceptions of health and illness. Individuals in good health exhibit an appropriate balance of hot and cold in their bodies, while illness may be caused or exacerbated by a poor balance of these qualities. The specifics of these classification systems vary across Southeast Asia, both in qualities assigned to specific foods and in how they are applied to dietary and health practices. The Malay classification of durian as heating probably acknowledges its high calorie content and is an exception to the common ascription of fruits as cold.

Some Westerners, too, have fallen in love with durian. One of the most famous of those who learned to appreciate the odoriferous fruit was Alfred Russel Wallace, who said:

> The pulp is the eatable part, and its consistence and flavour are indescribable. A rich custard highly flavoured with almonds gives the best general idea of it, but there are occasional wafts of flavour that call to mind cream-cheese, onion-sauce, sherry-wine, and other incongruous dishes. Then there is a rich glutinous smoothness in the pulp which nothing else possesses, but which adds to its delicacy. It is neither acid nor sweet nor juicy; yet it wants neither of these qualities, for it is in itself perfect. . . . In fact, to eat Durians is a new sensation worth a voyage to the East to experience. . . . If I had to fix on two only as representing the perfection of the two classes, I should

certainly choose the Durian and the Orange as the king and queen of fruits. (Wallace 1856:229)

Wallace was not alone. A friend of Edmund Banfield was quoted as reporting,

> I have been spending a small fortune in durians, they are relatively cheap and very good this season in Singapore. Like all the good things in Nature ... durian is indescribable. It is meat and drink and an unrivalled delicacy besides, and you may gorge to repletion and never have cause for penitence. It is the one case where Nature has tried her hand at the culinary art and beaten all the CORDON BLEUE out of heaven and earth. (Banfield 1911: chapter 5; capitalization follows the original)

Banfield adds the note that his friend was not an enthusiast in regard to tropical fruits (Banfield 1911:chapter 5), making his rapture all the more remarkable.

Despite these rave reviews, though, it is extraordinarily easy to find quotes from Westerners who did not like the odor or flavor of durian. Many of their descriptions use a death, decay, or scatological reference to describe the experience. Sir Stanford Raffles, founder of Singapore, told friends that when confronted by the smell, he held his nose and ran away (Rolnick 2003:541). The nineteenth-century naturalist Henri Mouhot said, "On first tasting it, I thought it like the flesh of some animal in a state of putrefaction" (quoted in Rolnick 2003:541). Bob Halliday, a food writer based in Bangkok, said, "To anyone who doesn't like durian it smells like a bunch of dead cats" (quoted in Fuller 2007: n.p.). Rob Walsh, a self-proclaimed veteran food writer who had successfully eaten a wide range of odd foods, was taken aback by his response to durian: "[T]he smell of rotten eggs is so overwhelming. I suppress a gag reaction as I take a bite" (Walsh 1999:76–77).

That gag reaction is a physiological manifestation of disgust, a culturally conditioned response to certain situations, including the thought of eating smelly foods (Rozin et al. 1997; Schiefhövel 1997). While the origins of disgust are in distaste, the latter is a purely physical reaction, whereas the former is a conceptual rejection of the food in question (Schiefhövel 1997; Rozin et al. 1997.) Walsh (1999:76–77) quoted Paul Rozin as saying, "this aversion [to a rotten smell] is not innate. I believe the disgust reaction comes from a universally acquired aversion that is probably taught in the toilet training process." Foods that resemble feces in smell or texture become disgusting through that socialization process. Yet, as Rozin points out (in Walsh 1999), in many cultures, a few rotten-smelling substances become favored foods. European aged cheeses, Inuit rotted whale meat, Southeast Asian fermented fish sauces, and durians are all examples of these culturally significant exceptions. Rozin posits that part of the enjoyment from eating these foods is the struggle between mind and body, where the mind tells the diner that it is okay and the body says no. Because the taste is much better than the smell, there is a payoff to this thrill-seeking. Rozin compares the strong appeal of this situation to riding a roller-coaster and other actions that are initially off-putting.

The popular guides for visitors traveling to Malaysia generally discourage tourists from trying durian. For example, a recent edition of *Frommer's Guide to Malaysia* says:

> Dare it if you will, the fruit to sample—the veritable king of fruits—is the durian, a large, green, spiky fruit that when open, smells worse than old tennis shoes. The "best" ones are in season. . . . In case you're curious, the fruit has a creamy texture and tastes lightly sweet and deeply musky. (Eveland 2005:98)

The Rough Guide to Malaysia, Singapore and Brunei is even more discouraging, stating:

> [o]ne of the most popular fruits in Southeast Asia, durians are also, for many visitors, the most repugnant, thanks to their unpleasant smell. . . . flesh, whose flavour has been likened to vomit-flavoured custard. (de Ledesma et al. 2006:66)

The *Lonely Planet* guide, often chosen by more adventurous travelers, is a bit more encouraging. It says, "Hold your nose and let your taste buds discover the reason for all the fuss about durian" (Richmond et al. 2007:20) in their mention of durian as one of the "Top 10 Eating and Dining experiences to try." On the whole, the lack of strong statements encouraging people to try durian as part of their travel experience is surprising. Being exposed to the new—new people, new customs, new smells, new places, and new foods—is an intrinsic aspect of the travel experience. This should make trying durian especially attractive simply because the flavor of this fruit is distinctly alien to a Western palate.

Durian is so closely associated with Southeast Asia by Europeans that the name graces the titles of a memoir (Wynward 1939) and at least two novels (Keon 1960; Linehan 1996). Both novels are set in Malaysia, and the memoir, while principally focused on the author's experiences in neighboring Thailand, also recounts visits to Malaysia.

TRYING DURIAN

I visited Malaysia (Figure 7.3) to attend a family wedding, but as an anthropologist, I was eager to see and experience as much of the local culture as possible. Noting that Malaysia promised a wonderful selection of new foods to try, I gratefully learned that most of peninsular Malaysia has reliably purified public

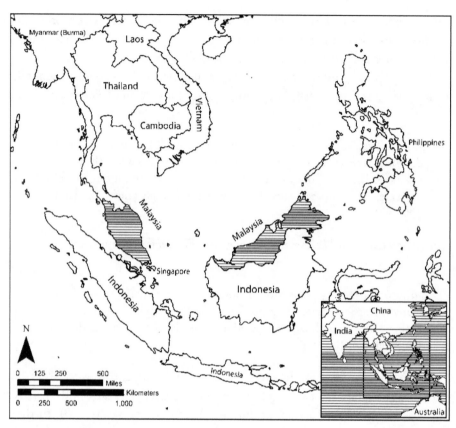

7.3. Map of Malaysia. (MAP BY MAXINE MCBRINN)

water. This is a boon for all tourists and is especially fortunate for adventurous eaters.

Malaysia is a food lover's delight. Because of its location and history, Malay, Indian, Chinese, and Thai cuisines are all easily and abundantly available. Most of these cuisines offer strongly flavored and spicy dishes. Malay food, in particular, uses chilies, lemongrass, coconut, and lime leaves and features a generous use of shrimp paste and dried fish. *Sambal*, a chili paste, is used in many dishes. Most towns have one or more areas where food venders congregate every evening in parks or markets with steam carts, creating a large temporary food court. Malay dishes like *asam kaksa*, a spicy noodle soup; *mee goring*, fried noodles; and *nasi lemak*, coconut-flavored rice served with greens and *sambal ikan bilis*, made from chilies and dried anchovies, are common and delicious.

Southeast Asia offers a wonderful and varied array of fresh fruit that can be bought in markets, and fruit juice venders at the food courts will squeeze fresh fruits to order. While many of the available fruits were familiar, like star fruit, lychee, banana, mango, papaya, passion fruit, watermelon, and pineapple, others, like jackfruit, mangosteen, rambutan, and pomelo were new to me. Rambutan was a special favorite. I could buy a bag of the red, fuzzy little fruit at street markets and then stroll along, using my thumbnail to loosen the peel and popping the fruit into my mouth. Even Malay desserts were an adventure. For example, *ais kacang* is made from shaved ice and red beans, often served with other toppings in luridly bright colors.

My husband, Ken, and I tried as many different dishes as we could find, dining at small local restaurants and from the ubiquitous food carts and playing many rounds of a favorite game that we call "menu roulette." To play, you point to any item on the menu that you do not recognize, and when it is served, you try it, no matter how it looks or smells. My cousin and her new husband looked on with a mix of excitement, enthusiasm, and disgust as we dined our way through many foods that they had not tried in more than a year in the country. The one Malaysian food that we were especially eager to try was durian. For that experience, we were prepared to make a special effort.

One evening, my cousin, Mary-Lyn, and David, her husband, drove us to an outdoor market in Petaling Jaya, the Kuala Lumpur suburb where they lived. Because of its pervasive odor, whole durian is not sold at most indoor markets or grocery stores, although prepackaged sections are often now available in many shops. Unbeknownst to us at that time, there is a ritual to buying a fresh durian. Interested buyers might examine the stem of the fruit to determine how long it had been separated from the tree—a dry stem means that the fruit is too old—or listen for the seeds moving inside when the fruit is shaken, or make sure the thorns are still sharp, another sign of freshness (Teo 2006). Buyers may demand a taste of the fruit they select as promising. The seller we watched took a small core from the flesh of the fruit, offering it to the customer for evaluation. If all is satisfactory, the seller and buyer negotiate an acceptable price. A couple was buying a durian from the fruit-seller when we found him, so we waited until they had finished and watched the transaction. We chose not to sample the fruit first ourselves, in part because we did not know how a durian should taste. Mary-Lyn, who is proud of her ability to find a good deal, had enthusiastically taken to bargaining during her stay in Southeast Asia, even dickering with shopkeepers in situations that I initially thought were not negotiable. She had become a fierce and skillful negotiator. Seeing that her skills were needed, she took the lead and bargained for a minimal price. As a piece of fruit, durians are quite expensive but not outrageously so. The cost of a durian at that time was comparable to the price of a casual dinner, although coveted varieties can be considerably more expensive (Teo 2006).

Once the transaction was complete, the seller handed us the durian in a plastic bag, and we headed back to the apartment, eager to taste our prize. Closed up in David's automobile, we were unaware of the increasing intensity of durian odor. We stopped briefly so that Mary-Lyn could make a quick purchase, with the rest of us staying in the car. When she returned, though, she could smell how the car stank and insisted that all the windows be opened—and left open for the rest of the trip home. In fact, she voted then and there to throw the durian away. Luckily for us, David agreed with our argument that we had to try it while we were in Malaysia. After more than a year in the country he also wanted to taste it, so we made it to their apartment with our durian treasure. Once we left the vehicle, however, the rest of us could detect the durian's scent, which was strongly reminiscent of a natural gas leak. It was not an appetizing scent, but we had been warned and were determined to persevere. Mary-Lyn forcefully told us that she would not try anything that smelled so disgusting, and so the durian eaters were reduced to three. On the way to the apartment, I absentmindedly swung the bag that contained the fruit and the thorns sticking through the plastic carved a few bloody scratches into my thigh before I realized the danger. Durian seemed even more formidable!

The fruit we had bought had been reduced in price because of a natural split in the hull, a good sign if the fruit is newly fallen as it indicates full ripeness but a bad omen if the fruit has sat too long. Being durian innocents, we were not aware of this subtlety, knowing only that the split created a bargain and would make it easier to break open the thick, hard rind. We carefully pried open the fruit, exposing the soft, pale-yellow flesh nestled around the large seeds. When open, a typical durian has five sections, each with flesh surrounding stones in the center (Rolnick 2003). Not sure how to proceed, we spooned the flesh off the seeds as they lay in the rind. The flesh was creamy and smooth with a strong flavor of something like garlic or onion. It had the texture of a ripe avocado and the flavor of onion ice cream. It was not bad, but was not immediately delicious, so that several mouthfuls were plenty. Our tongue and taste buds were saturated with the flavor and we did not want or need more. Mary-Lyn was still complaining loudly about the odor, so we regretfully threw the fruit over the balcony and into the drainage canal behind the apartment.

Then my newly married cousin kissed her husband and quickly backed away in horror. She said that David tasted just like the fruit smelled! Hmm, my husband and I thought smugly, it is a good thing that we both ate durian. Just as with garlic, having both partaken, we could not smell it on each other. We were sitting around the living room, catching up with family news when we realized that durian repeats badly. The first burp of what tasted like sewer gas was a rude surprise, and soon all three of us were belching distastefully. Having eaten the fruit apparently did not protect us from ourselves. Now we could smell and taste that durian scent, and there was no creamy texture or rich flavor to hide it. It was disgusting and continued far too long. We later learned that not everyone experiences this side effect, with perhaps only one in two suffering it, but all three of us did. At the time, it seemed clear that this was a standard result of eating durian.

Well, we thought, that was that. We had tried durian and were not impressed. But then we noticed durian-flavored ice cream for sale at the grocery store. Perhaps that would be better, perhaps it would not have the same side effects, and perhaps this time we would understand how people could be so enthusiastic about durian. The ice cream was delicious, since the richness of the ice cream strengthened that aspect of the durian flavor and muted the sewer-gas overtones. David and I were particularly greedy and each had a large serving, Ken had a smaller one, and Mary-Lyn once again declined. Again, however, we started burping a half hour or so after finishing. Regrettably the burps tasted just as bad as they had after the real durian.

A week later, during a visit to the Cameron highlands, my husband and I found durian-flavored hard candy for sale. Although the first two durian experiences had not been notable successes, how bad could candy be? It is sugar and fruit, and it is hard to go wrong with sugar and fruit. We bought a bag and eagerly sampled our treat. These sweets turned out to have what tasted like a sour molasses base with a durian overtone. The molasses flavor did not provide the creamy texture and flavor of the real fruit or the ice cream. Instead, the durian's natural-gas odor dominated the underlying bitter molasses taste. The candy was a great disappointment and our worst durian experience yet. And then came the crowning insult. The candies repeated, too, with that same sewer-gas effect! Three attempts to learn to love durian, three failures.

One redeeming feature of the candies, however, was that we were able to bring them home, so that we could share our durian experience with our friends. We were wickedly gleeful at the way people's faces screwed up with distaste; somehow their visible disgust justified our reaction. Unfortunately, once our friends were wise to us, we had a hard time giving away the remainder.

CONCLUSION

A fresh durian, unlike the candy version, has many flavors. A sample of some of the comparisons offered by others range from decayed onion, turpentine, garlic, limburger cheese, spicy resin (according to Otis Barrett as quoted in Walsh 1999 and Morton 1987:287), to Wallace's list of almond custard, cream cheese, onion sauce, and sherry wine (1856:435). Which flavors dominate the experience is probably the result of cultural training, training that also informs us which flavors are appreciated and which are repulsive. People who love durian find the aroma enticing (Fuller 2007; Sullivan 2007), probably the result of connecting the odor to the taste within. The reaction to both the taste and the smell of a durian will be the result of past personal experience and cultural training.

In addition, a truly fresh durian, one that is less than a day old, may offer a very different taste experience than one acquired in a city market, which may have been a number of days past perfection. Someday I hope to have the opportunity to try a fresh durian, which may offer more of the flavors I liked and less of the sewer-gas overtone. With practice I may be able to shrug off the durian-flavored burps as easily as I do the aftereffects of eating asparagus or garlic, or drinking coffee, all of which scent the body in one manner or another. I have not found the resultant odor a reason to not indulge in any of these foods, although some people in the United States abstain for just this reason.

I wonder if one of the reasons I did not immediately love durian is that it was always presented as a fruit, a classification that in the United States we reserve for sweet or sweet and tart fruits. The flavors of our fruits are acidic and refreshing rather than rich and complex, and we place non-sweet fruits, like tomatoes and avocados, in other food categories. This echoes Malaysians' classing durian as heating, while almost all other fruits and vegetables are considered cooling. Would my initial reaction have been more enthusiastic if I had not already formed a mental construct of durian as a fruit? What if I had thought of it as a new cousin to an avocado, which is similarly soft and oily? Would that have allowed me to concentrate on the more pleasing tastes within the wide range of durian flavors? I am disappointed with my reaction to this unique food. I know the value that Southeast Asians place on durian and badly want to be able to appreciate the fruit as much as they do. I continue to try durian when it is available but am honestly still mystified as to why it is so coveted. In the end, all I can say is that durian is an acquired taste, and I am still in the process of acquiring it.

REFERENCES

Banfield, Edmund James
    1911   *My Tropic Isle.* T. Fisher Unwin, London.

Brosius, J. Peter
    1999   The Western Penan of Borneo. In *The Cambridge Encyclopedia of Hunters and Gatherers*, ed. Richard B. Lee and Richard Daly, 312–316. Cambridge University Press, New York.

Corner, E.J.H.
    1976   *The Seeds of the Dicotyledons.* Cambridge University Press, New York.

De Ledesma, Charles, Mark Lewis, Richard Lim, Steven Martin, and Pauline Savage
    2006   *The Rough Guide to Malaysia, Singapore and Brunei.* Rough Guides, New York.

Dentan, Robert Knox
  1968   *The Semai: A Nonviolent People of Malaya*. Holt, Rinehart and Winston, New York.

Dunne, Niall
  2002   Durian: The Real Forbidden Fruit. *Plant and Garden News* 17:3 (Fall). http://www.bbg.org/gar2/topics/kitchen/2002fa_durian.html, accessed November 27, 2005.

Endicott, Kirk
  1999a   The Batak of Peninsular Malaysia. In *The Cambridge Encyclopedia of Hunters and Gatherers*, ed. Richard B. Lee and Richard Daly, 298–306. Cambridge University Press, New York.
  1999b   Introduction: Southeast Asia. In *The Cambridge Encyclopedia of Hunters and Gatherers*, ed. Richard B. Lee and Richard Daly, 275–283. Cambridge University Press, New York.

Eveland, Jennifer
  2005   *Frommer's Singapore and Malaysia*. Wiley Publishing, Hoboken, NJ.

Fuller, Thomas
  2007   Fans Sour on Sweeter Version of Asia's Smelliest Fruit. *New York Times* April 8, 2007. http://www.nytimes.com/2007/04/08/world/asia/08durian.html, accessed October 3, 2007.

Harris, Marvin
  1985   *The Sacred Cow and the Abominable Pig: Riddles of Food and Culture*. Simon and Schuster, New York.

Howell, Signe
  1984   *Society and Cosmos: Chewong of Peninsular Malaysia*. Oxford University Press, New York.

Keon, Michael
  1960   *The Durian Tree*. Simon and Schuster, New York.

Kostermans, A.J.G.H.
  1992   An Important Economical New *Duro* Species from Northern Sumatra. *Economic Botany* 46(3):338–340.

Laderman, Carol
  1981   Symbolic and Empirical Reality: A New Approach to the Analysis of Food Avoidances. *American Ethnologist* 8(3):468–493.
  1983   *Wives and Midwives: Childbirth and Nutrition in Rural Malaysia*. University of California Press, Berkeley.

Linehan, Fergus
  1996   *Under the Durian Tree*. Macmillan, London.

Manderson, Lenore
  1986   Food Classification and Restriction in Peninsular Malaysia: Nature, Culture, Hot and Cold? In *Shared Wealth and Symbol: Food, Culture, and*

Society in Oceana and Southeast Asia, ed. Lenore Manderson, 127–143. Cambridge University Press, New York.

McCarthy, John F.
    2005   Between Adat and State: Institutional Arrangements on Sumatra's Forest Frontier. *Human Ecology* 33(1):57–82.

McKay, David A.
    1980   Food, Illness, and Folk Medicine: Insights from Ulu Trengganu, West Malaysia. In *Food, Ecology and Culture: Readings in the Anthropology of Dietary Practices*, ed. J.R.K. Robson, 61–66. Gordon and Breach Science Publishers, New York.

Messer, Ellen
    1984   Anthropological Perspectives on Diet. *Annual Review of Anthropology* 13:205–249.
    1989   Methods for Determinants of Food Intake. In *Research Methods in Nutritional Anthropology*, ed. Gretel H. Pelto, Pertti J. Pelto, and Ellen Messer. United Nations University Press, Tokyo.

Mintz, Sidney W., and Christine M. DuBois
    2002   The Anthropology of Food and Eating. *Annual Review of Anthropology* 31:99–119.

Morton, Julia F.
    1987   Durian. In *Fruits of Warm Climates*, ed. C. F. Dowling, 287–291. New-CROP, Center for New Crops and Plant Products, Purdue University, West Lafayette, IN. http://www.hort.purdue.edu/newcrop/morton/durian_ars.html, accessed April 14, 2006.

Peluso, Nancy Lee
    2003   Fruit Trees and Family Trees in an Anthropogenic Forest: Property Zones, Resource Access, and Environmental Change in Indonesia. In *Culture and the Question of Rights: Forests, Coasts, and Seas in Southeast Asia*, ed. Charles Zerner, 184–218. Duke University Press, Durham, NC.

Richmond, Simon, Damian Harper, Tom Parkinson, Charles Rawlings-Way, and
    Richard Watkins
    2007   *Malaysia, Singapore and Brunei*. Lonely Planet Publications, Oakland, CA.

Rolnick, Harry
    2003   Durian. In *Encyclopedia of Food and Culture*, Vol. 1: *Acceptance to Food Politics*, ed. Solomon H. Katz, 541–543. Scribner, New York.

Roseman, Marina
    1998   Singers of the Landscape: Song, History, and Property Rights in the Malaysian Rain Forest. *American Anthropologist* 100(1):106–121.

Rozin, Paul, Jonathan Haidt, Clark McCauley, and Sumio Imada
    1997   Disgust: Preadaptation and the Cultural Evolution of a Food-Based Emotion. In *Food Preferences and Taste: Continuity and Change*, ed. Helen MacBeth, 65–82. Berghahn Books, Providence, RI.

Schiefhövel, Wulf
  1997   Good Taste and Bad Taste: Preferences and Aversions as Biologic Prin-
          ciples. In *Food Preferences and Taste: Continuity and Change*, ed. Helen
          MacBeth, 55–64. Berghahn Books, Providence, RI.

Simoons, Frederick J.
  1994   *Eat Not This Flesh: Food Avoidances from Prehistory to the Present*, 2nd ed.
          University of Wisconsin Press, Madison.

Soegeng-Reksodihardjo, Wertit
  1962   The Species of *Durio* with Edible Fruits. *Economic Botany* 16(4):270–
          282.

Sokolov, Raymond
  1991   *Why We Eat What We Eat: How the Encounter between the New World
          and the Old Changes the Way Everyone on the Planet Eats.* Summit Books,
          New York.

Sullivan, Michael
  2007   Ooh That Smell: Designing a Stinkless Durian. National Public Radio
          Weekend Edition, May 12, 2007. http://www.npr.org/templates/story/
          story.php?storyId=10016534, accessed October 3, 2007.

Teo, Pau Lin
  2006   Durian King. *The Strait Times Stomp.* ST Foodies Club. Singapore. http://
          www.stomp.com.sg/stfoodiesclub/taste/03/index.html, accessed October
          21, 2007.

Van Der Sluys, Cornelia M.
  1999   The Jahai of Northern Peninsular Malaysia. In *The Cambridge Encyclopedia
          of Hunters and Gatherers*, ed. Richard B. Lee and Richard Daly, 307–311.
          Cambridge University Press, New York.

Veevers-Carter, W.
  1984   *Riches of the Rainforest: An Introduction to the Trees and Fruits of the Indo-
          nesian and Malaysian Rain Forests.* Oxford University Press, Singapore.

Wallace, Alfred Russel
  1856   On the Bamboo and Durian of Borneo. From a letter to Sir Jackson Hooker
          and printed in *Hooker's Journal of Botany*, vol. 8. http://www.wku.edu/
          ~smithch/wallace/S027.html, accessed October 3, 2007.

Walsh, Rob
  1999   The Fruit I Can't Get Past My Nose. *Natural History* (September) 108(7):
          76–78.

Wilson, Christine S.
  1975   Nutrition in Two Cultures: Mexican-American and Malay Ways with
          Food. In *Gastronomy: The Anthropology of Food and Food Habits*, ed. Mar-
          garet L. Arnott, 131–144. Mouton Publishers, Paris.

1980   Food Taboos of Childbirth: The Malay Example. In *Food, Ecology and Culture: Readings in the Anthropology of Dietary Practices*, ed. J.R.K. Robson, 67–74. Gordon and Breach Science Publishers, New York.

1986   Social and Nutritional Context of "Ethnic Foods": Malay Examples. In *Shared Wealth and Symbol: Food, Culture, and Society in Oceana and Southeast Asia*, ed. Lenore Manderson, 259–272. Cambridge University Press, New York.

Wynward, Noel

1939   *Durian: A Siamese Interlude.* Oxford University Press, London.

Discussion Questions: Durian: The King of Fruits or an Acquired Taste?

1. Why would some love the durian fruit while others hate it? What are the cultural reasons behind this strong feeling?
2. Why is durian a difficult fruit to grow and sell in the local or international market?
3. Where does one find durian for sale? Why is it sold in the places where one can find it?
4. Why is durian considered an aphrodisiac? What are the effects of eating the fruit and what do we know about it in terms of content and chemical breakdown?

1 Fermented marine food products in Vietnam

Ecological basis and production

Kenneth Ruddle

Eastern mainland Asia is the realm of *umami* ('good taste'; cf. Kawamura and Kare 1987), where the amino acid and salty tastes of fermented products enter the cuisine. There, much of the salt intake is from either the daily consumption of fermented foods or condiments. It is also the principal region of irrigated rice cultivation. Generally, in most of East and Southeast Asia, where rice is the staple carbohydrate, there is a high consumption of fish and fish products. So the predominant dietary pattern is fish combined with rice, which provides vegetable protein, amino acids and energy. Thus in this dietary culture a side dish used to facilitate consumption of large amounts of rice is indispensable. Such dishes are characteristically small in quantity and highly salty. Fermented products are the most suitable items for this purpose. They also have the advantage of being simple to preserve and have a long shelf life. Further, they do not require elaborate cooking for each meal. Fermented products also impart *umami* and a salty taste to vegetable dishes, which inherently lack these flavours.

The seasonal pattern of the monsoon is the main ecological driving force of Southeast Asia, when seasons of abundance and scarcity of food resources alternate according to the stage of the monsoonal circulation. Fermentation of fish and other aquatic organisms is one ancient technique used throughout East and Southeast Asia to provide an animal protein as well as a savoury side dish and condimental complement to rice in the seasons when fresh fish is either scarce or unobtainable. Fermentation is used to produce soy and fish sauces, the dominant condiments throughout the region (Ishige and Ruddle 1987, 1990; Kimizuka *et al.* 1987).

Despite a long and close cultural association with China, fermented soybean products did not develop in Vietnam. Instead, fermented fish products have always been used. In Vietnam, as in the rest of the region, the marine fish species deliberately targeted for use in the fermentation industry share three basic characteristics. They are (1) readily available in large quantities to permit bulk, low cost fermentation; (2) caught easily and in safe locations, to reduce labour costs and hazard, respectively; and (3) require little highly specialized or expensive fishing gear to catch. In addition, all the species meet certain physical criteria to ensure easy and even bulk fermentation, and are inexpensive, with few if any more valuable economic uses. Therefore, most marine species routinely preserved by fermentation are small, of low economic value and are seasonally abundant in inshore marine and brackish waters, in large shoals, that are easily captured with relatively simple gear (Ruddle 1986). In contrast, at other times of the year they are scarce or absent in the same locations. Since, with few exceptions, the fish utilized are juveniles, they are of low economic value and, apart from conversion into animal feed, have few alternative economic uses.

Although any species of fish can be fermented to produce fish sauces and pastes, by preference, because of the inherent chemical characteristics of certain species, as well as biological rhythms that favour uniform harvesting in bulk, only relatively few species are used in Vietnam. There, apart from the Indo-Pacific mackerel (*Rastrelliger* sp.), Gizzard shads (*Anodontostoma chacunda* and *Nematolosa nasus*) and Round scad (*Decapterus* spp.), the fish fermented are all clupeoids (Round herring [*Spratelloides* spp.], sardines [*Sardinella* spp.] and anchovies [*Coilia* spp., *Setipinna* spp., *Stolephorus* spp. and *Engraulis* spp.]) (Ruddle 1986). Thus, the fish used are mostly planktivores that depend on the plankton blooms generated by the upwelling induced by the offshore monsoon. And most of the marine fish utilized to make fermented sauces and paste are either juveniles or young adults, since the length of those used is about 50 per cent of the total body length (TBL) of adults.

In all cases the species used and the size needed are abundant, at particular coastal locations, only during certain times of the year. I have demonstrated elsewhere that the fundamental biological rhythm exploited by this fishery is the feeding and recruitment migration of juvenile planktivores (Ruddle 1986), which depends on the seasonal location of coastal upwellings induced by the prevailing offshore monsoon winds that give rise to phytoplankton blooms (Ruddle 2005).[1] In other words, the seasonal and diel[2] behavioural characteristic exploited by the fisheries that supply the fermentation industry is the tendency of the juveniles of the finfish species utilized to aggregate in vast shoals in shallow inshore marine and brackish estuarine waters for feeding. In all cases, this behavioural characteristic permits large quantities of fish to be captured, using relatively simple fishing gear, and in relatively shallow, sheltered and safe inshore waters.

The ecological basis of the fishery

The ecological basis of the fermentation industry in Vietnam are the physical oceanographic factors associated with the monsoons that cause local upwelling and, therefore, increase primary productivity in marine waters, and the seasonality of their biological rhythms. The driving force is the pattern of monsoon seasonality.

The large-scale atmospheric circulation in Southeast Asia is characterized by the northeast monsoon, the southwest monsoon, and two inter-monsoonal periods. The northeast monsoon lasts from about mid-October until March, when air flows basically north to south across Southeast Asia. At this time of the year strong onshore winds and heavy precipitation are experienced along the coasts of Vietnam, apart from the southern and west-facing coasts in the south of the country. The southwest monsoon season lasts from mid-May until September, when wind and precipitation patterns are essentially the reverse of those prevailing during the northeast monsoon. The two inter-monsoonal periods are transitions between the two monsoons. One occurs from late-March through May, and the other from late-September through November. Inter-monsoonals are characterized by frequent changes in the direction of the prevailing winds, and by variations in duration; from three to twelve weeks with the March–May transition period generally being longer.

That pattern of monsoon seasonality drives the seasonal pattern of vertical water movements. A very simplified explanation of the mechanism is that the fish production of any sea area depends on the fertility of its water,[3] or on the level of primary production of phytoplankton, the photosynthesis of which in tropical seas occurs in a euphotic zone that extends to a depth of about 200 metres.[4] However, in tropical seas a strong and persistent thermocline usually inhibits the water mixing[5] and so limits primary production because dead organisms and excreta, which provide the nutrients for phytoplankton growth, sink into the deeper waters beneath the thermocline. Nutrients are therefore gradually depleted in the euphotic zone, the fertility and fish production of which declines.

Thus, upwelling or vertical water movements that seasonally disrupt the thermocline and restore the temporarily lost nutrients to the productive cycle in the euphotic zone are fundamental to the fertility of the sea and to fish production. When nutrient-laden waters are thus restored to the surface a 'burst' of phytoplankton growth occurs, followed by a growth in the zooplankton population, and, in turn, an increase in the population of both planktivorous fish and those piscivores that predate on them. The spawning and feeding patterns of fish are adapted to this seasonal sequence of the loss and restoration of nutrient levels. Thus the occurrence of upwelling, which is caused by a variety of physical factors, is of fundamental importance to both the fish production of an area and the fishery based on it (Figure 1.1).

In Southeast Asia coastal upwelling is caused mainly by the prevailing offshore monsoonal wind flow.[6] Thus the location of areas of coastal upwelling, and therefore of fishing activity, changes seasonally according to the prevailing direction of the monsoonal winds. During the season of the northeast monsoon upwelling occurs on western, southwestern and southern coasts, and during the southwest monsoon it occurs on eastern, northeastern and northern coasts.

Conversely, during the monsoon season with prevailing onshore winds the reverse process operates. At this time of the year nutrient-rich waters are kept below the thermocline by the piling-up of surface water against the coast, under the pressure of the prevailing wind. Thus, without replenishment from below the thermocline, the euphotic zone undergoes a decline in nutrients and a concomitant decline in populations of phytoplankton and fish.[7]

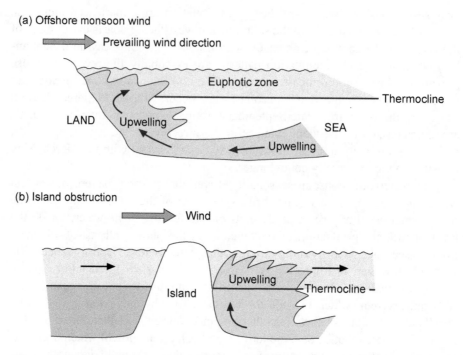

Figure 1.1 Principal causes of upwelling in the coastal waters of Vietnam (after Ruddle 1986).

The relationship between fishing season and monsoon seasonality

For the physical and biological reasons discussed above, most coastal fishing in Vietnamese waters is conducted during the monsoon, when the prevailing winds are offshore, when coastal upwelling, therefore, occurs, and during the inter-monsoonal (IM). In the coastal waters of Vietnam, anchovies (*Stolephorus* spp.) are taken from September until November, i.e. from the end of the offshore southwest monsoon (SW), through the inter-monsoonal, and into the beginning of the onshore northeast monsoon (NE). *Coilia* spp. and *Rastrelliger* spp. are caught for a somewhat longer period, from July to December. Anchovies of the genera *Setipinna* and *Engraulis* are caught only from July to September, i.e. only after the prevailing offshore winds of the southwest and the coastal upwelling that it induces are firmly established (Figure 1.2).

Hypothesis on monsoon seasonality and the biological rhythms of fish

Since most of the fish fermented are small, pelagic, schooling planktivores, their feeding behaviour depends on spatio-temporal variations in the location of plankton, which, in turn, depends on monsoonal seasonality. Further, since these fish are subject to high predation pressures it can be supposed that in their repro-

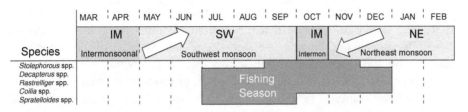

Figure 1.2 Relationship between the fishing season of selected fish species and monsoon seasonality in Vietnam (after Ruddle 1986).

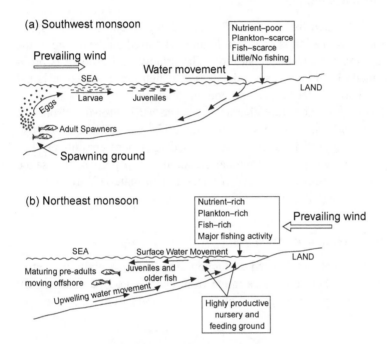

Figure 1.3 Hypothesis on fish behaviour and the monsoons (for a Western Coast) in Vietnam (after Ruddle 1986).

ductive strategy they migrate away from inshore zones, where predation rates are extremely high, to spawn in offshore areas where the pressure is less intense.

For the small pelagic fishes of concern here, however, I hypothesized (Ruddle 1986) that intense predation inshore leads to offshore spawning migrations at times and in places where the eggs and larvae are assured of being swept coastwards. They should also spawn at times and in locations where their eggs would not be flushed further offshore, and, on the contrary, when winds, currents and gyres would ensure a steady coastwards drift of eggs, larvae and post-larval forms. Thus at an early juvenile stage they would arrive at their plankton-rich inshore feeding grounds (Figure 1.3).

Thus, depending on the distance offshore of the spawning grounds, spawning of the migratory species should occur towards the latter part of the onshore monsoon. This would ensure that the post-larval forms reach inshore waters, where phytoplankton blooms are rich, as a consequence of the upwelling induced by the offshore monsoon, either before the winds of the offshore monsoon cause them to drift further out to sea, or just after they have developed the swimming ability as newly recruited juveniles. In the latter case they could swim against the wind-induced current and reach the inshore feeding grounds prior to the intense and persistent development of the monsoon (Ruddle 1986).[8]

Types of fermented fish product

A wide range of fermented fish product is produced in East and Southeast Asia. A simple generic classification is shown in Figure 1.4, based on the nature of the final product and the method of preparation. The prototypical product is probably *shiokara*, made by mixing fish and salt, and which preserves the original whole or partial shape of the fish. When comminuted *shiokara* yields *shiokara* paste, which has a condiment-like character. Fish sauce is prepared from the process of making *shiokara*. If no vegetable materials are added the salt-fish mixture eventually yields fish sauce, a liquid used as a pure condiment. The intent, however, particularly in commercial situations, is to prepare fish sauce and not *shiokara*. *Narezushi* is produced if cooked plant materials are added to the fish and salt mixture (Ishige and Ruddle 1987).

*Fish sauces (*nuoc mam*) in Vietnam*

Fish sauce is a condiment widely used throughout Asia, and especially in continental Southeast Asia, where processes range from simple procedures to satisfy household needs through large-scale factories using industrial techniques. In

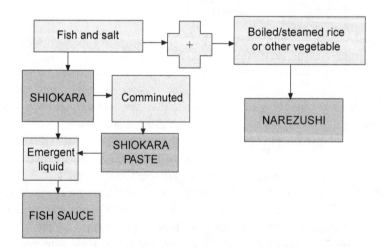

Figure 1.4 Generic classification of fermented fish products in Asia.

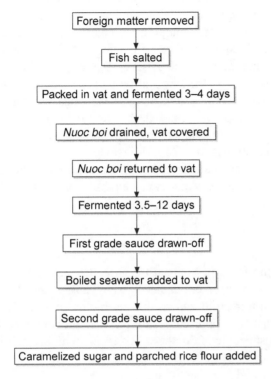

Foreign matter removed

Fish salted

Packed in vat and fermented 3–4 days

Nuoc boi drained, vat covered

Nuoc boi returned to vat

Fermented 3.5–12 days

First grade sauce drawn-off

Boiled seawater added to vat

Second grade sauce drawn-off

Caramelized sugar and parched rice flour added

Figure 1.5 The generic production process of marine fish sauce (*nuoc mam*) in Vietnam (adapted from information in Nguyen and Vialard-Goudou 1953).

Vietnam the mainstay of the fish sauce industry is large-scale production in specialized communities, using highly elaborate techniques, but household and cottage industry production is widespread and varied. The generic production process for fish sauce manufacture in Vietnam is shown in Figure 1.5. Three stages may be distinguished: (1) preliminary processing; (2) salting the fish and filling the fermentation container; and (3) drawing-off the sauce.

Where whole fish are used, preliminary processing consists just of removing all foreign matter. Elsewhere it is more complex. The fish are classified according to size and inherent salt content when a system of compression and just one salting is used. The different sizes and salt content types are treated differently. Further, the level of the inherent saltiness of fish varies by season, being higher in summer. The fish is also classified by the number of scales and thickness. Large ones are cut into pieces prior to salting.

Salting rates and the method of filling the container depend on the species used and their inherent salt content. When Round scad (*Decapterus* sp.), miscellaneous stolephorid and other anchovies (*Engraulis* spp.) are being used, the fermentation container is divided into three sections. In the bottom section the fish are salted (by weight) at 1:0.5, in the centre the rate is 1.5:1 and at the top 1.2:1.

The fish are left thus to disintegrate slowly. The time required for this varies according to species. *Dorostoma nasu* and miscellaneous species require 12 months, since they are bony and their flesh tough. But *Decapterus* requires four months and *Engraulis mystax* and *Stolephorus* sp. will disintegrate in 3.5 months. The precise length of the fermentation period depends on the seasonal climate. It is faster in summer. It also depends on the size and type of fish being used, as well as on the attention paid to the processing. Small, soft-boned fish ferment faster than large fish with many scales and thick flesh. The first grade of sauce (*nuoc mam nhi*) is drained from the container, then boiled seawater with salt added is poured in. This drains through the fish-salt residue and yields a lower grade sauce. Where there are many small fermentation containers in a factory, they are divided into groups of five. The water is passed through all five and so becomes enriched.

Conclusion

The principal ecological driving force in Southeast Asia is the seasonal pattern of the monsoon. In the physical environment this is clearly visible in the alternation of dry and wet seasons in terrestrial and freshwater biomes of the region, and in the alternating constraints and opportunities for resource procurement that this regime presents. Since most people in Southeast Asia remain highly dependent on primary industry, climate is of major importance in their daily lives and the seasonal round of economic and social activities.

That this monsoonal regime is of equal magnitude and socioeconomic importance in the marine environment of the region has been less than thoroughly appreciated, apart from a generally superficial interpretation of its impact on fishing schedules and the like. I have demonstrated here and on other occasions (e.g. Ruddle 1986, 1987) that in the aquatic environments of Southeast Asia, as in their terrestrial counterparts, seasons of abundance and scarcity of potential food resources follow each other according to the stage of the monsoonal circulation. To balance such extreme fluctuations in food availability, techniques were devised centuries ago to store and preserve at least the rice and fish staples. The fermentation of fish into various types of paste, sauce and other products is one such ancient technique that remains of vital culinary and economic importance in Southeast Asia.

The research on which this contribution is based began in the early-1980s, when I did a collaborative study of fish fermentation throughout East Asia. From the outset it was clear that attempts to account for the ecological basis of the fish fermentation were hampered by a paucity of marine biological research on the seasonal behaviour of the species involved, and the biological and physical bases for it. The occurrence of seasons in tropical environments, in general, is still little appreciated. So I was forced back to basic principles of physical oceanography and fisheries biology to make several hypotheses about the likely physical and biological basis for the fermentation industry (Ruddle 1986). About a decade later I was able to test these assertions over several weeks in the field by analysing the traditional fisheries management techniques and their basis in local marine ecological knowledge at Van Thuy Tu, Phan Thiet, a major and old-established fisheries base (Ruddle 1998). Extended and multiple interviews to elicit fishers' ecological knowledge on the seasonality of fish behaviour then provided the verification of the hypotheses (Ruddle 1998, 2005). I would commend this combination as a useful but time-consuming approach, particularly when scientific data are either absent or depauperate.

Acknowledgements

It is my pleasure to acknowledge the financial support of the Ajinomoto Co. Ltd (Tokyo) that permitted initial field research in 1984. Work on the whale shrine management system was conducted during the course of a three-year project (1995–1998) on the socio-economic aspects of coastal fisheries in Central Vietnam, funded by Japan International Cooperation Agency.

Notes

1 The constraints on this kind of study have been elaborated by Ruddle (1986, 2005).
2 Diel refers to a 24-hour cycle that includes a daylight and a night period.
3 Here, 'fish production' means 'biological production' as opposed to the 'yield of a fishery'. The latter obviously depends also on a variety of cultural, economic and technical factors.
4 A euphotic zone refers to the upper layers of a body of water into which enough sunlight penetrates to permit the growth of green plants.
5 A thermocline is a layer of water in a thermally stratified area that separates an upper, warmer, lighter and oxygen-rich zone from a lower, colder and oxygen-poor zone.
6 These vertical water movements in the marine environment are extremely complex. The discussion here has been greatly simplified. Local upwelling is also caused by obstructions such as islands or submerged raised areas of the seabed. They obstruct the surface current flow induced by the prevailing wind.
7 But those broad patterns of coastal upwelling are locally distorted by such phenomena as the impact of currents, a major influx of nutrients via discharge of rivers swollen by monsoon rains, and by the rain itself.
8 Thus, for example, if the hypothesis is correct, spawning on western coasts should occur at the end of the southwest monsoon so that juveniles can utilize the food supply at the inshore upwelling areas induced by the northeast monsoon, as is the case with the anchovies (*Stolephorus heterolobus* and *S. punctifer*) and slipmouths (*Leiognathus blochii*) in Manila Bay waters (see Ingles and Pauly 1984). The spawning of *Rastrelliger brachysoma* and *R. neglectus* off both the west coast of Thailand and the west coast of Peninsular Malaysia, together with *Decapterus* spp. off the latter, is also consistent with this hypothesis that seasonality in food availability influences reproductive seasonality and therefore the fishery (Ruddle 1986).

References

Ingles, J. and Pauly, D. (1984) *An Atlas of the Growth, Mortality and Recruitment of Philippine Fishes*, ICLARM Technical Report No. 13, Manila: ICLARM.
Ishige, N. and Ruddle, K. (1987) 'Gyosho in Southeast Asia – a study of fermented

aquatic products', *Bulletin of the National Museum of Ethnology*, 12 (2): 235–314 (in Japanese).

—— (1990) *Gysho to Narezushi no Kenkyu (Research on Fermented Fish Products and Narezushi)*, Tokyo: Iwanamishoten (in Japanese).

Kawamura, Y. and Kare, M.R. (1987) *Umami: A Basic Taste*, New York and Basel: Marcel Dekker.

Kimizuka, A., Mizutani, T., Ruddle, K. and Ishige, N. (1987) 'A chemical analysis of fermented fish products and discussion of fermented flavors in Asian cuisines', *Bulletin of the National Museum of Ethnology*, 12 (3): 801–864.

Nguyen, A.C. and Vialard-Goudou, A. (1953) 'Sur la nature de l'acidité volatile de la saumure vietnamienne "nuoc-mam"', *Comptes Rendues des Séances de l'Academie des Sciences*, 236: 2128–2130.

Ruddle, K. (1986) 'The supply of marine fish species for fermentation in Southeast Asia', *Bulletin of the National Museum of Ethnology*, 11 (4): 997–1036.

—— (1987) 'The ecological basis for fish fermentation in freshwater environments of continental Southeast Asia, with special reference to Burma and Kampuchea', *Bulletin of the National Museum of Ethnology*, 12 (1): 1–48.

—— (1998) 'Traditional community-based coastal marine fisheries management in Viet Nam', *Ocean and Coastal Management*, 40: 1–22.

—— (2005) 'The use and management of small clupeoids in Viet Nam', in N. Kishigami and J. Savelle (eds) *Indigenous Use and Management of Marine Resources* (Senri Ethnological Studies 67), Osaka, Japan: National Museum of Ethnology, pp. 215–236.

Discussion Questions: Fermented Marine Food Products in Vietnam

1. Why has fermentation been important in Southeast Asia?
2. What are some of the characteristics of the food items that are fermented in Vietnam?
3. What is the staple carbohydrate of Asia?
4. What does this article imply about the cuisine of Vietnam? Of Asian countries?

The Pink Revolution, or How Asia Is Getting Hooked on Meat, Fast

Marta Zaraska

As steak houses go, The Only Place is rather unassuming. The atmosphere is relaxed, the decor quite simple: square tables covered in red-and-white-checkered linen, alpine-style wooden chairs. Rows of Christmas lights blink lazily under the ceiling. The mustachioed waiters appear slightly bored in their crisp white shirts. In fact, little would be notable about The Only Place if not for its location. The steak house is hidden on one of the backstreets of downtown Bengaluru, India—the country where cows are so worshipped that killing one can get you in prison. In fact, their urine is considered sacred and is used to bathe sick kids. And yet the menu at The Only Place features Philly cheese steak, chateaubriand supreme, and double filet mignon. Beef, beef, and more beef.

My steak arrives on a simple white plate, in a cloud of succulent aromas. Although I take only a few bites (my husband polishes off the rest), it's enough to tell the meat is delicious. Sacred or not, Indian beef tastes good.

Whenever I tell this story, people (Westerners) usually react with shock: You had beef in India? Is it even legal? The answers are "yes" and "yes." The Only Place was a pioneer when it swung its doors open in 1970, but nowadays steak houses are all the rage in wealthy, metropolitan India. What's more, India has recently taken over Australia as the world's second-largest exporter of beef—after Brazil. That's right: the India of holy cows exports more dead bovines than almost any other nation on the planet.

Granted, India still has a very low meat intake—just 7 pounds per person per year to the US's astounding 275 pounds—but it's growing shockingly fast. By 2030, for example, poultry consumption in India's sprawling cities is projected to shoot up from 2000 levels by 1,277 percent. And the same thing is happening all across Asia. By 2030, Malaysia's beef consumption will likely be up 159 percent, Cambodia's 146 percent, and the urban dwellers in Laos will go through 1,049 percent more poultry. Meanwhile, China will gobble 22,050,000 tons more pork—that's about as much in weight as a hundred thousand fully loaded Boeing 787-8 Dreamliners. With 2.5 billion people in India and China alone, Asia's growing appetite for meat spells trouble not only for the animals that will be killed and eaten but also for the health of Asians—and of our planet.

What is happening in the nations of Asia and in developing countries on other continents, too, even if on a smaller scale, is what scientists refer to as the nutrition transition. There are five recognized patterns or stages of nutrition transition. First, a society goes from stage 1, collection of food (hunting and gathering), to stage 2, famine (which starts with agriculture). Then comes stage 3, receding famine, during which agriculture improves and severe hunger becomes a thing of the past but foods remain unprocessed and simple. Later, as time passes, societies go through an industrial revolution and enter stage 4, degenerative disease. That's where the West is now: eating poor diets loaded with cholesterol, sugar, and fat. But that's not the end of the path. Nutritionists predict that there is one more step to take: stage 5, behavioral change. Behavioral change means, in a way, moving back to eating foods similar to those consumed by stage 1 societies: much less meat, more fruits, veggies, and whole grains.

For now, what's going on in Asia is a transition from stage 3 (receding famine) to stage 4 (degenerative disease). The more money people in developing countries have to spend on food, the more meat they buy. One study showed that each increase in yearly income of US $1,000 boosts per capita meat consumption in Asian countries by 2.6 pounds, in Africa by 3.6 pounds, and in the Middle East by 8.8 pounds. Members of developing nations, which formerly comprised the world's least meathooked populations, have revealed that they're willing to spend their hard-earned wages on meat, which they may have no tradition of eating, and damage their health in the process. We're left with one question: Why?

The first East Asian country to develop an appetite for meat, and one that can offer a glimpse into the process of going from almost vegetarian to meat loving in a relatively short period of time, is Japan. As late as 1939 a typical Japanese ate just 0.1 ounce of meat per day. That's a yearly average, of course. Today, the daily meat portion of a typical Yamada Tarō (the Japanese equivalent of John Smith) is 4.7 ounces, and his favorite animal protein is pork, not tuna in a sushi roll. One reason behind this astounding change was the rise of Western influence.

Medieval Japan was practically vegetarian. The national religions, Buddhism and Shintoism, both promoted plant-based eating, but what was likely more key to keeping the Japanese off meat was the shortage of arable land on the islands. Growing livestock takes land away from more efficient plant agriculture, and already in medieval Japan, too many forests had been cleared for fields and too many draft animals were being killed for their flesh—which prompted Japan's rulers to issue meat-eating bans. The first such ban was announced in 675 CE and meant no beef, monkey, chicken, or dog in Japanese pots from late spring until early autumn. Later, more bans followed. For some time, the Japanese could still satisfy their meat cravings with wild game, but as the population increased and forests gave way to cropland, deer and boars disappeared and so did meat from the plates of the Yamada Tarōs.

The winds of change started blowing, at first mildly, in the eighteenth century. It was the Dutch who sowed in Japanese minds the idea that eating meat is good for health. The Japanese came to see the meat-loaded diets of the tall Europeans as a symbol of progress, of breaking with feudal, hierarchical society. In 1872, Japanese diets took a fast swerve toward meat. That year, on January 24, a feminine-looking, poetry-writing emperor Meiji publicly ate meat for the first time, giving the nation permission to follow his example. Over just five years, beef consumption in Tokyo shot up more than thirteen times (what made it possible were imports from Korea). Meiji and his government saw meat not only as a way to modernize Japan and boost the health of the average citizen but also as a way to bolster the strength of the Japanese army. Back then, typical conscripts were small and thin—over 16 percent of candidates failed to meet the minimum height of four feet eleven inches.

The American occupation after the Second World War gave another powerful boost to the Japanese hunger for meat. The Japanese observed the war victors stuffing themselves with hamburgers, steaks, and bacon. The words of Den Fujita, the chief of McDonald's Japanese operations, sum up the prevailing sentiment pretty well: "If we eat hamburgers for a thousand years, we will become blond. And when we become blond we can conquer the world."

The story of India's newfound taste for animal protein is in many ways similar to what had happened in Japan. It's a story of longing to become modern and powerful, a member of the "we've made it" club. And Bengaluru, this dusty tangle of humans and buildings and cars, this cacophony of a city, where the twenty-first century mixes with the distant past on every corner, is a perfect place to study India's ambivalent relationship with animal flesh.

Bengaluru used to be called the "garden city." But in recent years the trees and lawns have given way to offices and apartment buildings, to an outbreak of stores and potholed streets. Now Bengaluru is a city known for its pollution and congestion—but also for being the capital of the nation's IT industry, the silicon valley of India. It's loud. It's overwhelming. Expensive limousines maneuver between dirty, overcrowded buses and rusty auto rickshaws.

Renovated fancy boutiques at street level are housed in buildings that are otherwise crumbling. Loose wires hang over outdoor café tables, where middle-class patrons sip lattes. The air smells of perfumed women, of sweat, of gasoline and dust, the same dust that keeps pushing its way into my mouth and eyes.

The Only Place is much more peaceful. Behind its doors it is quiet enough so that I don't have to struggle to hear the story that Ajath

Anjanappa tells me over a beefsteak—the story of how so many young, middle-class Indians go about giving up vegetarianism.

Anjanappa is, in many ways, a typical successful Bengalurean. A thirty-something engineer with an MBA degree earned in the US, he now runs his own company, which provides energy-efficient lighting to local industries. He is easygoing and good-looking. And like many of his generation, he loves meat. These days, as Anjanappa explains, to eat steaks and burgers in India is to be modern and worldly. It is a sign that you belong to the group of people who jet around the planet and work for multinational corporations. "It can help you in your career," he tells me.

Anjanappa's affair with meat began the way it usually does for wealthy Indians: you grow up either in a family that is pure veg (Indian for "vegetarian") or one that consumes very little meat. You go to college, you make new friends. You start eating out in the many international restaurants that have sprouted all over Bengaluru, Mumbai, and Delhi. "All my non-veg friends were pushing me, saying I was missing out. If you are a vegetarian you don't belong to the same social circle. By the time we graduated, all my friends were meat eaters," Anjanappa says. Then you go to work for a Western corporation. "A lot of companies like Google or Apple have their own cafeterias where there is a lot of meat served, for free. So why not eat it?" Anjanappa tells me. As years pass, you travel for work outside India where there is often no decent vegetarian food to be had. You either eat meat, or you go hungry. So you eat it, and you start to like it. Those young Indians who work for multinational companies often make good money, and they spend it trying new things, including new cuisines. What makes pressure to eat meat harder to resist in India is the communal way in which meals are enjoyed there. As in many Asian countries, and not in the individualistic West, dishes in India are shared. There is a huge pressure to eat what others are having. To refuse food is to be antisocial.

Yet even in up-and-coming Bengaluru, steak houses are not a common sight. And many locals, when I ask them about their country's beef industry, are surprised to learn that India is the second-largest exporter of meat in the world. Unbeknownst to many, in 2013 and 2014, beef shipments from the subcontinent rose a staggering 31 percent. A big chunk of that meat goes first to Vietnam and later on to China. A lot ends up in the Gulf states and in North Africa. For the US and UK, there is only a trickle left, so the chances you are grilling Indian bovines on your barbecue are slim. But many Western producers are nevertheless worried about the competition. Indian beef is cheap and lean, and it's flooding the markets.

But at least officially, India is not killing off its holy cows. The beef it exports actually comes from water buffaloes, a species of bovine closely related to cows but not quite the same thing. Water buffaloes are not sacred. They do not spend their old age in senior houses or get buried in cemeteries—the way cows do in India. Instead, water buffaloes are overloaded on trucks, transported without food and water, and slaughtered in miserable conditions similar to the American meat industrial complex.

Officially, cow meat is not exported from India, but in reality, there exists an underground cow slaughter industry that labels the meat "buffalo" while it is still in India and relabels it "cow" once it crosses the border. According to a local chapter of the nonprofit organization PETA, there are about thirty thousand illegal slaughterhouses in India, many of them turning holy cows into steaks. As Anjanappa tells me: "As long as the money is coming in, they don't mind what they are killing."

For Western ethical vegetarians, who gave up meat for the sake of animals, such duality is often hard to comprehend. How is it possible that killing a holy cow is a horrible sin and often a crime, while butchering their close cousins, the buffaloes, is perfectly fine? How can young, wealthy Indians chuck their vegetarianism so fast—and seemingly with little regret? And yet, it does make sense. After all, in India, vegetarianism means a very different thing than it does in the West.

First and foremost, vegetarianism and the sacredness of cows don't necessarily go hand in hand. Millions of Indians who never touch beef have no problem at all eating chicken or pork. Meanwhile, even though cows have been considered holy in India for centuries, before 1000 CE the sacred animals were still slaughtered and eaten. The ban on eating holy cows crept into the culture slowly, over time. Today, devout Hindus believe that the body of every cow is inhabited by 330 million gods, and to become a cow, a soul has to transmigrate eighty-six times (that's a lot of lives to go through). Until recently, killing a cow carried the death penalty in the state of Kashmir. The fact that the ancestors of Indians ate the sacred animals is something that many in India are trying to forget: in 2006, mentions of ancient Hindus consuming beef were deleted from school textbooks.

Vegetarianism in India didn't arise from the veneration of cows. It developed independently, from a concept called *ahimsa*, or nonviolence. Basically, *ahimsa* means that all life is sacred and should not be destroyed. Nonviolence is a common thread linking the three Indian religions: Hinduism, Jainism, and Buddhism. But *ahimsa* doesn't necessarily imply that you cannot eat meat—not according to everyone's interpretation. *Ahimsa* is not about animals. It's about people. Just like Pythagoras in ancient Greece, Buddhism, Hinduism, and Jainism concentrate on what violence does to human souls and how it can degrade them. So if you didn't kill the animal yourself and didn't ask anyone to do it, there is no violence to stain your spirit, and you are OK. Buddha ate meat, and even the founder of Jainism, Mahavira, once ate a few pigeons that were killed by a cat.

For many in India *ahimsa* still means that meat should never be eaten because it comes from soul-polluting violence. Yet this form of vegetarianism is still all about humans and not about animals, which makes it easier for adherents to start eating meat once they cease being religious. There is very little discussion about the suffering of meat animals in Indian media, barely any at all. For most, vegetarianism is a way of life, a tradition taken as is. Those who consciously decide not to eat animals either for health or for ethical reasons stand out—so much so that they are called "out-of-choice vegetarians."

If vegetarianism in India is not a choice for most and often seen as conservative and even backward, meat eating stands for modernization and progress. Just like the Japanese poet-emperor Meiji, Mahatma Gandhi also, at some point in his life, believed that a meat-based diet could push India forward and upward. Yes, that Gandhi. Violence-abhorring, meat-abstaining Gandhi. But he wasn't always a vegetarian. Although he was born into a typical Indian religious pure-veg family, he soon came to regard meat eating as something that could help modernize the subcontinent. It was a common belief back in the late nineteenth century that to eat meat was a patriotic duty, a way for Indians to become as strong and powerful as the English so that they could drive the colonialists out. One comic poem became particularly popular: "Behold the mighty Englishman / He rules the Indian small, / Because being a meat-eater He is five cubits tall." And so, one day, Gandhi decided to start eating meat. He and his friend, already a meat eater, packed freshly baked bread and some cooked goat and hiked to a lonely spot by the river so that no one would see them. Once there, Gandhi took a bite of the meat and started to chew. He didn't like it, not at all. The meat was tough as leather. He just couldn't finish it. Later, at night, he was tormented by nightmares and felt as if "a live goat were bleating" inside him. But he kept reminding himself that eating meat was a duty, that he simply *had* to do it.

Soon after, when he moved to London, Gandhi began to eat meat in fancy restaurants and learned to enjoy the taste. He admitted in his autobiography that for a while he wished that "every Indian should be a meat-eater." But in time, Gandhi went back to vegetarianism. He became, as he said, a "vegetarian by choice." After reading many books on nutrition and ethics, he was convinced not only that vegetarianism was better from a moral perspective but also that a plant-based diet was advantageous for health. He started to see that meat eating wouldn't turn India into a powerful nation—and maybe just the opposite.

Today, you won't hear many Indians say that meat eating is a national duty and that it will help India rule the world, but the belief that animal protein makes individual people strong is still alive and well. In India, the media are rather quiet about all the studies that connect a meat-eating diet with cancer, diabetes, and heart disease; yet there are many articles that glorify meat eating as a key to good nutrition. The protein myth is particularly potent. The *Times of India*, a leading newspaper, writes: "Keep in mind that vegetarianism comes with its share of problems because plant foods tend to lack protein." On television, celebrity chefs whip up meat-based dishes, and male actors go non-veg to gain muscles for their roles. Salman Khan, the highest-paid Bollywood star, famed and beloved not only for his stage talents but also for his muscular body, is a proud meat eater, preaching the gospel of non-veg to the masses. And so it's hard to blame Anjanappa for believing that as a regular gym-goer he needs to eat meat—even though science clearly shows that that is not true. In fact, the traditional veg Indian fare is far from deficient in proteins. Just think about it: they have over fifty varieties of lentils, peas, and beans, all loaded with protein, and if paired with rice, the combination makes a complete protein. Vegetarianism could have taken root in India much easier than in Europe or North America precisely because of the culinary diversity and protein load that local plants could offer. A prominent Indian food historian, K. T. Achaya, went so far as to declare: "Perhaps nowhere else in the world except in India would it have been possible 3000 years ago to be a strict vegetarian."

Just as in Gandhi's times, though, consuming meat in India is still often a political act. Several beef-eating festivals organized at India's universities ended in violent clashes with more conservative groups. "Beef is a symbol of anti-Brahmanism," stated one student organization. And scientists agree: eating beef in India stands for modernization. It opposes the caste system, which is topped by beef-avoiding Brahmins, and thereby undermines authority. During the campaign for parliament in 2014, the conservative BJP party tried to win votes for its leader using a slogan: "Vote for Modi, give life to the cow." Narendra Modi, a stout man with white hair that connects via sideburns with his trim beard and perfectly circles his round face, coined the term *pink revolution* to describe India's growing hunger for meat—and for money made from exporting beef. Before the elections, Modi spoke of the meat industry's crimes against "mother cow" and suggested the beef trade should be banned. Yet months after he won and became prime minister, the pink revolution was still rolling. It seems that meat exports are just too good of a cash cow for India to shut down.

Beef may be the most politically sensitive of India's meats, but it's chicken that is the most often eaten. Girinagar, an upscale neighborhood of Kerala's twin city Ernakulam-Kochi, is leafy and green, with traffic subdued, almost calm. The air here is thick with foul vapors that rise from the area's many canals, green streams of trash and vegetation that crisscross this part of urban Kerala, but most houses are neat, over-sized, and obviously pricey. In the maze of unnamed, narrow streets, a small store is hidden. A store that embraces India's growing hunger for meat and what's behind it: hunger for modernity, for riches. The store belongs to a chain called Suguna Daily Fressh and offers hygienically packed, easy-to-prepare chicken. It may look like nothing special to a Westerner, but in India, a country where until recently to cook a chicken entailed buying it at an overcrowded market, plucking it, and cleaning its guts, the store is very different. Stores like Suguna Daily Fressh, with their conveniently packaged and expensive products, are for the upper classes, who are driving India's desire for meat. After all, people crave meat precisely because it is expensive. Who doesn't want to be like the beautiful, light-skinned, and obviously successful people who gorge themselves on animal protein in the advertisements for KFC, McDonald's, and the Meat Products of India? India wants to go up, and to go up means to eat meat.

Similar things are happening in China. In a country where the average person ate less than seven pounds of meat *per year* (in the early twentieth century), China is fast becoming a nation where many plates are overflowing with pork, chicken, and, to a lesser extent, beef. Since the 1980s, meat consumption in the People's Republic has quadrupled. China is already ingesting over half of Earth's pork, 20 percent of its chicken, and 10 percent of its beef. Soon, these numbers will be much higher. If China, with its population of 1.3 billion, ate as much animal flesh as Americans do today, they would be hogging (no pun intended) over 70 percent of the meat produced on the planet.

The themes behind China's growing appetite for meat are similar to those in India and Japan. The Chinese are eating more and more meat because they are finally starting to be able to afford it and because the many years in which there was not enough animal flesh to go around resulted in it symbolizing luxury and wealth, modernity, the West, and power. And as in India, to eat meat in China often means to reject old social hierarchies. This is one of the reasons why fast-food joints such as McDonald's and KFC thrive in the People's Republic. As anthropologist Yunxiang Yan once wrote: "Many people patronize McDonald's to experience a moment of equality." In Western fast-food chains, all customers are treated with similar respect, no matter their age, social status, or wealth. That's very different from traditional Chinese eateries, where—as Yan described—there is an ongoing competition among customers as to who will order the most expensive, luxurious meal. Say the guy sitting at the table next to you orders a chicken. Now, if you don't want to lose face, you can't just have veggies. To prove your social standing, you have to order meat, too, and preferably a more expensive dish. You are just about to ask the waiter for pork, when the guy at another table, to your left, beats you to it and places an order for pork dumplings. After mentally calculating how many yuans are left in your wallet, you order, with a slightly shaky voice, the most expensive pork on the menu. Face saved, money lost. At McDonald's or KFC, with their short, simple menus of similarly priced and standardized dishes, such dilemmas don't exist. What's more, in these restaurants, people are consuming not just food but also Western culture, so often associated with individualism and democracy. And, of course, McDonald's, KFC, Burger King, and the like are all about eating meat, so if you go there to experience the spirit of Western equality, as a side order you may get hooked on burgers and chicken.

Even though there may be many parallels between India's and China's growing desire for meat, there are quite a few important differences, too—differences that are the reason why China is already gorging on much more animal protein. Although the traditional Chinese diet is mostly plant based, vegetarianism never took root in China as deeply as it has in India. The Chinese ate so little meat in the past largely because they simply didn't have enough good land to grow feed for livestock. Famines were common, very common, so the people here learned to eat anything that was available (hence the donkey penises, grilled scorpions, and other unusual-for-Westerners foods on Chinese menus). In China, the seeds for its future love affair with meat were already present, buried deep in the culture, waiting for a good time to sprout.

For many centuries, most followers of Buddhism in China were not vegetarian. By the sixth century, though, meat eating evolved to become a no-no for devout Chinese Buddhists. Consuming meat, the holy scriptures said, inhibits the ability to feel compassion. It causes nightmares. And yet Buddhist vegetarianism in China never became as widely practiced as Hindu vegetarianism did in India. It was mainly the domain of monks, while the elites kept wolfing down meat—so much of it that they were dubbed "the meat eaters." The rich of China were at least as extravagant in their meat tastes as were their European counterparts and ate things like yak tails, bear paws, and leopard fetuses. And just like the medieval European peasants, who hungered for all the animal flesh heaped on the plates of the aristocracy, the Chinese masses dreamed of eating just like their nobles and equated wealth with meat. (By contrast, Indian nobility meant vegetarianism, and so that's what people aspired to.) What also played a role in keeping China carnivorous, despite the arrival of Buddhism, was its bureaucracy. To rise through the ranks of the imperial government, a civil servant basically *had to* eat meat. Vegetarianism was considered inappropriate for high officials because public occasions required sharing meat to ensure social harmony. Meat avoiders were looked upon with suspicion and sometimes even forced to eat pork to make certain they didn't belong to some radical vegetarian sect (heretics in Europe come to mind). And if that wasn't enough to ensure China didn't go completely veg, the beliefs of traditional Chinese medicine discouraged plant-based diets, too. Vegetables are generally "cold," according to traditional Chinese dietary therapy. That's fine if you are suffering from a fever, but if you have chills or fatigue, you need to nourish yourself with "hot" foods—such as meat. In traditional Chinese food therapy, meat is often necessary to balance your energy. If you don't eat it, you may end up in trouble.

And then there is the Mandarin language. Take the words *chicken* and *fish*, for example. These words, when spoken in Mandarin, have the same sound as the words for "prosperous" and "abundance." For this reason, people in China eat chicken and fish on Lunar New Year's Eve to ensure good luck. *Home* is another word that may help reinforce meat-based diets in China. To make the character for "home" you basically take the character for a pig and put the character for a roof over it: pig plus roof equals home.

I remember staring at the thicket of Chinese characters covering the menu in one of Beijing's sprawling restaurants. The room was bright and open and dotted with round tables. Everything seemed loud in there: the people, the smells of frying and roasting, the colors—a jumble of white, red, and gold. The plastic menu, sticky from too many hands touching it before me, was in Chinese only, and the pictures were quite blurred. When a waiter walked past me, I caught his attention. "What is that?" I asked, in my stiff, phrase-book Chinese. "Meat," I heard in reply. "What meat?" I pressed. "Meat," the waiter shrugged. I pointed to another dish, then another, and kept asking. But my understanding of the food on offer got only slightly better. It appeared that although some dishes were "chicken" or "fish" or even "donkey" (there was a donkey penis soup listed), lots of others were just "meat," period.

In time I came to learn that if something in China is described simply as "meat," it means pork. The Chinese love pork. Every other pig that is alive on this planet is being raised in China—and it will be slaughtered and cooked there. In the famine-ridden past, pigs were economic security. They were cheap to raise, feeding on household leftovers and even human excrement, and could be exchanged for political favors, given as wedding presents, and—of course—eaten. Today, China's swine are still seen as a measure of food security, even on a national scale. The Communist government makes sure people keep buying pig meat by handing out grants and subsidies to hog producers, waiving their taxes, and offering them insurance. For China's leaders, providing citizens with enough pork to fill their plates means progress and modernity. It means they've succeeded.

But there are problems. Asia's nutrition transition means the health of people there is going downhill. It's not all on account of meat, of course. The sodas, the sweets, the fries—all this has a role too, an ugly one. Still, there are plenty of studies that connect high intakes of meat with higher odds of cancer, diabetes, and heart disease. And that's what Asia is getting right now. There are already over sixty-one million people with type 2 diabetes in India, and by 2030 that number will likely double. In the twin city Ernakulam-Kochi, where hygienically wrapped Suguna Daily Fressh chicken is sold, almost one in five inhabitants is diabetic. The waists of Asia are expanding, too. Over 30 percent of Chinese adults are overweight. One hundred million are obese.

The poor nutrition and resulting poor health are only part of Asia's meat-related problems. In March 2013, the pale bodies of over sixteen thousand dead pigs floated down Huangpu River near Shanghai. The carcasses were swollen and rotting, the stench nauseating. The animals, which may have died either of a virus or of extreme cold, had been dumped into the water from industrial farms upstream. The "hogwash incident," as it was called in the media, is just one of many scandals that have plagued India's and China's booming meat business. There was the "instant chicken" scandal (China), when poultry were supposedly given eighteen different antibiotics to grow ultrafast. There was "Avatar meat" (China), when pork was said to be contaminated by phosphorescent bacteria and glowed blue in the dark. There has been one avian flu outbreak after another. It's the sheer scale of the industry's growth that causes these problems. When it comes to animal products, China in many respects has more stringent safety regulations than the US does. Take ractopamine, a drug that mimics stress hormones, which is given to as many as 80 percent of American pigs. But when the Chinese found out it was administered to their hogs, a scandal erupted (ractopamine is illegal as a feed additive in China).

Asia's burgeoning appetite for meat is not just its problem—it's our problem, too. The meat industry is international, and what happens in one part of the world often affects the others. The major challenge for the industry in China is land—as in, there's not enough of it. China has a mere 0.08 hectare of arable land per person—6.5 times less than the US, over 16 times less than Canada. The Chinese simply can't grow feed for all the animals they want to eat. India is also struggling with a land shortage and with a severe water shortage to boot. If China and India want to have a meat industry, which is enormously water intensive, on an American scale, they will be in trouble.

What do countries do that want meat but can't produce enough of it? They could issue meat-eating bans the way medieval Japan did, but that's highly unlikely these days, of course. Instead, they outsource. They import. And where are all these chops and burgers going to come from? The US, for one. In the last decade, the flow of pork from the States to China rose almost ten times. And that was before the biggest meat processor, Shuanghui International, purchased the American giant Smithfield Foods, to become the world's largest pork producer. Yes, the money is pouring into US coffers, but there is a dark side to the deal. While the Chinese are consuming the meat, we are consuming the pollution: the lagoons of manure, the dirty air, the antibiotic-resistant bacteria.

The Chinese also import vast quantities of feed for their domestic livestock—and again, export the pollution. Chinese meat producers are on the constant lookout for land to grow soy and corn to fill the stomachs of their livestock. A lot of it comes from the US, some comes from Africa, and some from Eastern Europe, but the majority comes from Latin America. Already over 80 percent of Brazil's soy exports are going to China, and the growth curve is nearly vertical. A slice of Brazil the size of Colorado is currently covered in soy crops destined for China; a similar thing is happening in Argentina. That's not exactly good news. Ninety-nine percent of the soybeans grown in Brazil are genetically modified, and they are intensely sprayed with herbicides and fungicides. In Argentina's soy-growing districts, such use of chemicals has already caused epidemic levels of cancers and birth defects.

It's easy to criticize Asia's meat hunger and point fingers at the trouble it's causing, but these nations are basically following the path Europe and North America took some time ago. They are getting hooked on meat for many of the same reasons we did: because of meat's taste, because of the meat industry's lobbying and marketing, and because of meat's symbolism. They want meat because they want to be modern, industrial, and rich. Often, they want to get rid of social hierarchies— and the West with its meat-laden cuisines stands for equality. The power of meat's symbolism is particularly clear in India: when the Brahmin elites sat on top of the Indian world, the masses aspired to be vegetarian. Now, there is the West to look up to as the ultimate "we've made it" people. And these "we've made it" people eat plenty of meat. The young upper classes, the IT workers, and those with MBAs from US schools don't want to be like the traditional villagers with their stomachs filled

307

with lentils. The media is selling the protein myth, and they buy it. Even when they were vegetarian, they didn't care for animals much, and they didn't choose their diets themselves anyway, which now can make going non-veg a bit easier.

The Chinese, meanwhile, have loved meat, and pork in particular, all along—they just didn't have enough land and resources to grow it. Now they can virtually "import" land from Brazil or the US, and they do. The Communist Party is all for it. Meat means prosperity, and the party wants the Chinese people to feel prosperous. The government distrusts vegetarianism because it is tied with religious movements of the past—something the government has worked hard to suppress. Asia is starting to eat more meat often not in spite of its vegetarian religions but precisely because of them—as a way to reject them and consign them to the past.

Of course, not everyone in India is an Ajath Anjanappa. Not everyone has money to dine on steaks in Western-style restaurants. In India, almost 70 percent of the population lives on less than $2 a day, while a Suguna chicken breast costs about $2.50 per pound. In China, millions can't afford to dine on KFC chicken, either. But this destitute people look up to the rich and take note of their growing appetite for meat. They see the butcher shops opening, the steak houses luring; they see the non-veg Bollywood stars flexing their muscles on TV. And they want meat, too.

But our planet simply can't afford Asia's hunger for meat. It can't afford the antibiotics loaded into livestock, the water that needs to be pumped into production. It can't afford the global warming that it is causing. Likewise, it can't afford the West's meat addiction, either. It is time for nutrition transition, stage 5: behavioral change. But is it likely that we will markedly cut down our meat consumption in the near future? And how exactly *can* we change?

Discussion Questions: The Pink Revolution or How Asia is Getting Hooked on Meat, Fast

1. Which countries are the first and second largest exporters of beef?
2. Why do Indians have a low beef intake compared to other countries? How does this contrast with the Chinese?
3. Where is the West in the 'nutrition transition'? What pattern characterizes the West at the present time?
4. What happens to a country's cuisine as the population becomes more affluent?

Paul S. Kinderstedt. *Cheese and Culture: A History of Cheese and Its Place in Western Civilization*
White River Junction, Vermont: Chelsea Green Publishing, 2012

Reviewed by Laina Farhat-Holzman

What began as a book that would be a resource for new artisan cheese makers turned into a book that tracks the history of western civilization, a history in which cheese plays a larger role that one would have ever guessed. Kinderstedt's research turned into an undergraduate course at the University of Vermont (a big cheese state) that would integrate cheese science and technology. Cheese has been an enormous part of our civilizations from Neolithic times to today.

I read this book because I am an artisan cheese lover, and have even made a pilgrimage to Parma, Italy, where Parmigiano Reggiano, called "the king of cheeses," has been produced for the past 1,000 years. This book made that journey even more significant for me.

Although almost all cultures have some sort of simple cheeses, such as the yogurt cheeses that the Mongols developed out of mares' milk, it is only in the West that the great technology of cheeses developed, a process begun in earliest human civilization after the domestication of ruminant animals.

Milk quickly spoils but cheese, a food transformed by technology, can keep, making it a value-added product. The history of this process began some 9,000 years ago in Southwest Asia, a region in which cattle, sheep, and goats had been domesticated. All of these animals provided a variety of useful products, particularly sheep and goats providing wool. But all of them in breeding seasons did have surplus milk, which our ancestors wanted to use around the year.

Beginning about 17,000 years ago, the post-glacial global warming began to establish what has come to be known as Mediterranean climate, hot dry summers and cool wet winters. Wild cereals such as wheat, rye, and barley, along with legumes such as beans, peas, and lentils, began to thrive. The extensive stands of wild cereals extended in an elongated swath from the Jordan River Valley northward through inland Syria and to what is now southeastern Turkey. This became, with the advent of hunter-gatherers, "the fertile crescent," mother of civilization for much of the Old World.

Between 11,000 and 9,500 BC, the earth had one last cycle of extreme cooling which wiped out these early settlements. But around 9,500 BC, there was a sudden intense episode of global warming, increasing the average annual temperature by as much as 13 degrees Fahrenheit over just a couple of generations. This was followed by slow but steady warming for the next two millennia, resulting in a global climate that we still have today.

As humans in the Fertile Crescent developed food crops, they found that such crops attracted sheep and goats, especially near mountains such as the Taurus Mountains of southwest Anatolia and the Zagros Mountains of western Iran. The farmers found an opportunity to begin herding these animals, taking them from the lowlands in the winter to the mountains in the summer, a pattern that still exists in the migrations of Iranian tribal peoples.

Mixed farming and rapid population growth brought profound cultural change: the blossoming of the Neolithic (New Stone Age) period. Architecture bloomed, as did a new widespread appearance of religious symbols and shrine building. Humans then had moved beyond the status of a slightly revised and more efficient version of the eating and breeding machines that had preceded them. To use biblical language, says the author, humans were made in the image of God.

The archeological record tells us that until 7,000 BC, animals were raised for meat. It took generations of careful breeding and handling until sheep and goats were developed to have more milk than just needed for their young, and for these animals to permit humans to milk them. At the same time, intensive grain cultivation and population explosion produced widespread environmental degradation and erosion. Pastoralism and milk production were probably a response to this disaster.

Adult humans in Neolithic times were almost universally lactose intolerant (as many Asians are today). But they found that cheese, a product made by boiling milk, made this foodstuff digestible. The invention of pottery enabled milk to be stored, transported, and cooked. Ceramic pots with drain holes were the first sieves for draining the whey from curds formed either by heat or by adding a small amount of rennet (from the intestines of animals). The entire agricultural and herding revolution was characterized by the ability to store food, a need that cheese met.

According to Kinderstedt, cheese and religion have a long relationship. There are many references in the Bible to cheese being a gift for the deity (or in polytheist societies, gods). Several chapters are devoted to all of the inventions that emerged in primeval times that had something to do with farming--ceramics, metallurgy, animal husbandry, and cheese-making-- and the uses of these products in trade and religion (temple gifts).

Kinderstedt traces cheese development across the world from the Fertile Crescent across to India. China, however, never developed a culture of cheese making.

The Mediterranean world was early in developing cheese and the various technologies that produce varieties, some of which we know today: feta and ricotta, and somewhat later, the dry grating cheese such as Pecorino. But it was in northern Europe that the amazing cheese culture that we know today had its origins. The north was more hospitable to raising cattle, the most favored herding animal of the Indo-European peoples. Of these, the Celts were the specialists among cheese makers, and their descendants, the French and north Italians, still are.

Very interesting chapters involve cheese in the Greek religions, with a good deal on the diet of the earlier (and hardier) Athenians (cheese, barley cake, ripe olives and leeks). There is much interesting material on the very elegant cheeses developed by the Romans which were important trade and luxury goods as well as a culinary boost to their diets.

Italians, beginning with the Etruscans, were always enthusiastic cheese makers. The Italian genius showed itself in the connection of cheese making and pigs, an important source of meat that can be smoked and preserved in other ways. The pigs would consume the whey extruded during cheese making, a symbiotic development still used. Parma is not only the source of Parmigiano Reggiano cheese, but the equally famous Parma hams (prosciutto). These foodstuffs have been raised together for millennia.

With the advent of Christianity throughout the late Roman world, systematic cheese making became the norm. The chapters on the manor, monastery, and age of cheese diversification are fascinating. Monasteries in France have always been known for their splendid cheese making. I visited one monastery in the Auvergne region of France that sold in its gift stores the most marvelous brie-type cheese and all sorts of honey confections. The ethic of work promoted by the monastic movement produced such wonders.

Over time, peasant cheese makers in northwestern France fine-tuned their simple practices and storage conditions in ways that rendered them predictable and desirable. This was a process that continues to this very day in the production of European and now American artisan cheeses.

The author covers the extensive cheese making in England and the Netherlands, and introduces the development of factory-produced cheese which began to replace artisan farm cheese. The industrialization movement came at the same time as other practices that replaced female practitioners. Medicine went through such a transformation too, eliminating the midwife practitioners and replacing them with male doctors and hospitals.

The one good element that emerged with the industrialization of cheese making was that, for the first time, standardized instructions (recipes) for specific cheese varieties could be reproduced anywhere. Dairy schools were created during the latter half of the nineteenth century.

However, both the transfer of cheese making to male industrialists and midwifery to medical doctors produced unanticipated consequences: terrible cheese and high maternal death rates. Both female practices have had a revival today, to the benefit of both cheeses and maternal outcomes.

The author may have been focused on the evolution of cheese, but its connection with other aspects of history figures substantially in this book. The section on Holland's role as cheese provisioner of all Europe was fascinating. Their cheeses, which were solid, round, and encased in wax, traveled well and brought in much revenue.

But more interesting than the cheese was the very fact of the identity of a country that would never have come into being without great human intervention. During the Middle Ages, much of Holland was uninhabited or sparsely populated, a wasteland consisting of waterlogged peat bogs and maritime salt pastures. It wasn't until the fifteenth century, writes Kinderstedt, that commercial dairying began to emerge in Holland as a significant element of the economy. Despite the unpromising and sodden terrain, cheese making figured from the late Neolithic in this area because one could not grow much food in the salt marshes, but in the ridges formed by oceanic activity on the coast, the people could raise cattle and survive on dairying.

The miracle of Holland began from the tenth century onward, when the Dutch undertook massive land reclamation. They laboriously drained the fields with drainage ditches, built low dikes, all despite having a chronic labor shortage (this was the period of recurring cycles of Black Death). The aristocrats and churchmen recruited the necessary labor force by offering serfs their freedom and almost absolute, exclusive property rights to the land that they reclaimed in return for their labor. (The labor shortages in other parts of Europe were treated in much the same way, changing the social pecking order for the better.)

But in Holland, there were unexpected consequences. The reclaimed lands were not good for grain raising. In the fourteenth and fifteenth centuries, the production of bread cereals collapsed, brought on by an ecological crisis of largely human making.

Draining the peat bogs produced the sinking of landmass, opening the country to devastating oceanic flooding, made worse by a gradually rising sea level. They were losing their country. However, in an amazing example of human determination and ingenuity, says Kinderstedt, many Dutch peasants chose to adapt their agriculture and fight the North Sea. They developed the polder system, enclosing their fields with dikes and pumping out surface water to create permanent dry lands. In 1408, the windmill, once used for grinding grain, was adapted to pump water from a polder.

The soil still was not good enough for wheat, but it was fine for barley and hops, and gave rise to artisan beer brewing. Other farmers dropped grain cultivation for dairy cattle. The Dutch created a lucrative trade (in exchange for wheat that they imported) in their hearty artisan cheeses and beers. In addition, the rise of Calvinism in Holland further encouraged the entrepreneurial spirit that was already part of their culture.

Between 1500 and 1700, Holland's economy expanded, probably more rapidly than any other in Europe. Kinderstedt shows the interrelationships of trade, religion, ethnic temperament, and the growth of the nation state. Holland has been an amazing case study of what determined human beings can do.

The rest of the book tracks the modern evolution of cheese making, beginning with factories and systematic production, but then going on to today's wonderful artisanal cheeses and the governmental rules for keeping them pure and safe. Who would have thought that cheese could be such an important part of human history?

Discussion Questions: Cheese and Culture: A History of Cheese and its Place in Western Civilization

1. At what time period do we have evidence for the making of cheese?
2. Why is it that cheese became so common around the world? What was common for people in the Neolithic regarding milk consumption and food preparation?
3. What are some of the world regions where cheese was produced and what kinds of cheese come from these regions?
4. Why was cheese more easily made in some regions of the world compared to others? Where was cheese never made or developed?

Topic VII: The Future of Food and Nutrition

Countdown to the Future of Food does as the title suggests—it reviews all of the trends, issues, and concerns as related to food and food production in the future. There are multiple factors that could change the diversity of the world's food-related cultures and practices. Yet few of us think about these issues, even based upon our own food needs and desires. With climate change, how do we ensure a sustainable food production system while maintaining biodiversity?

Countdown to the Future of Food

Sarah Elton

To take a look into the future, all you need do is head to the Baltimore waterfront. On a few dozen square metres of urban green space, Lewis Ziska, a USDA scientist with the Agricultural Research Service's Crop Systems and Global Change lab, found the same climatic conditions that climate models project will be the norm here on Earth sometime before the year 2050. That is, hot—about 1.5 to 2 degrees Celsius warmer than today's average temperature—and rich in carbon dioxide. Ziska used this small plot to watch in real time what effect climate change will have on the food we grow.

For his study, Ziska established two other test sites, one in the suburbs of Baltimore to simulate conditions expected in the 2020s or 2030s and another on an organic farm in Maryland to stand in for the present. (He couldn't build a laboratory to recreate these climates because funding for the kind of work he does had been cut by the federal government.) He introduced the same topsoil, with the same naturally occurring seeds, into these three landscapes and then waited to see how the different climates affected what grew. "The goal was to see what species were going to be favoured," he explained to me.

The results were unsettling. What Ziska found over the course of the six-year study was that on the steamy, carbon-dioxide-rich Baltimore waterfront, weeds grew tallest—in fact, they grew to be about two times larger than their rural counterparts. Lamb's quarters, a common leafy weed, grew to between 2.5 and 3 metres—about double the height of its cousins on that organic farm in Maryland. Ragweed also fared much better under these future-like conditions. "What we found," Ziska told me, "was that the warming winter temperatures and the high carbon dioxide were all associated with a much greater increase in the weeds. Weeds are going to be a large issue when thinking about how much food we can produce."

For those of us who don't farm, tall weeds might not sound like a big deal. But for a farmer, weeds that would tower over even an NBA player are terrifying. Their giant stalks would likely jam machinery, shade even the tallest crops, and turn farming into an all-out war between the food plants and the weeds. Farmers use herbicides today to eliminate weeds before they grow, but research shows that as carbon dioxide levels increase, these chemicals are no longer as effective. That leaves weeding by hand. "Of all the things that people do, that is the most time consuming and laborious aspect of growing food," said Ziska.

Giant weeds, resistant to herbicides, that must be pulled by hand: it's science fiction come to life. We can safely conclude that weeds stretching to three metres would compromise our food security.

"If we are concerned as a country for maintaining our national security, doesn't it make sense to remember food security?" asked Ziska. "It is an issue that is going to impact everyone's lives in the not too distant future." And by everyone, he means everyone—no matter where you live, what you choose to eat, how much you spend on groceries. In some way, every one of us will be affected. Dr. Ziska's study raises the important question of how we will feed ourselves this century.

How *will* we feed ourselves in 2050? In the next forty years, the world's population is expected to surpass nine billion. At the same time, climate change is transforming life on the planet. According to the scientists who look at these big-picture issues, in the space of about one generation, a messy combination of climate, population trends, and environmental change will profoundly affect the world as we know it. We need to figure out how to feed the world, dramatically reduce our greenhouse gas emissions, and cope with climate change.

So how *do* we best move forward? How do we ensure that everybody has enough to eat as we contend with a new climate? How do we do this without releasing even more greenhouse gases, thereby ruining the environment and further hampering the ability of future generations to feed themselves?

These pressing questions are forcing us to make a choice about how we want to tackle these problems, and a debate rages about which direction we should take. On one side of the debate is the route of sustainable food, with its organic farms and farmers' markets, seed-saving networks, short food chains, and slow food traditions. On the other side is the path of the industrial food system.

Those who believe that industrial agriculture with its worldwide economy of food will best feed the planet argue that only a global industrial food system can provide the quantity of food we need at a low enough price for people to afford. Advocates tend to conjure up a Malthusian scenario of population outstripping food supply. The image of hungry teeming masses is even used to trump the idea of sustainability—as if we as a species must make a choice between creating sustainable food systems and allowing children to die of hunger in Africa. In *Foreign Policy* magazine in 2010, Robert Paarlberg, a professor of political science at Wellesley College, slammed the sustainable food movement for what he called its elitist approach to food that excludes the poor. The subtitle summed it up: "Stop obsessing about arugula. Your 'sustainable' mantra—organic, local, and slow—is no recipe for saving the world's hungry millions." He concluded that only a globalized industrial food system can produce what we need, efficiently and cheaply, so that everyone is fed.

I disagree. I stand firmly on the other side of the debate and argue for sustainable food systems. While industrial food might provide ample quantities of cheap calories, if you want to feed people *and* protect their livelihoods given the state of the environment, the status quo doesn't cut it anymore. To feed the planet in a time of climate change, we need to build sustainable food systems. We must dramatically lessen the environmental burden of food production, encourage new economies of food that allow small-scale and family farmers to thrive in their rural communities, and nurture a food culture that connects us to the natural world on which we all depend. We must start to assemble these new, sustainable food systems immediately, because the rice, the bread, all the food we put on our plates, is at stake.

And without enough rice or bread, society starts to crack. Over the course of history, civilizations have fallen because their food systems have failed. In the Middle Ages, the Vikings disappeared from Greenland, where they had been living for several hundred years, because their farming methods eroded the topsoil and the climate changed, making it harder for them to grow food. In Central America, the Maya fled their cities, such as Guatemala's Tikal, when centuries of dry conditions, followed by drought, undermined their ability to sustain a dense urban population. The Roman Empire teetered into poverty and hunger after they overworked the soil on the plantations that supplied their busy cities. On Easter Island in the Pacific Ocean, as vividly described in Jared Diamond's book *Collapse,* the people who lived there cut down every last tree somewhere between the 1400s and the 1600s. Without trees, the Easter Islanders could no longer build the seafaring boats they had used to fish in deep waters;

they soon hunted land birds into extinction. And without trees to protect the soil from erosion, farming dwindled. They were left with few food sources other than the flesh of their human neighbours. Archaeologists have found human bones in domestic middens, their ends rounded from being boiled in a pot.

Evan Fraser is a geography professor at the University of Guelph who studies food security as it relates to climate change and economic globalization. He is also co-author of the book *Empires of Food,* which examines the role that failing food systems played in the collapse of several historical civilizations. "When we look back over ten thousand years as a species bringing food from farms to cities, the good years outweigh the bad," he explained to me. "Though history definitely reminds us that problems do emerge. History reminds us that changes do happen and happen quickly over a large scale. There are these reversals when societies do collapse very quickly.

"If you were a noble aristocrat, say, born around the year 1290, you would have been born into an affluent, confident society. You wouldn't have had any clue of what was coming unless you were paying attention to the price of wheat. Yet within two generations, 40 percent of Europe was dead. In 1315, bad rain mid-summer flattened the wheat crop and people starved. Rising demand and falling supply. The fate of society does hang in the balance."

For us, it is the year 2050 that is a bleak date in our future. That's the year when all of our environmental debts come knocking at our door, asking us to pay up. By then, the temperature of the planet will likely have risen an average of a little more than 2 degrees Celsius, with more warming at higher latitudes. That's two times more than it has risen already since 1899, around the early years of the Industrial Revolution. This warming is altering our earth's climate system. "In agriculture, the warmer it gets, the harder it will be to maintain productivity of the crops we currently consume," said David Lobell, a professor of environmental earth systems science at Stanford University who studies the impact of climate change on agriculture. There will be other effects too. Frequent droughts will reduce crop yields—as we witnessed in North America when a severe drought during the summer of 2012 limited production over a large area—and an expected increase in heavy rains will lead to floods that could destroy what we do grow. We will be forced to change the way we raise our crops, and where we grow them will be affected. A climate of extremes is bad for farming.

The results from Lewis Ziska's study in Baltimore, where weeds thrived in the heat and the high carbon dioxide levels, suggest that the way we've grown our food in the last decades—planting homogeneous rows of one crop—isn't going to fare well in a future of climate change. "Modern agriculture tends to be very large monocultures with very little genetic diversity," said Ziska. But the study demonstrates that species with the greatest genetic diversity—the ones that are the most able to produce seed and that don't rely on pollination—are the ones most able to adapt to sudden changes in climate. "Modern agriculture is the opposite," Ziska pointed out. "Is that model of agriculture good for a rapidly changing climate? Not so much."

The way we produce and consume our food in the industrial system is not only vulnerable to the effects of climate change, it is also worsening the problem. It draws heavily on fresh water (for irrigation) and fossil fuels (used to make fertilizers) and also is draining groundwater aquifers, polluting our oceans, and eroding our soils. Furthermore, the global food system is responsible for just under one-third of humanity's greenhouse gas emissions.

The predicted changes in global demographics worsen the picture. The nine billion humans that the United Nations calculates will populate the earth by 2050 is a number far greater than humanity has ever seen before. (To put it in context, in 1950, the global population was around 2.5 billion.) The majority of these people will live in cities, leaving the smallest ratio ever of farmers to eaters. As cities grow to accommodate industrial development and the rising population, as well as to cater to the housing wishes of the well-to-do who yearn for their own home and a patch of land, if things don't change we will continue to pave over the earth's best farmland, leaving ourselves with less soil on which to grow our food. At the same time, more and more people, in countries such as India and China, are embracing a Western diet, which demands more meat, hence more of nature's resources. We also depend on farmland to grow cotton and biofuels, which adds to the competition for arable land as well as the environmental burden of farming, since each industry has its own ecologically damaging practices. If we don't change our ways now, by 2050 we will struggle with the consequences of our actions.

"We are basically on the road, by the end of the century, to being like the Cretaceous period, when the dinosaurs roamed the planet, when there was no ice," earth system scientist Steven J. Davis of the University of California, Irvine, told me. By the end of the century, "we're probably talking about 6 degrees of warming. That's not enough to melt all the ice by 2100, evaporate the oceans, and drive all humans out of existence, but it is going to be unpleasant. Especially if you live in impoverished nations and at tropical latitudes."

With changing weather patterns around the world, everyone will be affected one way or another. "There will be millions of people suffering from changes in climate," said Davis. "Many will be dying from lack of food—and wars. It is plausible that the effects of climate change could cause major hits to our global economy. I don't want to sensationalize the apocalyptic scenario, but it is pretty easy to imagine that crop failures and wars in certain countries could cause the collapse of governments, and that could have an impact on the global economy."

Indeed, poor crop yields and bad weather have caused problems before. A study published in the journal *Nature* in 2011 posited that rapid changes in climate do affect farming and can be linked to conflict. Researchers at Columbia University compared incidences of civil strife during years of El Niño and La Niña, cyclic ocean-atmosphere phenomena. About every five years, the warming trends of El Niño cause droughts and torrential rains in tropical regions. The study looked at more than 200 incidents of conflict between 1950 and 2004 in 175 countries; it found that in El Niño years, there was twice the rate of conflict than in La Niña years. When turbulent weather reduces agricultural production, food prices rise and people are more likely to protest. A 2011 study by the New England Complex Systems Institute, an independent research organization, identified a point at which the price of food increases the possibility of protest. The report acknowledged that although protests are motivated by many factors, the rise in the cost of food is a likely component.

If climate already affects how we behave, what's going to happen when it becomes less predictable?

Those on the other side of the food debate say that it is precisely the industrial food system that will spare us from wars triggered by climbing food prices. Their faith in industrial food comes from the fact that it has already improved our lives. There is truth in this. There is quantitatively less poverty on earth this century than there ever has been. Far fewer of us toil in the fields as subsistence farmers, always one bad crop away from famine.

But unfortunately, industrial food has created grave problems, and now the system is sick. We have produced a world of "stuffed and starved," in the words of Raj Patel, author of the book by that name. A growing number of humans are no longer hungry—we are the stuffed. In fact, we are increasingly obese, consuming a high-fat, high-sodium, and high-sugar diet that has caused an increase in type 2 diabetes and other non-communicable diseases, as well as a childhood obesity crisis. Then there are the poor—the starved—who are chronically undernourished or who don't have enough to fill their stomachs despite the increase in yields provided by industrial food. The Food and Agriculture Organization of the UN reports that between 2010 and 2013 there were 870 million chronically undernourished people, with 98 percent of them living in developing countries. The UN's World Food Programme has found that hunger kills more people than malaria, AIDS, and tuberculosis combined. Since 2007, food prices have risen, and in 2011, the FAO's global food price index reached a historic peak. And as prices climb, more and more people go without nourishment. Food insecurity—which leaves people without access to nourishing food, or hungry, without enough to eat—is growing in the United States and Canada too. Clearly, the industrial food system has not solved our problems when it comes to feeding people. There is no salvation from the future in the status quo. If food and agriculture is the base of our civilization today, it is also the basis for its demise. Only sustainable food systems will help us to move forward.

I am not alone in this belief. Many important institutions and research bodies have reached the same conclusion that sustainable, locally centred food systems are the only way we can feed the world while reducing the damage we do to this planet. In 2009, the International Assessment of Agricultural Knowledge, Science and Technology for Development, a research project investigating the future of agriculture and funded in part by the World Bank and the United Nations, released the findings of the more than four hundred scientists, academics, and development workers it had convened from around the world. They concluded that sustainable food systems, which incorporate small-scale agriculture and traditional knowledge, should replace industrial food systems. In 2010, two more reports concurred. Olivier De Schutter, the United Nations special rapporteur on the right to food, wrote in a document he submitted to the UN Human Rights Council that policies are urgently needed to support the expansion of locally based sustainable agriculture in developing countries so that the poorest people on earth can find a better life, as well as food security, through small-scale farming. And in the United States, the National Research Council's Committee on Twenty-First Century Systems Agriculture wrote in its 2010 report that to ensure that agriculture can meet the needs of the future, farming in the United States could even require a "significant departure from the dominant systems of present-day agriculture."

But if food is the problem, it is also the solution. A new food revolution can save us. A movement is afoot that is fundamentally changing the way we produce our food and helping to provide for tomorrow. I travelled around the world to research this book, and wherever I looked, in big cities and in the smallest of villages, I found different manifestations of a similar desire to create a new way of feeding ourselves that is fair and just, that is rooted in local communities, and that doesn't have such a high environmental cost. In this book, you will read the stories of the people I met in India, China, and France, as well as in the United States and Canada. They offer us a look at what this new food order looks like.

The food system as we know it today drew on centuries of know-how, technology, and social change that allowed it to become the status quo in a mere handful of decades. If you start the count in 1945, when the Second World War ended and the industrial food system began to take shape, by 1995 food production was fully industrialized within a new worldwide agri-food economy. So if we could build it in five decades, we can replace it in about the same amount of time. To build the infrastructure and create the policies that support our ability to feed the world without damaging the environment by our deadline of 2050, we must act quickly. We must draw on the best of innovation, science, and traditional knowledge to make this new food system the new global status quo. It must be grounded in ethics, human rights, and, above all else, sustainability. Any food system we create must not hinder in any way the ability of future generations to feed themselves in a world in ecological balance.

To accomplish these goals, we must attempt to meet the following targets. The challenge for the first ten years is to stop industrial farming and make all our agricultural systems sustainable. This means an end to the widespread use of artificial pesticides and fertilizers as well as monocrops such as soybean, sugar cane, and oil palm in biodiverse regions. It also means an end to all factory-farmed meat and dairy and the transformation of the seasonless supermarket, with its endless supply of processed foods. We must localize our food markets, by closing the gap between eaters and the farmers who grow their food, to ensure that farmers can earn a living producing food and to encourage a new generation to pursue this career.

By 2030, we need to ensure that our seed supply is biodiverse. Biodiversity is the key to security; we need to preserve the genes of our food so that we can eat tomorrow. At the same time, we must support research into new varieties of crops that can survive in the new climatic conditions, and we must keep this research in the public domain so everyone around the world has access to this shared resource.

These radical changes will require a cultural shift. We need to reconnect to the planet through the food we eat. The target for 2040, then, is to embrace new food values, particularly those that appreciate seasonality and tradition and connect us to nature. To do this, we must educate the next generation as well as those who live in cities, where people are often divorced from the natural world. And this all has to happen by 2050, in time to meet the challenges of climate change, environmental damage, and population growth.

The good news is that we have already begun. From New York City to Beijing, from the Northern Hemisphere to the Southern, in rich countries and in poor, and everywhere in between, people from all walks of life are creating an alternative to the industrial food we have grown accustomed to piling into our shopping carts. This movement is about so much more than green roofs in cities or the rise of the farmers' market or the much-hyped growth in organic food's market share. This is about a rupture—a rupture with the social norms of our modern world. And the cracks this rupture is causing are already, quietly, being filled by the ingenuity of people everywhere.

An alternative is taking shape. Hundreds of thousands—probably millions—of people are devoting their lives to creating new, sustainable, and just food systems where they live. They are building on millennia worth of knowledge and practice, combining science with traditional know-how, and proving not only that the new food revolution is necessary but that it is the better way to feed us all without destroying the planet. These people offer the rest of us the opportunity to be optimistic about the possibility of change, despite the dire environmental predictions. They also invite us to join in so we can find the best solutions for feeding us all with what we have on our finite planet.

The year 2050 is just a blink away. The great unspooling of the food system must speed ahead to ensure that those who come after us can all find a place at a metaphorical global table in a world with limits.

Discussion Questions: Countdown to the Future of Food

1. What are some concerns for producing food in the future?
2. What has been responsible for civilizations and cultures collapsing in the past?
3. Why do farming systems that focus on one crop face difficulty in the future?
4. What are the positives and negatives of industrial food production?

Author Biography

Dr. **Mary S. Willis** is a Professor in the Department of Nutrition and Health Sciences at the University of Nebraska Lincoln (UNL), Lincoln, Nebraska. She earned an MA and PhD in Anthropology from Washington University in St. Louis, St. Louis, Missouri, in 1991 and 1995 respectively. A Science and Diplomacy Fellow with AAAS from 1995-1997, Dr. Willis worked within USAID's Office of Population, Health, and Nutrition providing technical assistance to programs worldwide. She has traveled and worked in Asia, Africa and South America for more than 40 years. Dr. Willis joined the UNL faculty in 2000 and moved to Nutrition and Health Sciences in 2013, broadening the scope of her teaching and research to include bio-cultural approaches to food and nutrition, as well as global food security. She has studied transitions of refugee populations from South Sudan to the US since 2000 and has led a study abroad program to Ethiopia and Zambia, training students in food security, health, and nutrition, and collecting data on the impact of under-nutrition on growth-related sequelae within rural farming populations, since 2014. Dr. Willis employs a holistic approach to food and nutrition research and teaching; hence, she studies whole body health and incorporates both biological and cultural, but also archaeological and linguistic, perspectives into of her academic approach.

Credit Lines

CPSIA information can be obtained
at www.ICGtesting.com
Printed in the USA
LVHW102249051218
599388LV00008B/26/P